STERNBERG'S DIAGNOSTIC SURGICAL PATHOLOGY REVIEW

by

PIER LUIGI DI PATRE, MD

Chef de Clinic
Department of Pathology
Neuropathology Unit
Geneva
Switzerland

DARRYL CARTER, MD

Professor of Pathology, Emeritus
Department of Pathology
Yale University School of Medicine
New Haven, Connecticut

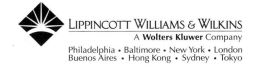

LIPPINCOTT WILLIAMS & WILKINS
A **Wolters Kluwer** Company

Philadelphia • Baltimore • New York • London
Buenos Aires • Hong Kong • Sydney • Tokyo

Acquisitions Editor: Jonathan Pine/Ruth Weinberg
Developmental Editor: Michelle LaPlante
Supervising Editor: Michael Mallard
Production Editor: Joanne Bowser
Manufacturing Manager: Ben Rivera
Compositor: TechBooks
Printer: Maple-Vail Press

Library of Congress Cataloging-in-Publication Data

DiPatre, Pier Luigi.
   Sternberg's diagnostic surgical pathology review / by Pier Luigi DiPatre, Darryl Carter.
      p. ; cm.
   Includes index.
   "This book is a thorough review of the textbook 'Sternberg's diagnostic surgical pathology'".
   ISBN 0-7817-4052-5 (pbk.)
   1. Pathology, Surgical—Examinations, questions, etc.   I. Carter, Darryl.
II. Sternberg, Stephen S.   III. Title.
RD57.D53   2004 Suppl.
617'.07'0076—dc22   2004013029

Care has been taken to confirm the accuracy of the information presented and to describe generally accepted practices. However, the authors, editor, and publisher are not responsible for errors or omissions or for any consequences from application of the information in this book and make no warranty, expressed or implied, with respect to the currency, completeness, or accuracy of the contents of the publication. Application of this information in a particular situation remains the professional responsibility of the practitioner.

The authors, editor, and publisher have exerted every effort to ensure that drug selection and dosage set forth in this text are in accordance with current recommendations and practice at the time of publication. However, in view of ongoing research, changes in government regulations, and the constant flow of information relating to drug therapy and drug reactions, the reader is urged to check the package insert for each drug for any change in indications and dosage and for added warnings and precautions. This is particularly important when the recommended agent is a new or infrequently employed drug.

Some drugs and medical devices presented in this publication have Food and Drug Administration (FDA) clearance for limited use in restricted research settings. It is the responsibility of the health care provider to ascertain the FDA status of each drug or device planned for use in their clinical practice.

10 9 8 7 6 5 4 3 2 1

CONTENTS

PREFACE

This manual is a collection of more than 600 multiple-choice questions with answers and explanations that provide a comprehensive review of the fourth edition of Sternberg Diagnostic Surgical Pathology—the "source book." The style of the questions is similar to that used in board examinations and "in-service" pathology tests. The material is organized in chapters that correspond to the chapters of the source book. The correct answers to all questions are given in a final section, where a concise, clear explanation is provided as to why a specific choice is correct. The explanatory notes review the topic by focusing on relevant pathological aspects, including not only morphology, but also issues of differential diagnosis, immunohistochemical features, pathogenesis, prognostic factors, and epidemiology.

Each explanation is referenced to the appropriate page(s) of the source book for more extensive reading. Approximately 150 questions are accompanied by pictures, reproduced in black and white from the source book. The pictures constitute the main clues to the correct answers and illustrate salient morphological aspects of common disorders. In addition, the "Answers and Explanations" section contains 18 original tables summarizing the features of major pathology issues.

This book is a learning guide that focuses on problem solving in differential diagnosis. We hope that it will serve as a study aid to residents in their first years of pathology training and a quick and effective review of surgical pathology for board examination and recertification.

STERNBERG'S DIAGNOSTIC SURGICAL PATHOLOGY REVIEW

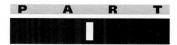

SKIN, SOFT TISSUE, BONE, AND JOINTS

1

NONNEOPLASTIC DISEASES OF THE SKIN

1. A skin biopsy from a 20-year-old man with eczematous dermatitis is submitted for histopathological examination. Which of the following changes would be most consistent with a diagnosis of *acute* spongiotic dermatitis?
   A. Acanthosis
   B. Epidermotropism
   C. Intraepidermal edema
   D. Papillomatosis
   E. Parakeratosis

2. Which of the following morphologic changes is most consistent with *allergic*, rather than *irritant*, contact dermatitis?
   A. Eosinophilic infiltration
   B. Lymphocytic exocytosis
   C. Papillary dermal edema
   D. Perivascular lymphocytes
   E. Spongiosis

3. A middle-aged patient presents with pruritic coin-shaped plaques over the extensor surfaces of upper and lower limbs. A biopsy shows acute and subacute spongiotic changes, without evidence of fungal organisms on special stains. Which of the following is the most likely diagnosis?
   A. Atopic dermatitis
   B. Dyshydrosis
   C. Irritant contact dermatitis
   D. Nummular eczema
   E. Seborrheic dermatitis

4. A 50-year-old patient with chronic eczematous lesions unresponsive to corticosteroid treatment undergoes a skin biopsy. Which of the following would favor a diagnosis of cutaneous T-cell lymphoma over that of subacute spongiotic dermatitis?
   A. Acanthosis
   B. Epidermotropism
   C. Lymphocytic exocytosis
   D. Papillomatosis
   E. Spongiosis

5. A skin biopsy shows changes of subacute spongiotic dermatitis. The clinical diagnosis is pityriasis rosea. Which of the following features would favor a diagnosis of syphilis over that of pityriasis rosea?
   A. Focal papillary hemorrhages
   B. Parakeratosis
   C. Perivascular lymphocytosis
   D. Plasma cell infiltration
   E. Spongiosis

6. A skin biopsy reveals spongiotic changes associated with acanthosis and parakeratosis. Neutrophils are found in the stratum corneum. The granular layer is of normal thickness. Which of the following diagnoses is most likely?
   A. Dermatophytosis
   B. Irritant contact dermatitis
   C. Pityriasis rosea
   D. Pustular psoriasis
   E. Stasis dermatitis

7. This photomicrograph depicts some of the most characteristic features of a common skin condition. Which of the following histopathologic features becomes prominent in the pustular variant of this condition?

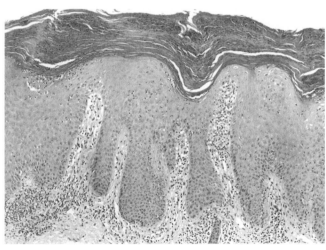

QUESTION 1.7

A. Confluent parakeratosis
B. Focal hemorrhages in the papillary dermis
C. Lymphocytic infiltration of the lower epidermis
D. Munro microabscesses
E. Suprapapillary thinning of epidermis

8. A skin biopsy of an erythematous lesion shows lymphocytic infiltration along the dermal-epidermal junction in a bandlike distribution. There are scattered colloid bodies in the basal layer, numerous melanophagocytes in the papillary dermis, and disruption of the basement membrane. Which of the following disorders should be considered in the differential diagnosis?

A. Arthropod bite reaction, gyrate erythema, urticaria
B. Contact dermatitis, atopic dermatitis, pityriasis rosea
C. Lichen planus, lichen nitidus, lichenoid drug eruption
D. Lupus erythematosus, dermatomyositis, graft versus host disease
E. Pemphigus vulgaris, pemphigus foliaceus, keratosis follicularis

9. The histopathological picture of a skin biopsy is shown in this picture. There are numerous Civatte bodies scattered immediately above and below the basement membrane. Which of the following is the most likely clinical presentation?

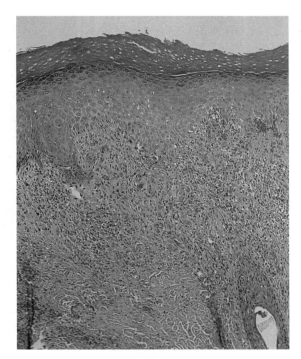

QUESTION 1.9

A. Erythematous plaques covered by silvery scale on extensor surfaces
B. Malar erythema in a butterfly distribution
C. Painful subcutaneous nodule on the anterior surface of the leg

D. Pruritic plaques with accentuation and thickening of skin markings
E. Pruritic purple papules on the flexor aspects of arms and legs

10. A 17-year-old female presents with bilateral malar rash in a butterfly distribution and signs of acute pleuritis. A skin biopsy shows liquefactive degeneration of the basal cell layer, variable epidermal atrophy, perivascular and periadnexal lymphocytic infiltration, and a thickened basement membrane. Which of the following patterns of immunofluorescence would be expected?

A. Deposits of IgA at the tips of dermal papillae
B. Granular deposits of IgG and C3 along the dermal–epidermal junction
C. Intercellular IgG deposition within the epidermis
D. Linear deposition of IgG and C3 along the dermal–epidermal junction
E. Smudgy IgG deposits around vessels of papillary dermis

11. A skin biopsy taken 4 weeks after bone marrow transplantation shows marked vacuolar degeneration of basal keratinocytes, a bandlike infiltration along the dermal–epidermal junction, and apoptosis of individual keratinocytes. In its chronic stage, this condition mimics which of the following disorders?

A. Actinic keratosis
B. Discoid lupus erythematosus
C. Late radiation dermatitis
D. Mycosis fungoides, plaque stage
E. Scleroderma

12. A 25-year-old man presents with target lesions, characterized by papules with central bullae and peripheral erythema. Histologic examination shows a lichenoid dermal infiltrate and vacuolar degeneration of the basal cell layer epidermis, with small subepidermal bullae. Within the epidermis, there are keratinocytes with bright eosinophilic cytoplasm and picnotic nuclei. Which of the following is the most common cause of this condition?

A. Herpes simplex virus
B. Histoplasma capsulatum
C. Mycoplasma pneumoniae
D. Nonsteroidal antiinflammatory drugs
E. Sulfonamides

13. An elderly patient presents with extensive areas of erosions and crusts on the trunk. Histopathological eamination of the lesions reveal acantholysis of the granular layer with formation of bullae containing scanty inflammatory cells, as shown in this picture. Which of the following is the most likely diagnosis?

A. Bullous impetigo
B. Erythema toxicum neonatorum
C. Pemphigus foliaceus
D. Pemphigus vulgaris
E. Staphylococcal scalded-skin syndrome

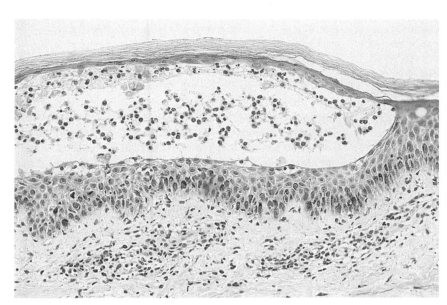

Pamphi. foliaceus :- Subcorneal blister
Pemph. vulgaris :- Suprabasal
Pemphegoid :- Subepidermal blister.

QUESTION 1.13

14. Which of the following bullous diseases is pathogenetically related to autoantibodies against antigens of epidermal intercellular junctions?
    A. Bullous pemphigoid
    B. Dermatitis herpetiformis
    C. Epidermolysis bullosa
    D. Erythema multiforme
    E. Pemphigus vulgaris

15. A 45-year-old man suffers from a skin disease characterized by chronic eruption of brown hyperkeratotic lesions on the neck and trunk. The lesions have a follicular distribution. Several family members on his father's side suffered from a similar disorder. Biopsies show suprabasal clefts containing acantholytic cells; dermal papillae are lined by a single layer of epidermal cells projecting into the clefts like villi. Many large dyskeratotic cells are present within the granular layer and stratum corneum. Which of the following is the most likely diagnosis?
    A. Benign familial pemphigus
    B. Keratosis follicularis
    C. Pemphigus vulgaris
    D. Transient acantholytic dermatosis
    E. Warty dyskeratoma

16. Which of the following skin conditions is most likely to be associated with subepidermal bullae accompanied by inflammatory infiltration?
    A. Bullous pemphigoid
    B. Epidermolysis bullosa
    C. Pemphigus foliaceus
    D. Pemphigus vulgaris
    E. Porphyria cutanea tarda

17. A patient with gluten intolerance complains of an itchy vesicular eruption on the back. A skin biopsy shows the histological changes in this photomicrograph whereas direct immunofluorescence demonstrates IgA deposition at the tips of dermal papillae. Which of the following is the most likely diagnosis?

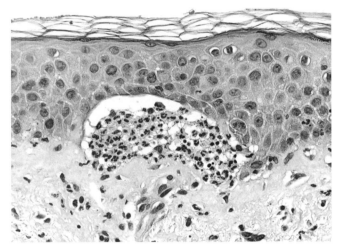

QUESTION 1.17

    A. Bullous pemphigoid
    B. Dermatitis herpetiformis
    C. Epidermolysis bullosa, junctional type
    D. Erythema multiforme
    E. Porphyria cutanea tarda

18. A patient with a history of a recent tick bite presents with a febrile illness characterized by skin lesions and lymphadenitis. The skin lesions are described as erythema chronicum migrans. Which of the following is the underlying etiology?
    A. *Borrelia burgdorferi*
    B. Cancer
    C. Group A streptococcus

D. *Rickettsia rickettsii*

E. *Treponema pallidum*

19. A 52-year-old woman presents with the recent onset of slowly enlarging brown-red plaques on her face. A biopsy shows a dense inflammatory infiltrate spanning the papillary and reticular dermis, consisting of lymphocytes, histiocytes, occasional neutrophils, and numerous eosinophils. There is a definite clear zone between the epidermis and the underlying dermal infiltrate. Which of the following is the most likely diagnosis?

   A. Granuloma annulare
   B. Granuloma faciale
   C. Infected insect bite
   D. Tumor stage of mycosis fungoides
   E. Wegener granulomatosis

20. Which of the following statements is correct concerning skin tuberculosis and leprosy?

   A. Acid-fast bacilli are easily demonstrated in tubercular granulomas
   B. Hansen bacilli are numerous in lepromatous leprosy
   C. Lepra (Virchow) cells are plentiful in tuberculoid leprosy
   D. Lupus vulgaris is most commonly associated with necrotizing granulomas
   E. Most cases of skin tuberculosis are due to primary infection

21. Which of the following histopathological lesions is most characteristic of conditions such as granuloma annulare, necrobiosis lipoidica, and rheumatoid nodules?

   A. Leukocytoclastic vasculitis
   B. Lobular panniculitis
   C. Palisading granulomas
   D. Sclerosis of upper dermis
   E. Septal panniculitis

22. A biopsy of atrophic and hypopigmented plaques from the perianal region of a 50-year-old woman shows the following microscopic changes: epidermal atrophy, loss of rete ridges, orthokeratotic hyperkeratosis, and plugging of keratin follicular orifices. Which of the following is the most likely diagnosis?

   A. Elastosis perforans
   B. Labial lentigo
   C. Leukoplakia
   D. Lichen sclerosus et atrophicus
   E. Morphea

23. A 33-year-old woman presents with painful red nodules on the anterior legs. A biopsy shows an infiltrate of neutrophils, lymphocytes, and histiocytes at the junction between dermis and subcutaneous tissue, spreading between fat lobules. A granuloma consisting of epithelioid cells arranged around a central cleft is also seen. Which of the following is the most common condition associated with this cutaneous lesion?

   A. Bacterial infections
   B. Drugs
   C. Inflammatory bowel disease
   D. Sarcoidosis
   E. Tuberculosis

2

NONMELANOCYTIC CUTANEOUS TUMORS

1. Verrucous hyperplasia in a nevus sebaceus of Jadassohn (organoid nevus) is associated with which of the following changes?
   - A. Basophilic cytoplasmic inclusions
   - B. Clearing of keratinocyte cytoplasm
   - C. Malformation of underlying adnexa
   - D. Prominence of horn cysts
   - E. Vacuolation of the granular layer (koilocytosis)

2. The paraneoplastic sign of Leser-Trélat is related to the sudden appearance of numerous skin lesions, whose characteristic histopathology is depicted in this low-power photomicrograph. This skin lesion is:

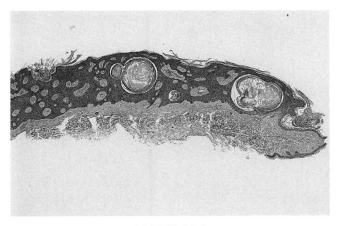

QUESTION 2.2

   - A. Acanthosis nigricans
   - B. Keratoacanthoma
   - C. Seborrheic keratosis
   - D. Subcorneal bullae
   - E. Xanthomas

3. In addition to keratinocyte atypia, which of the following is the most characteristic histological change of actinic keratosis?
   - A. Alternating columns of parakeratosis and orthokeratosis
   - B. Atrophy of the epidermis
   - C. Chronic inflammatory infiltrate in a lichenoid pattern

   - D. Loss of cohesion of keratinocytes
   - E. Marked pigmentation of basal melanocytes

4. The clinical condition known as Bowen disease of the skin is characterized histologically by:
   - A. Acantholytic suprabasal bullae
   - B. Epidermal atypia with koilocytosis
   - C. Low-grade squamous intraepithelial lesion
   - D. Melanocytic atypia
   - E. Squamous cell carcinoma *in situ*

5. This low-power photomicrograph shows a cutaneous neoplasm akin to squamous cell carcinoma. Which of the following is the most important morphological aspect in differentiating this neoplasm from squamous cell carcinoma?

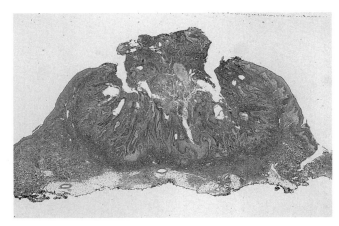

QUESTION 2.5

   - A. Architecture
   - B. Cytologic atypia
   - C. Mitotic activity
   - D. Nuclear features
   - E. Perineurial invasion

6. Which of the following microscopic types of basal cell carcinoma is associated with prominent cytologic atypia and a greater propensity for metastatic spread?
   - A. Basaloid
   - B. Clear cell
   - C. Fibroepithelial tumor of Pinkus

D. Sclerosing (morphealike)

E. Superficial

7. Which of the following statements is correct concerning squamous cell carcinoma of the skin?

A. The adenoid (pseudoglandular) variant is related to acantholysis

B. Most cases are poorly differentiated

C. The spindle cell variant occurs most commonly on sun-unexposed areas

D. Most cases do not express *Ulex europaeus* agglutinin I lectin-binding sites

E. Verrucous carcinoma is frequently associated with lymph node metastases

8. An ulcerated violaceous nodule is excised from the face of a 55-year-old man. As shown in this photomicrograph, the lesion is an intradermal tumor composed of small round cells with high mitotic activity. The chromatin pattern is finely granular. Which of the following immunohistochemical or ultrastructural features would favor a diagnosis of Merkel cell carcinoma?

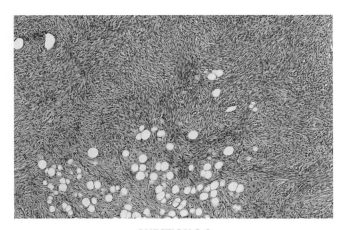

QUESTION 2.8

A. Diffuse cytoplasmic immunoreactivity for high molecular weight keratin

B. Identification of Birbeck granules on electron microscopy

C. Neuron-specific enolase immunoreactivity

D. Perinuclear dotlike immunoreactivity for low molecular weight keratin

E. Ultrastructural identification of melanosomes and premelanosomes

9. Sweat gland carcinomas are rare. These tumors are most likely to simulate histologically which of the following neoplasms?

A. Melanoma

B. Metastatic breast or renal cell carcinomas

C. Metastatic salivary gland tumors

D. Metastatic small cell carcinoma of the lungs

E. Metastatic thymoma

10. A 10-year-old child presents with flesh-colored papules around the nose and mouth. On biopsy, the lesions consist of islands of small basaloid cells with papillary fronds within a fibrotic stroma. There are scattered cystic spaces filled with laminated keratin. Retraction artifacts around tumor islands are absent. Which of the following is the most likely diagnosis?

A. Basal cell carcinoma

B. Inverted follicular keratosis

C. Trichilemmoma

D. Trichoepithelioma

E. Trichofolliculoma

11. Which of the following adnexal tumors is also referred to as "turban tumor"?

A. Chondroid syringoma

B. Cylindroma

C. Eccrine poroma

D. Sebaceous adenoma

E. Trichilemmoma

12. A painful nodule is excised from the lower leg of a young patient. Histologically, it shows extreme cellular density and a two-cell population, including a rich lymphocytic infiltrate within perivascular spaces and between tumor cells. Overall, its morphologic features are reminiscent of thymoma. Which of the following is the most likely diagnosis?

A. Cylindroma

B. Eccrine spiradenoma

C. Glomus tumor

D. Metastatic thymoma

E. Synovial sarcoma

13. Which of the following is the salient morphologic feature of pilomatricomas?

A. Abrupt keratinization with "ghost" cells

B. Extramedullary hematopoiesis

C. Foreign body giant cell reaction

D. Multiple foci of calcification

E. Ossification

14. Multiple small tan papular lesions on the lower eyelids of a female patient are biopsied, showing numerous small ducts with a two-cell epithelial lining and characteristic commalike extensions. Which of the following is the most likely diagnosis?

A. Chondroid syringoma

B. Cylindroma

C. Eccrine poroma

D. Syringoma

E. Trichoepithelioma

15. Which of the following adnexal tumors is morphologically similar to mixed tumors arising in salivary glands?

A. Chondroid syringoma

B. Cylindroma

C. Eccrine poroma

D. Syringoma

E. Trichoepithelioma

16. The immunohistochemical staining most helpful in differentiating a cellular dermatofibroma (fibrous histiocytoma) from dermatofibrosarcoma protuberans (DFSP) is:
    A. Actin
    B. CD34
    C. Factor XIIIa
    D. HMB-45
    E. Vimentin

17. A biopsy of a polypoid skin lesion on the back of 45-year-old man reveals a tumor characterized by a prominent "cartwheel" pattern as shown in this picture. On immunohistochemistry, tumor cells are positive for CD34 and negative for S100 protein. Which of the following is the most likely diagnosis?

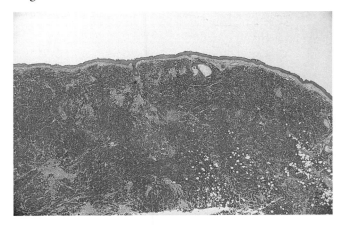

QUESTION 2.17

    A. Atypical fibroxanthoma
    B. Dermatofibrosarcoma protuberans (DFSP)
    C. Leiomyoma
    D. Neurofibroma
    E. Schwannoma

18. A 70-year-old man presents with a slowly growing, exophytic, reddish 1-cm nodule on the face. Excisional biopsy shows a poorly circumscribed, highly cellular tumor within the dermis, extending to, but not continuous with, the epidermis. It is composed of a mixture of fibroblast-like spindle cells and histiocyte-like cells. Many multinucleated giant cells are present. Mitoses are plentiful (including atypical ones), and cellular pleomorphism is marked. Neoplastic cells are variably immunoreactive for CD68, factor XIIIa, and occasionally S100, but negative for keratin and desmin. Which of the following is the most likely diagnosis?
    A. Atypical fibroxanthoma
    B. Cellular schwannoma
    C. Dermatofibroma
    D. Dermatofibrosarcoma protuberans
    E. Nodular fasciitis

19. Which of the following benign cutaneous tumors is often very painful?
    A. Atypical fibroxanthoma
    B. Fibrous histiocytoma
    C. Leiomyoma
    D. Neurofibroma
    E. Neurothekeoma

20. A rapidly growing red nodule on the lip of a pregnant woman shows a histologic pattern characterized by a vascular lobular architecture. It consists of a central branching vessel surrounded by proliferating endothelial and inflammatory cells. Mitotic activity is high. The most likely evolution of this lesion is:
    A. Hematogenous metastasis
    B. Local aggressive behavior
    C. Nodal metastasis
    D. Repeated recurrence after excision
    E. Spontaneous regression or stabilization

21. A patient with AIDS develops multiple nodular lesions in the skin. Biopsy shows a lobular proliferation of small blood vessels lined by plump epithelioid endothelial cells. The interstitium is infiltrated by clusters of neutrophils. Silver staining demonstrates the presence of small bacilli. Which of the following is the causative agent of this condition?
    A. *Bartonella bacilliformis*
    B. *Bartonella henselae*
    C. *Bartonella quintana*
    D. Herpes virus type 8
    E. *Treponema pallidum*

22. Which of the following descriptions concerning epithelioid (histiocytoid) hemangioma is correct?
    A. Benign vascular tumor with rich eosinophilic infiltration
    B. Intraluminal papillary growth due to organization of thrombus
    C. Vascular lesion related to *Bartonella henselae* infection
    D. Vascular lesion related to herpes simplex virus type 8
    E. Vascular tumor of borderline malignancy of deep tissues

23. Besides HIV, which of the following viruses is implicated in the pathogenesis of Kaposi sarcoma developing in patients with AIDS?
    A. Cytomegalovirus
    B. Herpesvirus type 8
    C. Human papillomavirus type 16
    D. Human papillomavirus type 18
    E. JC (papova) virus

24. Which of the following microscopic features is most characteristic of mycosis fungoides?
    A. Formation of lymphoid follicles in the dermis
    B. Intraepidermal collections of atypical lymphocytes
    C. Intraepidermal collections of neutrophils
    D. String-of-pearl distribution of lymphocytes along the dermal–epidermal junction
    E. Wedge-shaped dermal lymphocytic infiltrate in a perivascular pattern

3

MELANOCYTIC LESIONS

1. Which of the following histopathologic features is characteristic of benign melanocytic proliferations?
   A. Lack of neurotization
   B. Nuclear atypia
   C. Pagetoid spread
   D. "Shoulder" of junctional melanocytic hyperplasia
   E. Symmetric growth pattern

2. Which of the following is true about congenital melanocytic nevi?
   A. Junctional pattern is the most common
   B. Maturation and senescence are typically absent
   C. Occur in 50% of neonates
   D. Often involve the subcutaneous fat
   E. Smaller and more regular in contour than acquired nevi

3. A 0.4-cm dome-shaped red nodule is found on the neck of a 15-year-old male. An excisional biopsy demonstrates a neoplasm with a roughly triangular shape and a broad base corresponding to the epidermis. It consists of a mixture of atypical spindly and epithelioid cells with prominent nucleoli, as shown in this high-power photomicrograph. The spindle-cell component is arranged in fascicles perpendicular to the epidermis, whereas epithelioid cells are interspersed at random. Pigment is scanty, although small vessels are abundant. Mitoses are seen. Which of the following would favor a diagnosis of malignant melanoma?

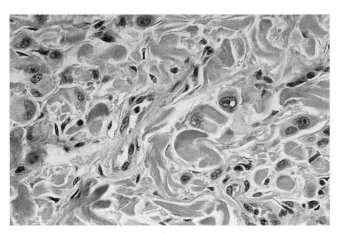

QUESTION 3.3

   A. Cellular atypia
   B. Mitotic activity
   C. Pagetoid spread
   D. Scarcity of melanin
   E. None of the above

4. Which of the following histologic features is most characteristic of a common blue nevus?
   A. Compound nevus with admixture of spindly and epithelioid cells
   B. Compound nevus with cytologic and histologic atypical features
   C. Intradermal spindly or dendritic melanocytes without junctional activity
   D. Nevus extending into reticular dermis and subcutaneous tissue
   E. Nevus with deep dermal infiltration but bland cytological features

5. According to the Clark system, which of the following is the level of invasion of a melanoma that fills the papillary dermis and extends to the interface with the reticular dermis?
   A. Level I
   B. Level II
   C. Level III
   D. Level IV
   E. Level V

6. Which of the following is the appropriate method of measuring the thickness of a melanoma according to the Breslow system?
   A. From the top of the squamous layer to the deepest point of invasion
   B. From the top of the granular layer to the deepest point of invasion
   C. From the dermal–epidermal junction to the deepest point of invasion
   D. From the top of the dermal papillae to the deepest point of invasion
   E. From the highest level of melanoma to the deepest point of invasion

7. The microscopic stage of a rather thick melanoma is evaluated by Breslow's and Clark's systems. It fills the papillary dermis, but stops at the border between the papillary and

reticular dermis. Its tumor thickness estimated from the top of the granular layer to its deepest level of invasion is 2.1 mm. Which of the following is the correct combination of microstage according to Clark's level and, respectively, the risk category according to Breslow's system?

	Clark's level	Breslow's category
A	I	Low risk
B	II	Intermediate risk
C	III	High risk
D	IV	Intermediate risk
E	V	High risk

8. Which of the following is the most frequent form of melanoma in white persons?
  A. Acral lentiginous melanoma
  B. Hutchinson freckle (lentigo maligna)
  C. Nodular melanoma
  D. Superficial spreading melanoma
  E. None of the above

9. A 65-year-old Caucasian female presents with a slowly growing, slightly raised, tan-brown patch on the right cheek. Histologically, it is composed of atypical melanocytes distributed singly or in small nests along the dermal–epidermal junction. Which of the following is the most likely diagnosis?
  A. Acral lentiginous melanoma
  B. Dysplastic nevus
  C. Lentigo maligna
  D. Nodular melanoma
  E. Superficial spreading melanoma

10. Which of the following is the most common form of melanoma in Asians and Blacks?
  A. Acral lentiginous melanoma
  B. Hutchinson freckle (lentigo maligna)
  C. Nodular melanoma
  D. Superficial spreading melanoma
  E. None of the above

4

MUSCLE BIOPSY IN NEUROMUSCULAR DISEASES

1. A 45-year-old woman undergoes muscle biopsy because of progressive weakness of unclear etiology. Which of the following microscopic changes would favor a myopathic process versus denervation atrophy?
   A. Degeneration and regeneration of myofibers
   B. Fibrosis of the endomysium
   C. Increased number of internal nuclei
   D. Myofiber splitting
   E. All of the above

2. A 55-year-old man undergoes electromyographic (EMG) studies because of slowly progressive weakness in the lower extremities and muscle atrophy. EMG shows a pattern suggestive of neurogenic atrophy. A muscle biopsy is performed. Which of the following alterations is most likely to be seen, if EMG findings were correct?
   A. Chronic inflammatory infiltration of the endomysium
   B. Group atrophy and fiber type grouping
   C. Hyaline fibers and endomysial fatty infiltration
   D. Internalization of nuclei and myofiber splitting
   E. Ragged red fibers on modified Gomori trichrome

3. On Gomori trichrome staining, frozen sections of a muscle biopsy show numerous myofibers with a ragged profile and red subsarcolemmal deposits, as shown in the picture at top of page. This finding suggests which of the following muscle conditions?
   A. Glycogenoses
   B. Immune-mediated myopathies
   C. Lipid storage diseases
   D. Mitochondrial myopathies
   E. Muscular dystrophies

4. A 4-year-old male presents with a history of progressive awkwardness and frequent falls. A clinical diagnosis of Duchenne muscular dystrophy can be confirmed or ruled out by:

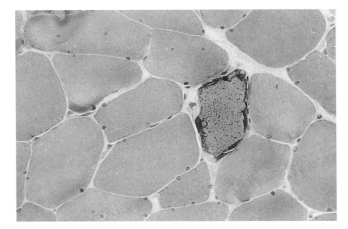

QUESTION 4.3

   A. Biochemical studies of mitochondrial metabolism
   B. Genetic analysis for detection of trinucleotide repeats
   C. Immunohistochemistry for dystrophin on muscle biopsy
   D. Measurement of blood creatine kinase
   E. Ultrastructural study of neuromuscular junctions

5. A 58-year-old man comes to medical attention with progressive distal weakness and markedly increased blood levels of creatine kinase. A muscle biopsy reveals myopathic changes, mild endomysial lymphocytic infiltration, and numerous rimmed vacuoles within myofibers. Furthermore, many atrophic angular myofibers are seen. Which of the following is the most likely diagnosis?
   A. Dermatomyositis
   B. Inclusion body myositis
   C. Limb-girdle dystrophy
   D. Neurogenic atrophy
   E. Polymyositis

5

DISORDERS OF SOFT TISSUE

1. In the microscopic evaluation of a soft tissue mass, which of the following is the most important *initial* question to answer?
   A. Is the lesion neoplastic?
   B. Is the lesion a malignant tumor?
   C. Is the lesion a sarcoma?
   D. What is the histogenesis?
   E. What is the mitotic rate?
2. Which of the following parameters strongly favors a diagnosis of malignancy in a soft tissue mass?
   A. Bizarre nuclei
   B. High vascularity
   C. Lobular architecture in a vascular lesion
   D. Presence of "floret" cells
   E. Rapid growth
3. A biopsy of a mass infiltrating a peripheral nerve shows a sarcoma-like lesion composed of spindly and epithelioid cells. There is brisk mitotic activity, focal necrosis, and marked nuclear pleomorphism. Fascicles of neoplastic cells are separated by dense fibrous bands. A differential diagnosis of desmoplastic melanoma versus malignant peripheral nerve sheath tumor (MPNST) is considered. Which of the following would favor melanoma?
   A. Absent HMB-45 immunoreactivity
   B. Desmoplastic reaction
   C. Diffuse immunoreactivity for S100 protein
   D. Pericellular reticulin network
   E. Strong HMB-45 expression
4. Which of the following soft tissue tumors (STTs) is strongly immunoreactive for CD34?
   A. Atypical fibroxanthoma
   B. Desmoplastic melanoma
   C. Solitary fibrous tumor
   D. Spindle cell carcinoma
   E. Synovial sarcoma
5. A 3-cm nodule is excised from the right forearm of a 40-year-old man, who says that it grew rapidly over 2 weeks. Histologically, it is densely cellular and mitotically active. The stroma is myxoid, and there are collagen bundles lined by spindle cells. Its architecture is shown in this low-power photomicrograph. Which of the following is the most likely diagnosis?

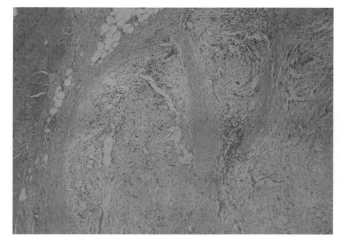

QUESTION 5.5

   A. Fibrosarcoma
   B. Keloid scar
   C. Myxoid liposarcoma
   D. Myxoid malignant fibrous histiocytoma
   E. Nodular fasciitis
6. Which of the following forms of lipoma is most likely to mimic a sarcoma?
   A. Angiolipoma
   B. Fibrolipoma
   C. Myxolipoma
   D. Pleomorphic lipoma
   E. Spindle cell lipoma
7. A review of slides of a tumor excised from the upper extremity of a 2-year-old child and previously diagnosed as myxoid liposarcoma reveals a neoplastic lesion composed of lipoblasts. The architecture is distinctly lobular, with a myxoid background containing a plexiform vascular network. Which of the following is the most likely diagnosis?
   A. Angiolipoma
   B. Hibernoma
   C. Lipoblastoma
   D. Myxoma
   E. Well-differentiated liposarcoma
8. The *fetal* form of rhabdomyoma may develop in the

vulvovaginal region of middle-aged women. Which of the following is the most common location in children?
  A. Extremities
  B. Head and neck
  C. Mediastinum
  D. Perineal region
  E. Retroperitoneum

9. Which of the following vascular lesions is thought to arise as a florid form of organized and recanalized thrombus?
  A. Capillary hemangioma
  B. Intravascular papillary endothelial hyperplasia
  C. Malignant endovascular papillary angioendothelioma
  D. Spindle cell hemangioendothelioma
  E. Symplasmic hemangioma

10. A poorly circumscribed nodular mass is removed from the right subscapular region of a 65-year-old man. The lesion lies beneath the latissimus dorsi muscle. Histologically, it consists of thick bundles of collagen intermixed with eosinophilic cylindrical structures removed by elastase digestion. Which of the following is the most likely diagnosis?
  A. Elastofibroma
  B. Fibroma of the tendon sheath
  C. Fibromatosis
  D. Keloid scar
  E. Nodular fasciitis

11. A small subcutaneous nodule removed from the wrist of a 13-year-old male consists of spindly, fibroblast-like cells with spotty calcifications. The cells surrounding calcific foci resemble chondrocytes. Cytologic atypia and mitotic activity are absent. Peripheral infiltration of muscle is seen. Which of the following is the most likely diagnosis?
  A. Calcifying aponeurotic fibroma
  B. Fibroma of the tendon sheath
  C. Fibromatosis
  D. Rheumatoid nodule
  E. Schwannoma

12. Ultrastructural and immunohistochemical studies indicate that the principal cell constituents of fibromatosis are:
  A. Fibroblasts
  B. Histiocytes
  C. Myofibroblasts
  D. Schwann cells
  E. Smooth muscle cells

13. One of the most characteristic morphologic features of fibrosarcomas is:
  A. Herringbone pattern
  B. Multinucleated giant cells
  C. Palisading of cells
  D. Serpentine nuclei
  E. Storiform pattern

14. Which of the following microscopic patterns is most characteristic of dermatofibrosarcoma protuberans (DFSP)?
  A. Cartwheel/storiform pattern with no significant atypia

  B. Long spindle cell fascicles in a herringbone pattern
  C. Parallel strands of keloidlike collagen
  D. Spindle cell tumor with giant rosettes
  E. Zonal architecture

15. A soft tissue tumor is excised from the lower limb of a 68-year-old man. It is attached to the muscular fascia, appears well circumscribed but not encapsulated, and measures 8 cm in greatest diameter. Histologically, the tumor appears as a mixture of large bizarre cells and spindle-shaped cells with a vague storiform arrangement, as shown by this medium-power view. The intercellular matrix shows focal myxoid changes. Mitotic activity is brisk. Tumor cells are immunoreactive for vimentin, but negative for keratin, S100 protein, desmin, myoglobin, smooth muscle actin, and CD34. Which of the following diagnoses is most likely?

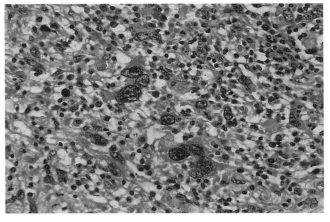

QUESTION 5.15

  A. Dermatofibrosarcoma protuberans
  B. Fibromatosis
  C. Fibrosarcoma
  D. Malignant fibrous histiocytoma
  E. Poorly differentiated rhabdomyosarcoma

16. Which of the following variants of malignant fibrous histiocytoma (MFH) shows prominent lymphocytic aggregates occasionally simulating a lymph node?
  A. Angiomatoid
  B. Giant cell
  C. Inflammatory
  D. Myxoid
  E. Storiform-pleomorphic

17. Which of the following variants of lipoma is frequently associated with local pain?
  A. Angiolipoma
  B. Angiomyolipoma
  C. Chondroid lipoma
  D. Fibrolipoma
  E. Myxolipoma

18. This photomicrograph shows an example of the most common type of liposarcoma. Which of the following is it?

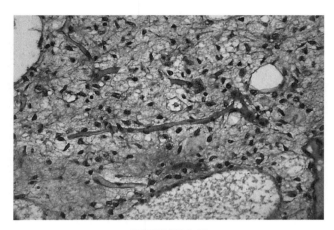

QUESTION 5.18

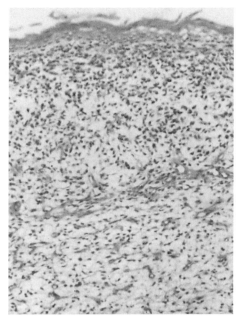

QUESTION 5.20

A. Dedifferentiated
B. Myxoid
C. Pleomorphic
D. Round cell type
E. Well differentiated

19. Which of the following is a correct statement regarding leiomyosarcomas of soft tissue?
  A. Histologic criteria for malignancy depend on site
  B. Most cases are associated with Epstein-Barr virus
  C. Most cases arising from large veins affect males
  D. Most cases arising in the skin affect females
  E. Superficial tumors have a worse prognosis than deep tumors

20. A highly anaplastic soft tissue neoplasm from a 5-year-old child consists of undifferentiated small cells with no distinctive features. Neoplastic cells tend to gather in dense aggregates beneath epithelial surfaces and around blood vessels, as seen in this picture. Which of the following is the most likely diagnosis?
  A. Extraskeletal Ewing sarcoma
  B. Intraabdominal desmoplastic small cell tumor
  C. Lymphoma
  D. Neuroblastoma
  E. Rhabdomyosarcoma

21. Which of the following forms of rhabdomyosarcoma has the worst prognosis?
  A. Alveolar
  B. Embryonal
  C. Rhabdoid
  D. Pleomorphic
  E. All have equally poor prognosis

22. Which of the following tumors is usually associated with tuberous sclerosis *and* displays HMB45 immunoreactivity?
  A. Epithelioid hemangioendothelioma
  B. Glomus tumor
  C. Hemangiopericytoma
  D. Lymphangiomyoma
  E. Rhabdomyoma

23. On histological examination, a soft tissue tumor reveals a spindle cell population with a widespread staghorn vascular pattern. Immunohistochemistry demonstrates small clusters of epithelioid cells reactive for cytokeratin and epithelial membrane antigen (EMA). Which of the following is the most likely diagnosis?
  A. Fibrosarcoma
  B. Hemangiopericytoma
  C. Peripheral nerve sheath tumor
  D. Solitary fibrous tumor
  E. Synovial sarcoma

24. A tumor with a biphasic spindle cell and glandular pattern, spotty calcifications, and chromosomal translocation t(X;18) develops most commonly in the proximity of the:
  A. Head and neck
  B. Hip joint
  C. Knee and ankle
  D. Mediastinum
  E. Retroperitoneum
  F. Shoulder and elbow

25. A soft tissue tumor shows a spindle cell population arranged in hypercellular areas alternating with paucicellular areas. Occasional Verocay bodies are found. The cells are immunoreactive for S100 protein. Which of the following ultrastructural features will support a light microscopic diagnosis of schwannoma?
  A. Continuous basement membrane
  B. Cytoplasmic aggregates of intermediate filaments
  C. Dense core granules
  D. Nuclear strangulations and cytoplasmic microfilaments
  E. Ruffled border

26. A 2-cm poorly circumscribed tumor is excised from the tongue. Histologically, the tumor consists of plump cells with granular cytoplasm. The cells are immunoreactive for S100 protein. Which of the following is present in the cytoplasmic granules?

    A. α_1-antitrypsin
    B. Glycogen
    C. Hydrolytic enzymes
    D. Neutral lipids
    E. Phospholipids

27. A soft tissue tumor with a gelatinous cut surface is excised from the upper extremity of a 25-year-old man. Histologically, it consists of a predominantly spindle cell population immunoreactive for S100 protein. Neurofilament immunohistochemistry reveals axons running through the neoplasm. Which of the following is the most likely diagnosis?

    A. Dermatofibroma
    B. Nerve sheath myxoma
    C. Neurofibroma
    D. Schwannoma
    E. Traumatic neuroma

28. A malignant spindle cell tumor with a fascicular pattern shows focal palisading, perivascular aggregates of plumper cells, and large gaping vascular channels. A focus of pseudopalisading necrosis is also identified. Which of the following is the most likely diagnosis?

    A. Malignant fibrous histiocytoma
    B. Malignant peripheral nerve sheath tumor
    C. Spindle cell hemangioendothelioma
    D. Spindle cell liposarcoma
    E. Spindle cell melanoma

29. The histologic examination of a soft tissue mass from the thigh of a 25-year-old woman reveals a neoplasm with an alveolar pattern as shown in this photomicrograph. The neoplastic cells have granular cytoplasm, vesicular nuclei, and prominent central nucleoli. PAS-positive needlelike cytoplasmic inclusions are identified. Electron microscopy reveals membrane-bound crystalloid inclusions with an orderly linear or crossed pattern. Current hypotheses on the histogenesis of this neoplasm favor a derivation from:

    A. Fibroblasts
    B. Muscle
    C. Primitive neuroectodermal precursors
    D. Schwann cells
    E. Synovial epithelium

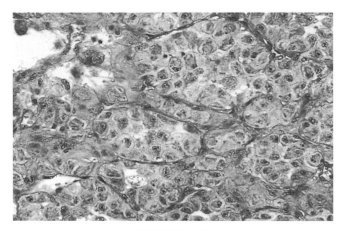

QUESTION 5.29

30. Which of the following is the most characteristic ultrastructural feature of the cells of soft tissue rhabdoid tumors?

    A. Crystalloid inclusions
    B. Paranuclear aggregates of intermediate filaments
    C. Long and slender microvilli
    D. Numerous lysosomes
    E. Numerous mitochondria

31. Which of the following neoplasms is generally considered the soft tissue equivalent of melanoma?

    A. Alveolar soft part sarcoma
    B. Clear cell sarcoma
    C. Epithelioid sarcoma
    D. Granular cell tumor
    E. Pigmented neuroectodermal tumor of infancy

32. A 22-year-old male presents with abdominal pain. A large tumor is found by computed tomography (CT) scan studies within the right pelvis. Smaller peritoneal implants are also described. The tumor is surgically resected. Histologically, it is composed of nests of uniform small cells surrounded by a fibroblastic reaction. Tumor cells are immunoreactive for desmin, which is expressed as dotlike spots in a perinuclear location. Additionally, tumor cells are positive for keratin. Which of the following is the most likely diagnosis?

    A. Desmoplastic small cell sarcoma (DSCS)
    B. Ewing sarcoma
    C. Mesothelioma
    D. Metastatic carcinoma
    E. Peripheral neuroectodermal tumor (PNET)

6

JOINT DISEASES

1. Fibrillation of the cartilaginous matrix and degeneration of chondrocytes are early pathological changes of which of the following conditions?
    A. Ankylosing spondylitis
    B. Degenerative joint disease
    C. Gouty arthritis
    D. Psoriatic arthritis
    E. Rheumatoid arthritis

2. A 50-year-old woman with a systemic disease involving small joints develops subcutaneous nodules in the forearms. One of these is biopsied and shows the histological features demonstrated in this low-power picture. Which of the following is the most likely diagnosis?

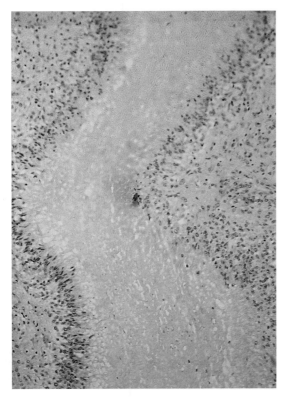

QUESTION 6.2

A. Amyloidosis
B. Degenerative joint disease
C. Gout
D. Rheumatoid arthritis
E. Sarcoidosis

3. A biopsy of a destructive lesion in the foot of a patient with a history of gout is submitted for pathologic examination. Which of the following is the most appropriate manner to handle this specimen?
    A. Fixation in alcohol
    B. Fixation in formalin
    C. Fixation in glutaraldehyde
    D. Formalin fixation followed by 3% potassium chromate
    E. Microscopic examination of unstained frozen tissue

4. A 48-year-old patient develops acute swelling and pain of the knee. A synovial aspirate from the affected joint leads to identification of rhomboid crystals, which are blue when parallel and yellow when perpendicular to the axis of a red compensator. These crystals are composed of:
    A. Calcium oxalate
    B. Calcium pyrophosphate
    C. Cholesterol
    D. Homogentisic acid
    E. Urate

5. In *Hoffa's disease*, the most characteristic pathologic alteration is:
    A. Accumulation of crystals within joint space
    B. Degeneration of cartilage matrix
    C. Formation of pannus over the articular surface
    D. Necrosis of subsynovial bone
    E. Subsynovial fatty infiltration

6. A 25-year-old female presents with swelling and mild pain in the volar aspect of the right wrist. A portion of the synovium is excised. Its macroscopic features are shown in this photograph. Histologically, it consists of sheets of polygonal and occasionally multinucleated cells. Papillary fronds arise from the adjacent synovial lining. Foamy histiocytes, hemosiderin-laden macrophages, and multinucleated giant

cells are abundant at the periphery. These features are most consistent with:

A. Baker cyst
B. Ganglion cyst
C. Hemosiderotic synovitis
D. Pigmented villonodular synovitis
E. Primary synovial chondromatosis

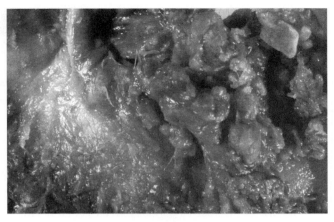

QUESTION 6.6

7

NONNEOPLASTIC DISEASES OF BONES

1. X-ray studies of a patient with osteogenesis imperfecta show bilateral expansion of the distal ends of the femurs with numerous round calcifications, resulting in the radiologic appearance shown in this picture. The pathologic correlate of this radiologic finding is:

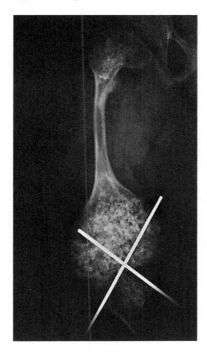

QUESTION 7.1

A. Abnormal mineralization of growth plate
B. Fragmentation of growth plate
C. Increased density of bone
D. Premature fusion of growth plate
E. Thinning of bone trabeculae

2. Which of the following bones is preferentially involved by bone lesions of osteitis fibrosa cystica?
   A. Clavicle
   B. Femur
   C. Mandible
   D. Ribs
   E. Vertebral bodies

3. Which of the following viral agents is suspected of playing a pathogenetic role in Paget disease?
   A. Epstein-Barr virus
   B. Herpes simplex virus
   C. Human papillomavirus
   D. JC virus (papovavirus)
   E. Paramyxovirus

4. A 20-year-old football player undergoes excision of a recently developed mass in the flexor aspect of the right arm. There is a history of recent trauma. H&E sections show a central region of highly cellular pleomorphic stroma, surrounded by osteoid deposition and a peripheral rim of bone trabeculae. These features are consistent with:
   A. Extraneous osteosarcoma
   B. Juxtacortical osteosarcoma
   C. Myositis ossificans
   D. Nodular fasciitis
   E. Proliferative fasciitis

5. Of the pathogens causing acute osteomyelitis, which of the following is most frequently associated with hemoglobinopathies such as sickle cell disease?
   A. Coagulase-negative staphylococci
   B. *Pseudomonas*
   C. *Salmonella*
   D. *Staphylococcus aureus*
   E. *Streptococcus pyogenes*

8

BONE TUMORS

1. The stage of a high-grade bone tumor limited to the femur and without evidence of distant metastasis is:
    A. Stage IA
    B. Stage IB
    C. Stage IIA
    D. Stage IIB
    E. Stage IIIA
    F. Stage IIIC

2. Which of the following is the most common primary malignant neoplasm of bone?
    A. Chondrosarcoma
    B. Lymphoma
    C. Metastatic carcinoma
    D. Multiple myeloma (MM)
    E. Osteosarcoma

3. The most typical x-ray bone change due to multiple myeloma is:
    A. Codman triangle
    B. Expansion of bone and thickening of cortex
    C. Onionskin appearance
    D. Punched-out osteolytic lesions
    E. Radiolucent nidus and sclerotic rim

4. A 16-year-old male presents with swelling and pain in the right arm and fever. A mass expanding the right humerus with an onionskin pattern is identified on x-rays. A biopsy reveals the tumor shown in this high-power photomicrograph. There is no evidence of osteoid formation. Special stains demonstrate intracytoplasmic glycogen and immunoreactiv-

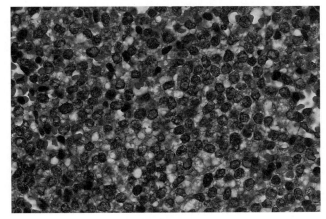

QUESTION 8.4

ity of tumor cells for CD99. All other immunostains are negative except for vimentin. Following resection of the tumor, which of the following steps should be carried out to support this diagnosis?
    A. Place the mass in decalcifying solution
    B. Save tissue for cytogenetic studies
    C. Save tissue for electron microscopic studies
    D. Send specimen for culture studies
    E. No further investigation is necessary

5. Which of the following microscopic features is most consistent with a diagnosis of osteochondroma?
    A. Chondroblasts with osteoclast-like giant cells and chicken-wire calcification
    B. Core of normal bone trabeculae capped by mature cartilage
    C. Misshapen trabeculae of woven bone without osteoblastic rimming
    D. Osteoid lined by fibroblasts within a cellular stroma
    E. Well-differentiated cartilage in a lobular pattern

6. A lobulated tumor is removed from the third proximal phalanx of a 25-year-old man. Histologically, it consists of mature cartilage with a lobular architecture. The tumor expands from the metaphyseal bone and produces thinning of the cortex. A condition characterized by numerous cartilaginous tumors such as this one and soft tissue hemangiomas is known as:
    A. Albright syndrome
    B. Gardner syndrome
    C. Maffucci syndrome
    D. Ollier disease
    E. Osteochondromatosis

7. A 15-year-old male has a bone tumor in the proximal epiphysis of his right tibia. A biopsy shows the following: high cellular density, polygonal cells with well-demarcated borders and thick cell membranes, abundant cytoplasmic glycogen, scattered multinucleated giant cells, delicate microcalcifications in a chicken-wire pattern, and reticulin fibers around each cell. Which of the following is the most likely diagnosis?
    A. Chondroblastoma
    B. Chondroma
    C. Chondrosarcoma
    D. Chordoma
    E. Giant cell tumor of bone

8. A 15-year-old boy comes to medical attention because of persistent dull pain in the lower right thigh, not relieved by aspirin or other antiinflammatory drugs. X-rays reveal a well-demarcated peripheral radiolucent lesion in the distal femur. Excised, the lesion appears composed of islands of hyaline cartilage with stellate and spindle cells within a myxoid matrix. These islands are separated by cellular fibroblastic bands, giving rise to a biphasic pattern. Scattered osteoclast-like giant cells are present. Mitotic figures are not found. Which of the following is the most likely diagnosis?
  A. Chondroblastoma
  B. Chondromyxoid fibroma
  C. Chondrosarcoma
  D. Giant cell tumor
  E. Osteoid osteoma

9. A correct statement concerning chondrosarcoma is:
  A. The Codman triangle is a characteristic radiologic feature
  B. Grading is very important for prognosis
  C. It is immunoreactive for vimentin and negative for S100
  D. It is most commonly located in the long bones of limbs
  E. Young adults and children are most frequently affected

10. The designation of *dedifferentiated* chondrosarcoma applies to a chondrosarcoma with:
  A. Chordoma-like growth within myxoid background
  B. Cords and nests of cells with clear cytoplasm and sharp borders
  C. Dimorphic pattern with poorly and well-differentiated areas
  D. Tumor arising from previous osteochondroma
  E. Well-differentiated central region surrounded by poorly differentiated sarcoma

11. A 14-year-old male presents with a history of pain in the right leg that manifests at night and is promptly relieved by aspirin. A 1.5-cm radiolucent focus surrounded by diffuse osteosclerosis is identified in the right tibia and excised. This

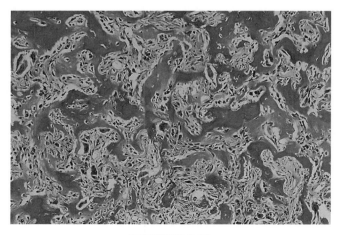

QUESTION 8.11

photomicrograph demonstrates its histological appearance. Which of the following is the most likely diagnosis?
  A. Fibrous dysplasia
  B. Osteoblastoma
  C. Osteochondroma
  D. Osteoid osteoma
  E. Osteosarcoma

12. In which of the following syndromes are multiple osteomas found?
  A. Familial adenomatous polyposis (FAP)
  B. Gardner syndrome
  C. Maffucci syndrome
  D. McCune-Albright syndrome
  E. Ollier disease

13. Which of the following features is most important in supporting a diagnosis of osteosarcoma in an otherwise poorly differentiated mesenchymal tumor?
  A. Foci of cartilage
  B. Osteoclast-like giant cells
  C. Osteoid production
  D. Immunoreactivity for S100 protein
  E. Immunoreactivity for vimentin

14. Which of the following conditions is responsible for most cases of osteosarcomas arising in patients older than 45 years?
  A. Fibrous dysplasia
  B. Infections
  C. Paget disease
  D. Prior radiation
  E. Trauma

15. A variant of osteosarcoma manifests as a slow-growing, extracortical, lobulated mass arising from the metaphyses of long bones in older patients. Its radiologic appearance is shown in this photograph. Which variant is it?
  A. Gnathic
  B. Juxtacortical (parosteal)
  C. Paget associated
  D. Periosteal
  E. Telangiectatic

16. MRI scans show an osteolytic tumor within the distal epiphysis of the right femur of a 25-year-old female. The tumor is resected. On macroscopic examination, the lesion contains multiple cysts and brown deposits. Histologically, it is composed of sheets of mononuclear cells with uniformly scattered multinucleated giant cells and multifocal deposits of hemosiderin. These features are most consistent with:
  A. Brown tumor of hyperparathyroidism
  B. Chondroblastoma
  C. Giant cell reparative granuloma
  D. Giant cell tumor
  E. Pigmented villonodular synovitis

17. A 15-year-old male presents with a pathologic fracture of the distal fibula. A spongy hemorrhagic mass is excised. Its gross appearance is shown in the picture. Histologically, the lesion is composed of blood-filled spaces separated by septa containing fibroblasts, hemosiderin-laden macrophages, and

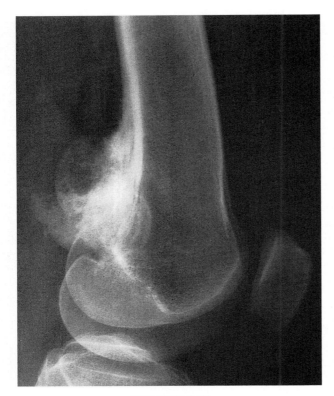

QUESTION 8.15

occasional giant cells. There is no endothelial lining. The most likely diagnosis is:

A. Aneurysmal bone cyst
B. Giant cell reparative granuloma

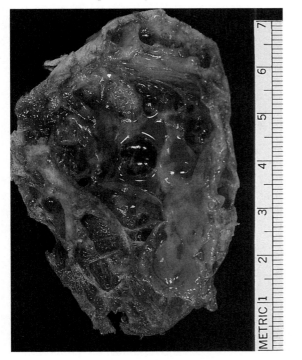

QUESTION 8.17

C. Giant cell tumor
D. Hemangioma
E. Telangiectatic osteosarcoma

18. X-ray studies reveal a unicameral cystic lesion in the proximal metaphysis of the humerus in a 14-year-old male. It contains brown fluid, and its wall is composed of vascular fibrous tissue with hemosiderin-laden macrophages and cholesterol clefts. These features are consistent with:

A. Aneurysmal bone cyst
B. Ganglion cyst of bone
C. Massive osteolysis (Gorham disease)
D. Metaphyseal fibrous defect
E. Solitary bone cyst

19. Which of the following is the most common location of ganglion cysts?

A. Dorsal aspect of the carpal area
B. Dorsal surface of feet
C. Knee
D. Volar aspect of the wrist
E. Volar surface of metacarpophalangeal joints

20. A 30-year-old man presents with swelling of the right mandible. X-ray studies demonstrate an ill-defined and sclerotic focus. Histologic examination reveals irregularly shaped trabeculae of immature bone within moderately cellular fibrous stroma. The bone trabeculae are not surrounded by osteoblasts or psammoma-like structures. This lesion is most consistent with:

A. Cementifying fibroma
B. Cementoossifying fibroma
C. Fibrous dysplasia
D. Juvenile ossifying fibroma
E. Ossifying fibroma

21. An 8-year-old female presents with precocious puberty, numerous café au lait spots on the right side of the body, and hyperthyroidism. X-ray studies show multiple bone lesions in the skull, femur, ribs, and mandible, which are also located on the right side. A biopsy of one of these lesions reveals trabeculae of woven bone with a fishhook appearance without osteoblastic rimming. This patient has:

A. Albright syndrome
B. Gardner syndrome
C. Hand-Schüller-Christian disease
D. Neurofibromatosis
E. Ollier disease

22. A 12-year-old boy complains of pain in the right thigh. X-ray studies show a radiolucent defect in the distal metaphysis of the right femur. On biopsy, this consists of a fibroblastic population arranged in a storiform pattern. Hemosiderin-laden macrophages and clusters of giant cells are also found. These features are most consistent with:

A. Brown tumor of hyperparathyroidism
B. Giant cell tumor
C. Massive osteolysis (Gorham disease)
D. Metaphyseal fibrous defect
E. Osteosarcoma

23. A well-demarcated osteolytic lesion in the parietal bone of a 23-old-female is biopsied, showing aggregates of cells with lobulated nucleus, lymphocytes, histiocytes, and numerous eosinophils. Ultrastructural studies reveal rodlike, tubular structures with expanded racket-shaped ends. The diagnosis is:

A. Chronic osteomyelitis
B. Infectious granuloma
C. Langerhans cell histiocytosis
D. Metastatic carcinoma
E. Sinus histiocytosis with massive lymphadeno-pathy

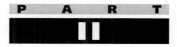

BREAST

9

THE BREAST

1. A biopsy of a breast nodule from a 25-year-old pregnant woman reveals the histologic features depicted in this photograph. Rare foci of necrosis are identified. These findings are most consistent with:

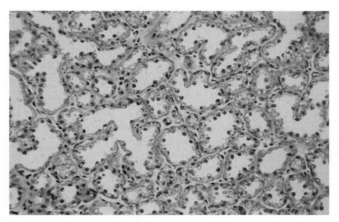

QUESTION 9.1

A. Ductal *in situ* carcinoma
B. Epithelial hyperplasia
C. Fibrocystic changes
D. Pregnancy-related changes
E. Tubular adenoma

2. The term *adenosis* refers to which of the following changes?
A. Increased number of epithelial cells within preexisting glands
B. Increased number or enlargement of glandular elements
C. Dilated sacs containing fluid
D. Formation consisting of an epithelial-lined fibrovascular core
E. Transformation of one type of epithelium into another

3. Which of the following elements in fibrocystic change is related to increased risk of breast cancer?
A. Adenosis
B. Apocrine metaplasia
C. Cyst formation

D. Epithelial hyperplasia
E. Papillomatous growth

4. Mammographic and gross examination of a breast mass reveal a stellate-shaped lesion containing a central core of fibrosis, as shown in this gross picture. Histologically, on low-power examination the lesion resembles the head of a flower. The central fibrotic core contains distorted tubules and lobules and is surrounded by glandular elements showing varying degrees of dilatation, hyperplasia, adenosis, and occasional papillomatous formations. Which of the following is it?

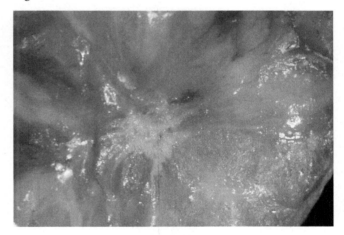

QUESTION 9.4

A. Atypical ductal hyperplasia
B. Fat necrosis
C. Infiltrating lobular carcinoma
D. Sclerosing adenosis/radial scar
E. Tubular carcinoma

5. Which of the following breast lesions lacks a myoepithelial lining in spite of its benign nature?
A. Intraductal papilloma
B. Microglandular adenosis
C. Radial scar
D. Sclerosing adenosis
E. Tubular adenoma

6. A breast biopsy shows alterations of the lobular architecture diagnosed as blunt duct adenosis. Which of the

following changes is most likely to be associated with this condition?

    A. Columnar cell metaplasia
    B. Loss of myoepithelial cells
    C. Papillomatosis
    D. Squamous metaplasia
    E. Stromal hyperplasia

7. A breast biopsy shows foci of extensive epithelial hyperplasia, with obliteration of the ductal lumina. Some of these foci are suspicious for ductal carcinoma *in situ* (DCIS). Which of the following morphologic features favors a diagnosis of DCIS?

    A. Indistinct cell borders
    B. Monotonous epithelial cell population
    C. Peripheral slitlike spaces
    D. Presence of apocrine metaplasia
    E. Streaming of nuclei

8. A biopsy of a breast nodule shows preservation of the lobular architecture, but several lobules are filled with sheets of large and pleomorphic cells, as shown in this photomicrograph. The change shown here is referred to as:

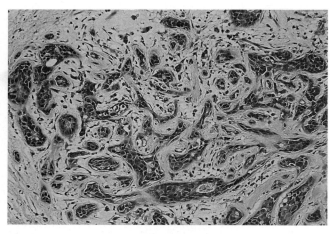

QUESTION 9.8

    A. Ductal carcinoma *in situ,* high grade
    B. Ductal carcinoma *in situ,* low grade
    C. Invasive ductal carcinoma
    D. Lobular cancerization
    E. Lobular carcinoma *in situ*

9. Which of the following biological markers is most consistent with low-grade (well-differentiated) DCIS?

    A. Expression of c-*erb*-B2 oncoprotein
    B. Expression of p53 oncoprotein
    C. High proliferative index
    D. Increase in stromal vessels
    E. Positivity for estrogen/progesterone receptors

10. A 35-year-old female presents with bloody nipple discharge and an ill-defined subareolar nodule. This photomicrograph demonstrates the low-power architecture of the lesion. All of the following histological features are consistent with a diagnosis of solitary intraductal papilloma, *except:*

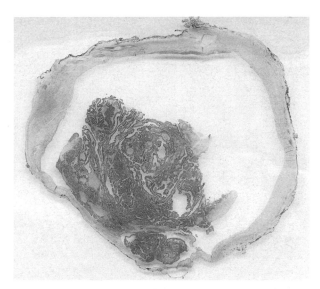

QUESTION 9.10

    A. Apocrine metaplasia
    B. Fibrovascular core
    C. Hyperplasia of luminal epithelium
    D. Infarction
    E. Single-cell layer

11. A breast biopsy shows histopathological changes diagnostic of lobular carcinoma *in situ* (LCIS). This diagnosis implies that:

    A. Changes are probably present in contralateral breast
    B. Long-term follow-up is not necessary
    C. Magnitude of cancer risk is proportional to extent of changes
    D. Metastatic spread has already occurred
    E. There is no increased risk of cancer development

12. A breast biopsy shows several acini filled with sheets of malignant cells that expand and distort the lobular architecture. Neoplastic cells are immunoreactive for E-cadherin and negative for high-molecular-weight keratin. Besides the immunohistochemical profile, which of the following features is most helpful in the differential diagnosis of this change?

    A. Cytological features
    B. Fibroplasia
    C. Lobular architecture
    D. Mitotic activity
    E. Necrosis

13. Which of the following breast changes is associated with a relative risk of developing cancer four to five times that of the general population?

    A. Atypical epithelial hyperplasia
    B. Benign intraductal papilloma
    C. Mild epithelial hyperplasia
    D. Sclerosing adenosis
    E. Severe epithelial hyperplasia

14. Histological evaluation of a breast cancer demonstrates an infiltrating ductal carcinoma. Neoplastic cells form solid trabeculae, whereas tubule formation is negligible. Nuclear

pleomorphism is minimal, and the mitotic rate is 3/high-power field. Which of the following is the grade according to the criteria of Bloom-Richardson system?

- A. Grade 1
- B. Grade 2
- C. Grade 3
- D. More information is necessary

15. Which of the following is the most significant *predictive* factor in breast carcinoma?

- A. Expression of hormone receptors
- B. Ki-67 labeling index
- C. Lymphatic invasion
- D. Lymph node status
- E. Tumor grade
- F. Tumor size
- G. Tumor type

16. A breast lesion is composed of malignant cells distributed as shown in this picture. The most likely diagnosis is:

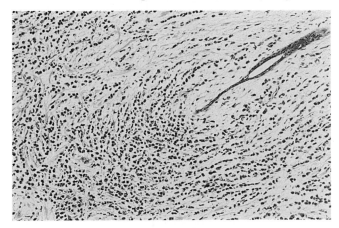

QUESTION 9.16

- A. Infiltrating ductal carcinoma
- B. Infiltrating lobular carcinoma
- C. Medullary carcinoma
- D. Sclerosing adenosis
- E. Tubular carcinoma

17. A 40-year-old woman presents with a breast nodule. After excision, histological examination reveals a lesion composed of well-developed tubular structures with an angulated profile within a desmoplastic stroma. Apical snouts are noted in epithelial cells. No metastases are found in axillary lymph nodes. Markers for myoepithelial cells are negative. Which of the following is the most likely diagnosis?

- A. Invasive ductal carcinoma, not otherwise specified (NOS)
- B. Invasive lobular carcinoma
- C. Microglandular adenosis
- D. Sclerosing adenosis
- E. Tubular carcinoma

18. Mucinous carcinoma of the breast is characterized by:

- A. Absence of hormone receptor expression
- B. Better prognosis than ductal carcinoma of no special type
- C. More frequent occurrence in younger women
- D. Strong association with BRCA-1 mutations
- E. Worse prognosis than ductal carcinoma of no special type

19. Foci of mucinous differentiation are not infrequent in infiltrating ductal carcinoma NOS. Which of the following percentages of mucinous pattern should be present for a breast carcinoma to have a good prognosis?

- A. 50%
- B. 60%
- C. 70%
- D. 80%
- E. 100%

20. The *medullary* variant of breast carcinoma is characterized by:

- A. Expression of hormone receptors
- B. Frequent association with BRCA-1 gene mutations
- C. Low mitotic activity
- D. Marked desmoplastic reaction
- E. Worse prognosis than invasive ductal carcinoma

21. Which of the following patterns of differentiation is associated with a pronounced tendency for lymphatic invasion and a poor prognosis?

- A. Apocrine
- B. Metaplastic
- C. Micropapillary
- D. Mucinous
- E. Tubular

22. Of the breast tumors similar to neoplasms of salivary glands, which of the following is the most common?

- A. Adenoid cystic carcinoma
- B. Adenomyoepithelioma
- C. Adenosquamous carcinoma
- D. Mucoepidermoid carcinoma
- E. Pleomorphic adenoma

23. A 14-year-old female presents with a well-circumscribed 0.8-cm breast nodule. Fine-needle aspiration shows evidence of malignancy. Which of the following tumor types is most likely to be found on biopsy?

- A. Ductal infiltrating, NOS
- B. Medullary
- C. Mucinous
- D. Secretory
- E. Tubular

24. Upon histological examination, an infiltrating breast tumor shows large cell size, prominent cytoplasmic eosinophilia, conspicuous nucleoli, and apical snouts. These changes are homogeneously present throughout the neoplasm. EM reveals abundant mitochondria. Which of the following is the most likely diagnosis?

- A. Apocrine carcinoma
- B. Ductal carcinoma of no special type
- C. Lobular carcinoma
- D. Medullary carcinoma
- E. Mucinous carcinoma

25. Which of the following is the pathological substrate underlying the clinical appearance of inflammatory breast carcinoma?
    A. Abscess formation in ductal carcinoma
    B. Chronic inflammatory infiltration surrounding the tumor
    C. Epidermal extension of neoplastic growth
    D. Florid neovascular proliferation
    E. Neoplastic invasion of dermal lymphatic vessels

26. A biopsy of an ulcerated, crusted skin lesion of the nipple shows large cells infiltrating the epidermis. Which of the following is characteristic of this lesion?
    A. Cells are immunoreactive for HMB-45
    B. Cells are immunoreactive for S100 protein
    C. Cells are of epidermal origin and immunoreactive for high-molecular-weight keratin
    D. Prognosis depends on extent of skin involvement
    E. Underlying carcinoma is present in up to 60% of cases

27. Which of the following statements applies to carcinoma of the male breast?
    A. Accounts for at least 10% of all breast cancers
    B. Gynecomastia is the most common risk factor
    C. Klinefelter syndrome is a well-recognized predisposing condition
    D. Occurs in young males
    E. Usually negative for estrogen/progesterone receptors

28. Which of the following histological features or patterns are associated with increased risk of malignancy in fibroadenomas?
    A. Cysts greater than 3 mm, sclerosing adenosis, epithelial calcification
    B. Infarction
    C. Multinucleated giant cells
    D. Myxoid hyaline stroma
    E. Presence of heterologous stromal components

29. This low-power photomicrograph demonstrates the salient histological features of a large (14-cm) mass excised

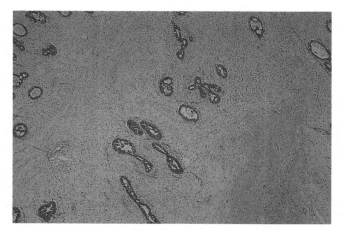

QUESTION 9.29

from the breast of a young woman. The most likely diagnosis is:
    A. Fibroadenoma
    B. Hamartoma
    C. Infiltrating ductal carcinoma
    D. Juvenile fibroadenoma
    E. Phyllodes tumor

30. A breast tumor from a 46-year-old woman shows the features in this low-power photomicrograph. Which of the following is the most likely diagnosis?

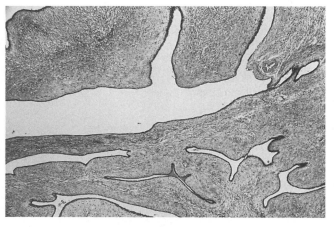

QUESTION 9.30

    A. Adenomyoepithelioma
    B. Fibroadenoma
    C. Fibrosarcoma
    D. Phyllodes tumor
    E. Radial scar

31. A breast angioma is usually an incidental microscopic finding. Its most typical histologic feature is:
    A. Anastomosing vascular channels
    B. Frequent cellular atypia and mitoses
    C. Intralobular invasion
    D. Perilobular arrangement
    E. Subcutaneous location

32. Which of the following is the most common predisposing factor for lymphangiosarcomas?
    A. Chronic lymphedema
    B. Foreign bodies
    C. Polyvinyl chloride
    D. Radiation
    E. Thorotrast

33. A 40-year-old woman undergoes resection of a poorly circumscribed nodule of the subareolar region. Histologically, the lesion appears round and consists of aggregates of tubular structures that extend up to the epidermis, where the junction with the squamous epithelium is abrupt. The stroma is fibrous and focally sclerotic. The glands have irregular outlines and a two-cell layer. The most likely diagnosis is:
    A. Benign intraductal papilloma
    B. Juvenile (small duct) papillomatosis

C. Nipple adenoma

D. Syringomatous adenoma

E. Tubular carcinoma

34. H&E sections of a small freely movable breast nodule show a lesion composed of cuboidal cells with clear cytoplasm admixed with tubular epithelial elements. The clear cells are immunoreactive for smooth muscle antigens. Which of the following is the most likely diagnosis?

A. Adenomyoepithelioma

B. Adenosquamous carcinoma

C. Melanoma metastasis

D. Metaplastic carcinoma

E. Mucoepidermoid carcinoma

35. Breast abscesses are most frequent in:

A. Adolescence

B. Gynecomastia

C. Oral contraceptive use

D. Postmenopausal age

E. Postpartum state

36. A 50-year-old woman with a history of recent trauma to the left breast presents with a nodule, which on biopsy shows numerous large foamy cells with small, sometimes multiple nuclei. The most likely diagnosis is:

A. Acute mastitis

B. Fat necrosis

C. Fibrocystic changes

D. Granulomatous mastitis

E. Mammary duct ectasia

37. A 45-year-old woman presents with nipple discharge and retraction in the right breast. An ill-defined nodule is biopsied. It shows ducts filled with inspissated fluid and surrounded by a plasma cell–rich chronic inflammatory infiltrate and fibrosis. Which of the following is the most likely diagnosis?

A. Abscess

B. Fat necrosis

C. Infiltrating ductal carcinoma

D. Mammary duct ectasia

E. Radial scar

38. A 50-year-old woman with a long history of type I diabetes mellitus presents with ill-defined bilateral breast nodules, which are painful. The most likely histopathologic substrate in this setting consists of:

A. Dilated ducts filled with eosinophilic material with periductal inflammation

B. Granulomas with Langhans-type giant cells around lobules

C. Lobular carcinoma *in situ*

D. Necrotic fat with chronic inflammation and calcification

E. Perilobular and perivascular lymphocytosis with fibrosis and lobular atrophy

39. A breast lesion is shown in this photomicrograph. Cells lining the slitlike spaces are immunoreactive for vimentin and CD34 and negative for factor VIII–related antigen. Which of the following is the most likely diagnosis?

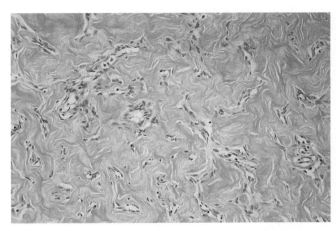

QUESTION 9.39

A. Angiosarcoma

B. Fibroadenolipoma

C. Lymphocytic lobulitis

D. Perilobular hemangioma

E. Pseudoangiomatous hyperplasia

40. Of the following immunostains, which would be most strongly positive on the "collagen balls" of collagenous spherulosis?

A. Actin

B. Collagen type I

C. Collagen type IV

D. Desmin

E. Keratin

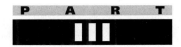

CENTRAL NERVOUS SYSTEM

10

THE BRAIN, SPINAL CORD, AND MENINGES

1. Rosenthal fibers are eosinophilic, corkscrew-shaped structures that are pathognomonic of:
   A. Alexander disease
   B. Pilocytic astrocytoma
   C. Reactive astrocytosis around infarcts
   D. Reactive astrocytosis around tumors
   E. None of the above

2. CT studies show bilateral hemorrhagic lesions in the temporal lobes of a 35-year-old male with fever and mental status changes. A biopsy reveals perivascular lymphocytic cuffing and Cowdry type A inclusion bodies. Which of the following is the most likely etiologic agent?
   A. Arboviruses
   B. Cytomegalovirus (CMV)
   C. Herpes simplex virus (HSV)
   D. Human immunodeficiency virus (HIV)
   E. Rabies virus

3. Progressive multifocal leukoencephalopathy (PML) is most common in immunocompromised patients, especially those with AIDS. Which of the following is the etiologic agent of this condition?
   A. Arbovirus
   B. Cytomegalovirus (CMV)
   C. Herpes simplex virus (HSV)
   D. Herpes zoster
   E. Papovavirus

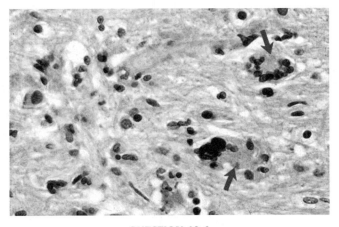

QUESTION 10.4

4. Autopsy investigations on a 42-year-old HIV-positive male reveal mild cerebral atrophy without focal lesions. Histologically, there are multifocal lymphohistiocytic infiltrates and clusters of inflammatory cells such as those shown in the picture. Which of the following is the most likely diagnosis?
   A. CMV encephalitis
   B. HIV encephalitis
   C. Nonspecific findings
   D. Progressive multifocal leukoencephalopathy
   E. Rasmussen encephalitis

5. A 40-year-old female presents with seizures of recent onset. MRI investigations show a ring-enhancing mass in the right parietal lobe. A primary neoplasm or infectious process is suspected. Which of the following tumors shows no increased association with HIV infection?
   A. Gliomas
   B. Kaposi sarcoma
   C. Leiomyosarcoma
   D. Non-Hodgkin lymphoma
   E. Squamous cell carcinoma of the cervix

6. A patient with seizures undergoes surgery for resection of a right frontal lesion. On H&E stained sections, the lesion is composed of thin-walled (capillary-like) vessels with little intervening parenchyma. Some hemosiderin deposits and Rosenthal fibers are noted around it. Elastic stains do not reveal elastic tissue within the vessel walls. Which of the following is the most likely diagnosis?
   A. Arteriovenous malformation
   B. Berry aneurysm
   C. Capillary hemangioma
   D. Cavernous angioma
   E. Vascular teleangiectasia

7. A CT scan shows an intracerebral hemorrhage located superficially within the right frontal lobe of a previously healthy 75-year-old man. After surgical evacuation of the hematoma, histologic evaluation demonstrates cortical and leptomeningeal arterioles similar to those shown in this photomicrograph. Which of the following is the most likely underlying cause of the hemorrhage?
   A. Amyloid angiopathy
   B. Berry aneurysm

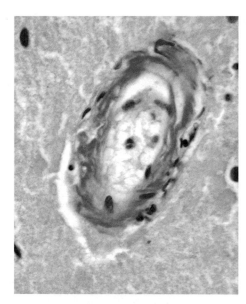

QUESTION 10.7

C. Coagulopathy

D. Hypertension

E. Trauma

8. Which of the following is the most frequent primary malignant tumor of the central nervous system?

  A. Anaplastic oligodendroglioma

  B. Ependymoma

  C. Glioblastoma multiforme

  D. Lymphoma

  E. Medulloblastoma

9. A tumor is resected from the right cerebellar hemisphere of a 15-year-old patient. Histologically, it is composed of spindly cells and shows a biphasic pattern, with alternating compact and microcystic areas. Rosenthal fibers are numerous in the compact areas. Cells are positive for GFAP immunohistochemistry. According to the WHO grading system, this tumor is:

  A. Grade 1

  B. Grade 2

  C. Grade 3

  D. Grade 4

  E. Grading not applicable

10. A 33-year-old male presents with seizures. MRI scans show an ill-defined area of T2 hyperintensity in the white matter of the left frontal lobe. A biopsy of the lesion shows a glial population with slightly increased cellularity compared with normal white matter, and mild nuclear pleomorphism. No mitotic activity, necrosis, or vascular hyperplasia is detected. Neoplastic cells express GFAP. Which of the following is the most likely diagnosis?

  A. High-grade astrocytoma

  B. Low-grade astrocytoma

  C. Metastatic lesion

  D. Normal brain parenchyma

  E. Reactive astrogliosis

11. A biopsy of a subependymal mass shows a glial tumor diagnosed as subependymal giant cell astrocytoma. The patient is affected by:

  A. Neurofibromatosis type 1

  B. Neurofibromatosis type 2

  C. Sturge-Weber syndrome

  D. Tuberous sclerosis

  E. von Hippel-Lindau syndrome

12. A brain biopsy reveals homogeneous cellular composition, which is shown in this photomicrograph. The neoplastic cells are negative for GFAP immunohistochemistry. These features are most consistent with:

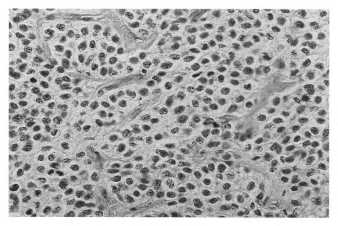

QUESTION 10.12

  A. Ganglioglioma

  B. High-grade astrocytoma

  C. Low-grade astrocytoma

  D. Oligodendroglioma

  E. Primitive neuroectodermal tumor

13. The biopsy of a ring-enhancing tumor in the left parietal lobe of a 60-year-old patient reveals an astrocytic tumor (GFAP-positive) that displays marked cellular atypia, mitotic activity, areas of pseudopalisading necrosis, and multifocal microvascular hyperplasia. The diagnosis is:

  A. Astrocytoma, grade 1

  B. Astrocytoma, grade 2 (well-differentiated astrocytoma)

  C. Astrocytoma, grade 3 (anaplastic astrocytoma)

  D. Astrocytoma, grade 4 (glioblastoma multiforme)

  E. Pilocytic astrocytoma

14. Histological examination of a well-circumscribed mass involving the cerebellum and fourth ventricle of an 18-year-old male reveals a tumor. Which of the following is the most likely diagnosis?

  A. Cerebellar liponeurocytoma

  B. Ependymoma

  C. Hemangioblastoma

  D. Medulloblastoma

  E. Pilocytic astrocytoma

15. Myxopapillary ependymoma occurs most commonly in:
    A. Cervical/thoracic spinal cord
    B. Conus medullaris
    C. Fourth ventricle
    D. Lateral ventricles
    E. Third ventricle

16. Histological examination of a midline (vermis) cerebellar tumor from a 5-year-old child shows sheets of monotonous small cells with a high nucleocytoplasmic ratio and "molding" nuclei. There is mitotic activity as well as numerous apoptotic bodies. Neoplastic cells are GFAP-negative but show multifocal immunoreactivity for synaptophysin. Which of the following is the most likely diagnosis?
    A. Ependymoblastoma
    B. Ependymoma
    C. Medulloblastoma
    D. Pilocytic astrocytoma
    E. Pineoblastoma

17. A dural-based tumor is resected. Light microscopic features are shown in this picture. Neoplastic cells are immunoreactive for EMA and negative for S100 protein. Which of the following is the most frequent and characteristic chromosomal abnormality of this tumor?

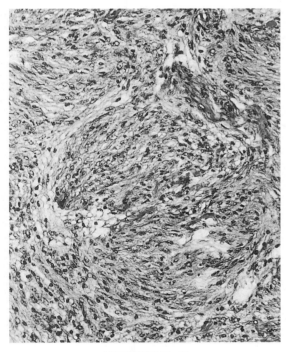

QUESTION 10.17

A. Chromosome 1p deletion
B. Isochromosome 17q
C. Loss of heterozygosity of chromosome 19q
D. Loss of heterozygosity of 10q
E. Monosomy of chromosome 22

18. A tumor composed of physalipherous cells and immunoreactive for keratin, EMA, and S100 is a(n):
    A. Astrocytoma
    B. Chondrosarcoma
    C. Chordoma
    D. Hemangioblastoma
    E. Metastatic adenocarcinoma

19. Which of the following is correct about sacrococcygeal germ cell tumors?
    A. Associated with spina bifida
    B. Mature teratoma is the most common type
    C. Seminoma is the most common type
    D. Up to 90% occur in males
    E. Usually malignant if present at birth

20. A cystic-solid mass is excised from the cerebellar hemisphere. The tumor is composed of cells with finely vacuolated cytoplasm dispersed between a rich capillary network. Foamy cells are negative for epithelial markers, whereas the capillary component is positive for factor VIII–related antigen. This tumor most typically develops in patients with:
    A. Lhermitte-Duclos disease
    B. Neurofibromatosis type 1
    C. Neurofibromatosis type 2
    D. Tuberous sclerosis
    E. von Hippel-Lindau syndrome

21. Of the metastatic tumors listed below, which of the following has a pronounced tendency to manifest with intracerebral bleeding?
    A. Choriocarcinoma
    B. Melanoma
    C. Renal cell carcinoma
    D. All of the above

22. The wall of a third ventricular cyst consists of a single layer of mucin-producing ciliated columnar epithelium. Which of the following is the most likely diagnosis?
    A. Colloid cyst
    B. Craniopharyngioma
    C. Cysticercus
    D. Ependymal cyst
    E. Rathke cleft cyst

23. Which of the following groups of brain neoplasms are characterized by a gross appearance of "cyst with a mural nodule"?
    A. Ependymoma, schwannoma, epidermoid cyst
    B. Hemangioblastoma, ganglioglioma, pilocytic astrocytoma
    C. Medulloblastoma, pineoblastoma, retinoblastoma
    D. Oligodendroglioma, low-grade astrocytoma, glioblastoma multiforme
    E. Chordoma, dysgerminoma, lymphoma

24. Autopsy investigations are performed on a patient with a clinical history of dementia. Silver staining of sections of the hippocampus, frontal, temporal, and parietal cortex reveals numerous intraneuronal flame-shaped inclusions that

are immunoreactive for *tau* protein. Which of the following lesions will be most likely found in the same regions?

 A. Lewy bodies
 B. Microglial nodules
 C. Pick bodies
 D. Rosenthal fibers
 E. Senile plaques

25. Autopsy investigations would confirm a clinical diagnosis of Parkinson disease by finding loss of pigmented neurons in the substantia nigra. Which of the following microscopic alterations would also be detected?

 A. Granulovacuolar degeneration
 B. Hirano bodies
 C. Lewy bodies
 D. Marinesco bodies
 E. Negri bodies

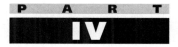

PART IV

ENDOCRINE SYSTEM

11

THE NEUROENDOCRINE AND PARACRINE SYSTEMS

1. Neuroendocrine neoplasms can be identified by several techniques. Dense core granules measuring 50 to 400 nm are characteristic features that represent the storage of peptide hormones. Because ultrastructural examination is not always available on a given case, the demonstration of general and specific antigens by immunohistochemistry may be of great value. The following antigens are considered general markers of neuroendocrine differentiation. Which of the following is *not* considered a general marker of neuroendocrine activity:

    A. Neuron-specific enolase
    B. Chromogranin A
    C. Bombesin
    D. Leu-7
    E. Adrenocorticotropic hormone (ACTH)

THE PITUITARY AND SELLAR REGION

1. A reticulin-stained section of a 0.8-cm pituitary lesion removed by transphenoidal resection is shown in this photomicrograph. Which of the following is the most common clinical presentation of this tumor?

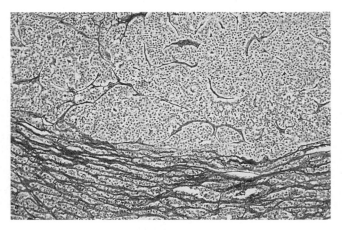

QUESTION 12.1

A. Acromegaly/gigantism
B. Cushing syndrome
C. Hyperprolactinemia
D. Panhypopituitarism
E. Visual field deficits

2. A 23-year-old female undergoes transphenoidal resection of a prolactinoma after receiving prolonged treatment with bromocriptine. Which of the following are morphological effects of bromocriptine on the pituitary tumor?

A. Apoplexy
B. Degeneration and necrosis
C. Increase in cellular atypia

D. Interstitial fibrosis
E. No morphological effect

3. An intracranial tumor characteristic of childhood is shown in this photomicrograph. This tumor is most likely to arise from which of the following regions?

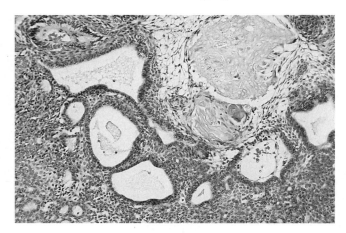

QUESTION 12.3

A. Cribriform lamina of ethmoid
B. Petrous portion of temporal bone
C. Posterior fossa
D. Suprasellar region
E. Temporal lobe

4. Which of the following factors accounts for the *primary* form of empty sella syndrome?

A. Compression by herniated arachnoid
B. Irradiation to sellar tumors
C. Pituitary apoplexy
D. Postpartum pituitary necrosis
E. Surgical intervention

13

PATHOLOGY OF THYROID AND PARATHYROID DISEASE

1. Which of the following is the most common location of heterotopic thyroid tissue?
   A. Perihyoid bone
   B. Prelaryngeal
   C. Sublingual
   D. Substernal
   E. Tongue

2. Which of the following forms of thyroiditis is thought to be caused by a viral infection?
   A. Graves disease
   B. Hashimoto thyroiditis
   C. Lymphocytic thyroiditis
   D. Riedel thyroiditis
   E. Subacute (granulomatous) thyroiditis

3. A thyroid specimen reveals marked lymphocytic infiltration and scattered lymphoid follicles with germinal centers on histological examination. Follicular cells exhibit oxyphilic change, with numerous Hürthle cells. Which of the following is the mechanism accounting for this condition?
   A. Type 1 hypersensitivity reaction
   B. Type 2 hypersensitivity reaction
   C. Type 3 hypersensitivity reaction
   D. Type 4 hypersensitivity reaction
   E. Viral infection

4. A patient with Graves disease receives antithyroid drugs and propranolol prior to subtotal thyroidectomy. Which of the following histopathological aspects will *regress* following such treatment?
   A. Follicular hyperplasia
   B. Glandular enlargement
   C. Lymphocytic infiltration
   D. Presence of Hürthle cells
   E. Presence of lymphoid follicles

5. *Riedel thyroiditis* is a pathological process akin to:
   A. Amyloidosis
   B. De Quervain thyroiditis
   C. Hashimoto thyroiditis
   D. Progressive systemic sclerosis
   E. Retroperitoneal fibrosis

6. Fine-needle aspiration of a thyroid nodule shows psammoma bodies. This finding suggests a diagnosis of:
   A. Follicular carcinoma

   B. Hashimoto thyroiditis
   C. Hürthle cell tumor
   D. Papillary carcinoma
   E. Squamous cell metaplasia

7. Which of the following variants of thyroid papillary carcinoma is associated with the most aggressive behavior?
   A. Diffuse sclerosing
   B. Encapsulated
   C. Follicular
   D. Microcarcinoma
   E. Tall cell variant

8. Which of the following is true about dominant nodule of goiter and thyroid adenoma?
   A. Both dominant nodule and adenoma are monoclonal
   B. Both dominant nodule and adenoma are entirely surrounded by a capsule
   C. Dominant nodule is monoclonal; adenoma is polyclonal
   D. Dominant nodule consists of variably sized follicles; adenoma of uniform follicles
   E. Dominant nodule compresses the surrounding parenchyma; adenoma does not

9. This photomicrograph demonstrates the histologic features of an isolated thyroid nodule. The most important step in pathologic examination of this specimen is:

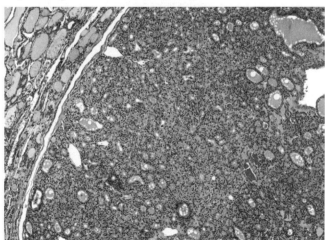

QUESTION 13.9

A. Determination of MIB-1 labeling index
B. DNA ploidy analysis
C. Identification of areas of oncocytic change
D. Measurement of main diameter
E. Microscopic evaluation of capsule

10. Which of the following is a true statement regarding follicular carcinoma of the thyroid?
 A. The brain is the most common target of hematogenous metastasis
 B. Lymphatic metastasis is the usual route of spread
 C. It is most commonly multiple and occult
 D. Prognosis is related to capsular and vascular invasion
 E. Prognosis is related to the presence of *ras* mutations

11. The cytoplasm of the neoplastic cells in Hürthle cell tumors is filled with:
 A. Glycogen
 B. Lipids
 C. Lysosomes
 D. Mitochondria
 E. Thyroglobulin

12. A thyroid biopsy reveals the tumor shown in this photomicrograph. Congo red staining is positive on the stroma surrounding cell nests. Which of the following immunohistochemical markers is likely to be positive in neoplastic cells?

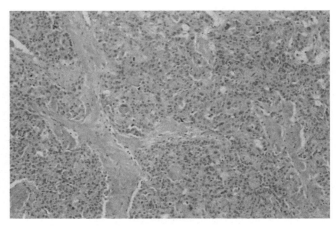

QUESTION 13.12

A. Calcitonin
B. Carcinoembryonic antigen (CEA)
C. Keratin
D. Synaptophysin
E. All of the above

13. The so-called *insular carcinoma* of the thyroid is most probably a/an:
 A. Atypical carcinoid of the thyroid
 B. Equivalent to anaplastic carcinoma
 C. Poorly differentiated follicular or papillary carcinoma
 D. Salivary gland–like neoplasm
 E. Well-differentiated follicular or papillary carcinoma

14. An elderly patient undergoes surgery because of a thyroid mass. The surgical specimen reveals a poorly circumscribed hemorrhagic tumor extending beyond the thyroid. The histological appearance of the tumor is demonstrated by this picture. Areas of increased vascularity and others with a prominent storiform pattern are seen.

Immunohistochemical studies demonstrate diffuse vimentin and focal keratin reactivity. These findings are most consistent with:

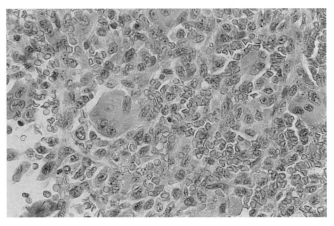

QUESTION 13.14

A. Anaplastic carcinoma
B. Angiosarcoma
C. Giant cell tumor
D. Hemangiopericytoma
E. Malignant fibrous histiocytoma

15. Which of the following is true regarding normal histological features of parathyroids?
 A. All parathyroid cells are morphological variants of chief cells
 B. Amount of adipose tissue keeps increasing throughout life
 C. Amount of adipose tissue shows little interindividual variation
 D. Oxyphil cells have abundant secretory granules
 E. Water-clear cells are predominant in childhood

16. A 35-year-old woman with a history of hypercalcemia and recurrent urinary stones undergoes surgery for resection of a parathyroid adenoma. Histologically, the lesion is encapsulated and composed of a mixture of cell types with a predominance of chief cells. There are foci of cells with bizarre hyperchromatic nuclei, scattered clusters of lymphocytes, and occasional mitoses. Which of the following histological parameters suggests a diagnosis of parathyroid carcinoma rather than adenoma?
 A. Bizarre nuclei
 B. Capsular invasion
 C. Diffuse growth pattern
 D. Lymphocytic infiltration
 E. Occasional mitoses

17. Which of the following criteria is most useful in differentiating parathyroid adenoma from chief cell hyperplasia?
    A. DNA ploidy studies
    B. Identification of at least one normal gland
    C. Proliferative indices such as Ki-57
    D. Proportion of cell types
    E. Size of lesion

18. Which of the following parathyroid lesions may lead to massive enlargement of parathyroid glands and does not occur in association with multiple endocrine neoplasia syndromes?
    A. Chief cell hyperplasia
    B. Lipoadenoma
    C. Oxyphil adenoma
    D. Oxyphil cell hyperplasia
    E. Water-clear cell hyperplasia

19. This high-power picture shows a representative region of a parathyroid mass weighing 13 g Upon resection, the mass appeared to be adherent to adjacent structures. Which of the following is the most likely diagnosis?

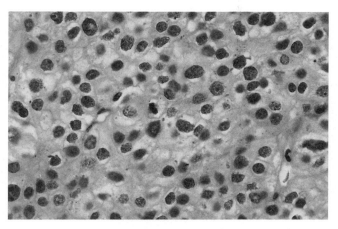

QUESTION 13.19

A. Chief cell hyperplasia
B. Oxyphil adenoma
C. Parathyroid adenoma
D. Parathyroid carcinoma
E. Water-clear cell hyperplasia

14

THE ADRENAL GLANDS

1. *Primary pigmented nodular adrenocortical disease* (PPNAD) is a form of adrenocortical hyperplasia most probably due to:
   A. ACTH-producing pituitary adenoma
   B. Autoimmune mechanism
   C. Ectopic production of ACTH or corticotropin-like factors
   D. Genetic defects
   E. Hypothalamic stimulation by corticotropin-releasing hormone (CRH)

2. Surgical excision of an adrenal gland is performed because of a 2-cm well-demarcated tumor. This tumor has a homogeneous, tan-yellow cut surface without hemorrhage or necrosis. Histologically, it is composed of cells with vacuolated cytoplasm in a trabecular arrangement. Large bizarre nuclei are scattered throughout the tumor, but mitotic figures are not appreciated. There is neither vascular nor capsular invasion. The cells are immunoreactive for low-molecular-weight keratin and vimentin, but not epithelial membrane antigen (EMA). Which of the following is the most likely diagnosis
   A. Adrenal cytomegaly
   B. Adrenocortical adenoma
   C. Adrenocortical carcinoma
   D. Metastatic renal cell carcinoma
   E. Pheochromocytoma

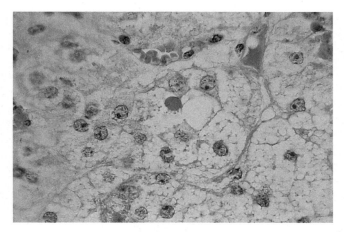

QUESTION 14.3

3. A patient suffering from secondary hypertension undergoes surgical excision of an adrenal tumor. Histological examination reveals intracytoplasmic eosinophilic inclusions similar to that present in the center of this picture. On closer examination, these bodies consist of concentric laminations. The presence of such inclusions indicates:
   A. Aggressive behavior of tumor
   B. Hyperproduction of androgens
   C. Hyperproduction of cortisol
   D. Nonfunctioning adenoma
   E. Prior treatment with spironolactone

4. By the time of clinical diagnosis, adrenocortical carcinoma is usually associated with which of the following features?
   A. Homogeneous cut surface without necrosis or hemorrhage
   B. Lymph node and/or distant metastases in over 50% of cases
   C. Paucity of mitotic figures or atypical mitoses
   D. Presence of glandular formations
   E. Small size (less than 100 g) on clinical diagnosis

5. The factors influencing the prognosis of neuroblastomas are diverse. Which of the following is associated with a better prognosis?
   A. Age younger than 1 year
   B. Chromosome 1 deletions
   C. Diploidy
   D. Low expression of high-affinity nerve growth factor (NGF) receptors (TRK-A)
   E. MYCN amplification

6. Ganglioneuroblastoma and ganglioneuroma are tumors that most frequently develop in the:
   A. Adrenal gland
   B. Cervical region
   C. Intracranial space
   D. Intravertebral, epidural space
   E. Retroperitoneum and mediastinum

7. Which of the following is the only reliable criterion for distinguishing benign from malignant pheochromocytomas?
   A. Metastasis
   B. Mitotic rate
   C. Number of sustentacular cells

D. Tumor size

E. Vascular and capsular invasion

8. In which of the following familial syndromes is pheochromocytoma most likely to develop?

   A. Li-Fraumeni syndrome

   B. Multiple endocrine neoplasia (MEN) type 1

   C. Multiple endocrine neoplasia (MEN) type 2

   D. von Hippel-Lindau syndrome (VHL)

   E. von Recklinghausen disease

15

PARAGANGLIOMAS

1. A 40-year-old man comes to medical attention with a slowly growing, painless mass near the angle of the left mandible. On physical examination, his heart rate is

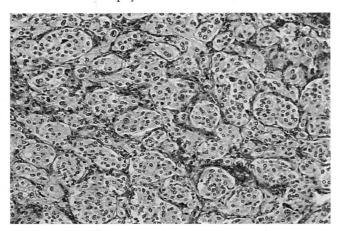

QUESTION 15.1

45 beats/min. The tumor is excised. This picture shows its typical histological appearance. Cells express neuroendocrine markers such as chromogranin and synaptophysin. Scattered cells are immunoreactive for S100 protein. Which of the following is the single most reliable marker of malignancy in this type of neoplasm?

    A. Cytological atypia
    B. Evidence of metastasis
    C. Immunohistochemical profile
    D. Mitotic index
    E. Vascular/neural invasion

2. Extraadrenal paragangliomas arise most frequently in which of the following regions?

    A. Gallbladder
    B. Neck
    C. Pelvis
    D. Posterior abdomen
    E. Posterior thorax

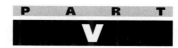

HEMATOPOIETIC AND LYMPHATIC SYSTEMS

16

DISORDERS OF BONE MARROW

1. A bone marrow biopsy from a 40-year-old patient with AIDS shows hypocellularity, shrinkage of adipocytes, and expansion of the interstitial tissue by an amorphous eosinophilic substance. Besides AIDS, this characteristic change is associated most commonly with:
   A. Bone marrow transplantation
   B. Cachexia
   C. Drug toxicity
   D. Parvovirus B19 infection
   E. Rheumatoid arthritis

2. A bone marrow biopsy from a 30-year-old male with fever of unknown origin reveals several nonnecrotizing granulomas. Culture studies and special stains for infectious organisms are carried out. The most common etiology of granulomas in bone marrow biopsies is:
   A. Idiopathic: no apparent etiology
   B. Infectious: fungal or mycobacterial
   C. Non-Hodgkin or Hodgkin lymphomas
   D. Q fever
   E. Sarcoidosis

3. A bone marrow biopsy is performed in a patient with clinical and hematological findings suggestive of acute leukemia. Which of the following morphological features allows distinguishing acute myeloid leukemia (AML) from acute lymphocytic leukemia (ALL)?
   A. Auer rods
   B. Blast size
   C. Chromatin pattern
   D. Cytoplasmic features
   E. Presence and number of nucleoli

4. A 58-year-old male undergoes bone marrow examination because of blood cytopenia without apparent cause. The bone marrow is hypercellular with an increased number of myeloid precursors and marked erythroid hyperplasia. Clusters of immature myeloid precursors are seen in an abnormal location, far from bone trabeculae. Which of the following is the most likely diagnosis?
   A. Chronic idiopathic myelofibrosis
   B. Chronic myeloid leukemia
   C. Essential thrombocythemia
   D. Myelodysplastic syndrome
   E. Polycythemia vera

5. In the stage referred to as "obliterative myelosclerosis," *chronic idiopathic myelofibrosis* is characterized by:
   A. Hypercellular marrow with expansion of erythroid precursors
   B. Hypercellular marrow with expansion of granulocytic and megakaryocytic lines
   C. Marrow hypercellularity and increased reticulin network
   D. Splenomegaly and normal to increased blood counts
   E. Splenomegaly, extramedullary hematopoiesis, and teardrop elliptocytes

6. Systemic mast cell disease is clinically suspected in a 65-year-old female patient. A bone marrow biopsy is carried out to confirm the diagnosis. Large clusters of histiocyte-like and fibroblast-like cells are identified. Which of the following special techniques is most useful to confirm bone marrow involvement by mast cell disease?
   A. CD1 immunohistochemistry
   B. Myeloperoxidase histochemistry
   C. Tartrate-resistant acid phosphatase (TRAP) histochemistry
   D. Tryptase immunohistochemistry
   E. Ultrastructural studies

7. A bone marrow biopsy is performed for staging of a non-Hodgkin lymphoma (NHL). Histologic examination reveals a focal paratrabecular pattern of marrow involvement. This pattern is most consistent with:
   A. Burkitt lymphoma
   B. Follicular lymphoma
   C. Lymphoblastic lymphoma
   D. Small lymphocytic lymphoma
   E. Splenic marginal zone lymphoma

8. With respect to evaluation of bone marrow involvement by Hodgkin lymphoma (HL), which of the following is correct?
   A. Aspiration smears are more sensitive than trephine biopsies
   B. "Dry taps" imply lack of bone marrow involvement
   C. HL type can be correctly classified in bone marrow
   D. Leukocyte common antigen (LCA; CD45) is useful in identifying Reed-Sternberg cells
   E. Marrow biopsies are usually performed for staging

9. A bone marrow biopsy of a 60-year-old woman contains a lymphocytic cluster such as that shown in the photomicrograph. This finding is commonly associated with:

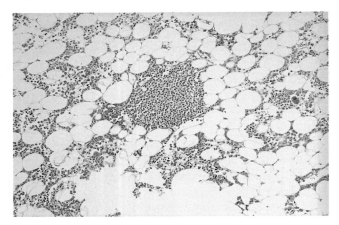

QUESTION 16.9

A. Acquired immunodeficiency syndrome (AIDS)
B. Rheumatoid arthritis
C. Small lymphocytic lymphoma
D. Splenic marginal zone lymphoma
E. No specific disorder

10. A bone marrow examination is performed in a 58-year-old man with multiple osteolytic lesions and a monoclonal spike in the serum protein electrophoresis. The biopsy reveals several focal aggregates of slightly atypical plasma cells. The percentage of plasma cells in the smear is 8%. Immunohistochemistry for Ig light chains shows that the ratio between κ and λ expression is in excess of 16:1. Which of the following is the most likely diagnosis?
A. Immunoblastic lymphoma
B. Monoclonal gammopathy of undetermined significance (MGUS)
C. Multiple myeloma
D. Plasmacytoma
E. Reactive plasmacytosis

11. A patient with monoclonal gammopathy, organomegaly, polyneuropathy, and multiple bone lesions is most likely to have which of the following forms of plasma cell dyscrasia?
A. Monoclonal gammopathy of undetermined significance
B. Nonsecretory myeloma
C. Osteosclerotic myeloma
D. Plasma cell leukemia
E. Smoldering myeloma

12. A bone marrow aspirate from a 25-year-old woman of Jewish descent with hepatosplenomegaly and pancytopenia reveals the cells shown in the picture. The most likely diagnosis is:

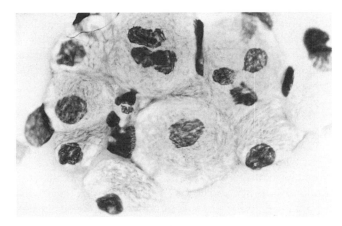

QUESTION 16.12

A. Deficiency of α_1-antitrypsin
B. Gaucher disease
C. Niemann-Pick disease
D. Pompe disease
E. Tay-Sachs disease

13. A trephine biopsy shows entirely necrotic tissue. Which of the following conditions is the most frequent cause of necrosis in bone marrow biopsies?
A. Hodgkin lymphoma
B. Metastatic disease
C. Myelofibrosis
D. Non-Hodgkin lymphoma
E. Sickle cell anemia

17

LYMPH NODES

1. Low-power examination is most helpful in the diagnosis of which of the following types of lymphomas?
   A. Anaplastic large cell lymphoma, CD30 +
   B. Diffuse large cell lymphoma
   C. Lymphocyte depletion and mixed cellularity Hodgkin lymphoma
   D. Nodular-sclerosing Hodgkin lymphoma and follicular center cell lymphoma
   E. T-lymphoblastic lymphoma/leukemia

2. A diagnosis of rheumatoid arthritis is made in a 40-year-old woman with fever, weight loss, joint pains, and generalized lymphadenopathy. A biopsy of a lymph node is performed. Which of the following patterns should be expected?
   A. Follicular hyperplasia and interfollicular plasmacytosis
   B. Follicular hyperplasia with paracortical necrosis
   C. Large germinal centers with a serpentine shape and thin mantle zone
   D. Small follicles centered on vessels with hyalinized walls
   E. Subcapsular granulomas with necrosis and neutrophils

3. A young woman presents with fever, enlarged cervical lymph nodes, and leukopenia on the cell blood count. A lymph node biopsy reveals the following changes: extensive areas of necrosis with nuclear debris, lymphocytes and histiocytes surrounding necrotic areas, and large numbers of plasmacytoid monocytes. Which of the following is the most likely diagnosis?
   A. Angiofollicular hyperplasia (Castleman disease)
   B. Cat-scratch disease
   C. Histiocytic necrotizing lymphadenitis (Kikuchi disease)
   D. HIV infection
   E. Syphilis

4. The most characteristic histological changes of regional lymphadenopathy developing 2 to 3 weeks after a cat bite or scratch include:
   A. Capsulitis, subcapsular necrotizing granulomas, and follicular hyperplasia
   B. Emperipolesis and expansion of sinuses by histiocytes
   C. Follicular hyperplasia and interfollicular plasmacytosis
   D. Germinal centers with ragged margins and marked interfollicular hyperplasia
   E. Nonnecrotizing granulomas

5. A biopsy of a large mediastinal mass reveals numerous atretic lymphoid follicles, at the center of which lies a hyalinized vessel surrounded by concentric layers of lymphocytes. A high-power view of this finding is shown in the picture. Which of the following is true about this condition?

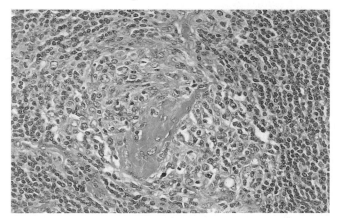

QUESTION 17.5

   A. Human herpes virus-8 (HHV-8) is associated with all cases
   B. Necrosis is a constant feature of lymph node involvement
   C. Plasma cell population is monoclonal
   D. Plasma cell variant is more likely associated with systemic involvement
   E. Prognosis is the same for both localized and systemic forms

6. A lymph node biopsy from a patient with a febrile disease, cervical lymphadenopathy, and splenomegaly shows the following histopathologic changes:

   ■ marked interfollicular expansion
   ■ mixed cellular infiltrate within sinuses, including numerous immunoblasts with conspicuous nucleoli but only a few plasma cells

■ partial preservation of the follicular architecture

Which of the following is the most likely diagnosis?
A. Angiofollicular hyperplasia
B. Angioimmunoblastic lymphadenopathy
C. Cat-scratch disease
D. Immunoblastic lymphadenopathy
E. Infectious mononucleosis

7. Posttransplantation lymphoproliferative disorder (PTLD) is one of the most frequent long-term complications of liver transplantation. Which of the following is thought to play a critical pathogenetic role in PTLD?
A. Cytomegalovirus
B. Epstein-Barr virus
C. Hepatitis B virus
D. Hepatitis C virus
E. Hepatitis D virus

8. Which of the following features is most characteristic of sinus histiocytosis with massive lymphadenopathy (Rosai-Dorfman disease)?
A. Emperipolesis
B. Interstitial Alcian blue–positive material
C. Interstitial proteinaceous deposits
D. Numerous immunoblasts
E. Melanin pigment

9. A 25-year-old man presents with cervical node enlargement. A biopsy of an affected lymph node shows effacement of lymph node architecture by a nodular growth, a thin rim of compressed normal node, and a predominantly small lymphocytic population with admixed histiocytes and scattered large cells like those seen in this picture. The latter are immunoreactive for CD45 and CD20 and negative for CD15. One cell with features of Reed-Sternberg cells is identified in two histological sections. The diagnosis is:

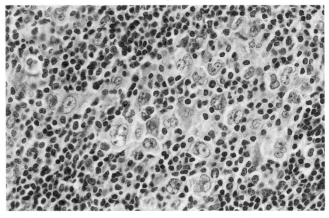

QUESTION 17.9

A. Lymphocyte-depleted Hodgkin lymphoma (HL)
B. Lymphocyte-predominant HL
C. Lymphocyte-rich classic HL
D. Mixed-cellularity HL
E. Nodular-sclerosing HL

10. A lymph node biopsy in a case of suspected lymphoma reveals a nodular pattern of growth with broad bands of collagen. A mercuric chloride–fixed section shows a mixed lymphohistiocytic, plasmacellular, and eosinophilic infiltrate, along with the cells shown in the picture. These cells are CD15 and CD30-positive and CD45-negative. Which of the following is the most likely diagnosis?

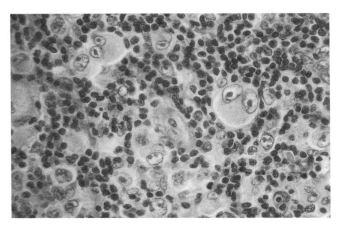

QUESTION 17.10

A. Diffuse large B-cell lymphoma
B. Follicular center lymphoma
C. Lacunar variant of Reed-Sternberg cells
D. L and H variant of Reed-Sternberg cells
E. Small lymphocytic lymphoma

11. A diagnosis of mixed-cellularity Hodgkin lymphoma (MCHL) is most likely when:
A. Broad bands of birefringent collagen result in a nodular pattern
B. Classic Reed-Sternberg (RS) cells are rare
C. Lacunar cells are abundant
D. RS cells are easily found in a mixed T-cell–rich infiltrate
E. Variants of RS cells are immunoreactive for CD45 but negative for CD15

12. Which of the following is true about lymphocyte-depleted Hodgkin lymphoma (LDHL)?
A. Accounts for more than 50% of HL cases
B. Bone marrow involvement is rare
C. Most patients present with localized cervical lymphadenopathy
D. Reed-Sternberg (RS) cells are CD45 + and CD15 −
E. Reticular LDHL has a worse prognosis than diffuse-fibrosis LDHL

13. A lymph node biopsy from a 60-year-old man with peripheral lymphocytosis and generalized lymphadenopathy reveals complete effacement of the nodal architecture. This is replaced by diffuse sheets of small lymphocytes with round nuclei and scanty cytoplasm. Mitotic figures are rare. Which of the following immunocytochemical, cytogenetic,

or molecular findings would support a diagnosis of chronic lymphocytic leukemia/small lymphocytic lymphoma (CLL/SLL)?

A. Immunoreactivity for CD5 and CD19
B. Immunoreactivity for CD10 and CD20, negativity for CD5
C. Strong immunoreactivity for surface immunoglobulin and CD43
D. Translocation t(8;14) with overexpression of c-*myc*
E. Translocation t(14;18) resulting in *bcl-2* overexpression

14. The entity known as lymphoplasmacytic lymphoma (LPL) is often associated with leukemia and:

A. Bence-Jones protein in the urine
B. Isolated bone mass
C. Primary amyloidosis
D. Richter syndrome
E. Waldenström macroglobulinemia

15. A 45-year-old patient suffers from a lymphoma involving lymph nodes, bone marrow, and spleen. Histologically, the lymph nodes display a vaguely nodular architecture, with striking expansion of the mantle zone around small residual follicles. Neoplastic lymphocytes are small with a slightly indented (cleaved) nucleus. Mitotic figures are easily found, but transformed lymphocytes are absent. Which of the following genotypic abnormalities characterizes this type of lymphoma?

A. t(8;14)
B. t(11;14)
C. t(14;18)
D. Trisomy 12
E. Trisomy 18

16. A non-Hodgkin lymphoma characterized by CD10-positive and CD5-negative lymphocytes with high levels of cytoplasmic IgG and a nodular pattern of growth will most likely have:

A. t(8;14)
B. t(11;14)
C. t(14;18)
D. Trisomy 12
E. Trisomy 18

17. So-called *nodal marginal zone lymphoma* (NMZL) is characterized by:

A. Features similar to mucosa-associated lymphoid tissue (MALT) marginal zone lymphoma
B. Lymphocytes closely resembling follicular center lymphocytes
C. Rapid progression to high-grade lymphomas
D. Translocation resulting in overexpression of bcl-1 protein (cyclin D1)
E. All of the above

18. A lymphoma diagnosed as *diffuse large B-cell lymphoma* (DLBCL) is most likely to express:

A. Bcl-2
B. CD5

C. CD10
D. CD19 and CD20
E. Surface immunoglobulin

19. Which of the following subtypes of diffuse large B-cell lymphoma (DLBCL) is associated with human herpes virus 8 (HHV-8)?

A. Immunodeficiency associated
B. Intravascular
C. Primary effusion (body cavity related)
D. Primary mediastinal
E. T-cell–rich B cell

20. Histological examination of an ileocecal mass reveals a lymphoma that appears as in this photomicrograph. The main population is composed of intermediate-sized lymphocytes with amphophilic cytoplasm and round nuclei with small nucleoli. Mitotic figures are numerous. Immunohistochemistry for MIB-1 shows a labeling index close to 100%. The majority of cases of this NHL are associated with translocations or rearrangements involving:

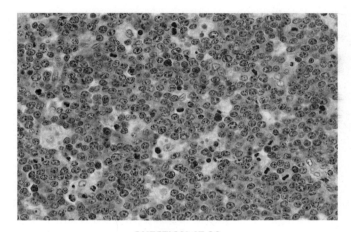

QUESTION 17.20

A. bcl-1 gene
B. bcl-2 gene
C. c-myc
D. PAX5
E. TAL1 gene

21. A 20-year-old male undergoes a biopsy of an anterior mediastinal mass. Histological examination reveals a diffuse lymphomatous infiltrate characterized by cells with angular irregular nuclei, blastlike dispersed chromatin, and inconspicuous nucleoli. Mitotic figures are plentiful. Immunohistochemical studies show neoplastic cells to be positive for CD3 and CD7. Which of the following markers is expressed in virtually 100% of this type of lymphoma?

A. CD10
B. CD20
C. CD30
D. Surface Ig
E. TdT

22. A lymph node biopsy reveals a diffuse lymphomatous growth. Neoplastic cells are intermediate in size and have clear cytoplasm. They express pan-T-cell antigens, CD4, and CD8, but are negative for TdT (terminal deoxytransferase), CD1, and CD30. The patient is a 50-year-old woman with generalized lymphadenopathy, night sweats, and pruritus. Which of the following is the most likely diagnosis?
    A. Anaplastic large cell lymphoma
    B. Angioimmunoblastic T-cell lymphoma
    C. Mycosis fungoides
    D. Natural killer cell lymphoma
    E. Peripheral T-cell lymphoma, unspecified

23. A lymph node biopsy reveals a diffuse T-cell lymphomatous population effacing nodal architecture within a meshwork of PAS-positive small vessels. Which of the following is the most likely diagnosis?
    A. Anaplastic large cell lymphoma
    B. Angioimmunoblastic lymphoma
    C. Large granular lymphocytic leukemia
    D. Natural killer cell lymphoma
    E. Precursor T-cell lymphoblastic lymphoma/leukemia

24. A lymph node from a 25-year-old patient with lymphadenopathy shows sheets of highly pleomorphic, cohesive, large cells with bizarre nuclei and prominent nucleoli. Neoplastic cells infiltrate sinuses and paracortical regions, while sparing follicles. They display cytoplasmic immunoreactivity for CD30 and EMA. Expression of which of the following antigens would have the greatest impact on prognosis?
    A. B-cell markers
    B. Cytotoxic granule-associated protein
    C. Epithelial membrane antigen (EMA)
    D. Fusion protein deriving from t(2;5)
    E. T-cell markers

25. Adult T-cell leukemia/lymphoma (ATLL) is caused by:
    A. Epstein-Barr virus (EBV)
    B. Human herpes virus-8 (HHV-8)
    C. Human immunodeficiency virus (HIV)
    D. Human papillomavirus (HPV)
    E. Human T-cell lymphotropic virus type I (HTLV-I)

26. The presumed cell of origin of *mycosis fungoides/Sezary syndrome* (MF-SS) is:
    A. CD-4 positive T-cell
    B. CD-8-positive T-cell
    C. Histiocyte
    D. Langerhans cell
    E. Natural killer cell

18

THE SPLEEN

1. A splenectomy specimen from a patient with clinically diagnosed idiopathic thrombocytopenic purpura (ITP) is submitted for pathological examination. In addition to reactive follicular hyperplasia, the most characteristic histological change associated with this disorder consists of:
   A. Arteriolar thrombi
   B. Ceroid-laden histiocytes in the red pulp
   C. Congested red pulp cords
   D. Hemophagocytosis
   E. Immunoblastic proliferation

2. This photomicrograph shows characteristic changes associated with a common type of primary lymphoma of the spleen. Which of the following is it?

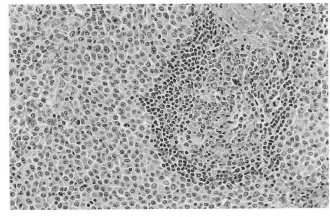

QUESTION 18.2

   A. Hairy cell leukemia
   B. Hodgkin disease
   C. Large cell lymphoma
   D. Marginal zone lymphoma

   E. Small lymphocytic lymphoma/chronic lymphocytic leukemia (SLL/CLL)

3. The distinguishing morphologic hallmark of myeloid metaplasia in the spleen is:
   A. Follicular atrophy
   B. Infiltration of red pulp by lipid-laden histiocytes
   C. Infiltration of red pulp by mast cells
   D. Presence of all three hematopoietic cell lines
   E. Severe congestion of sinusoids

4. A 55-year-old man comes to clinical attention with a very large spleen and pancytopenia. A bone marrow aspirate does not yield any material (dry tap). A splenectomy is performed. The cut surface of the removed spleen is homogeneous without nodular lesions. Histologically, there is widespread infiltration of the red pulp by a monotonous population of mononuclear cells with scanty mitotic activity. These cells are positive for tartrate-resistant alkaline phosphatase (TRAP) and immunoreactive for CD11c and CD22 antigens. Ultrastructural studies demonstrate cells with cytoplasmic villous projections. The diagnosis is:
   A. Chronic monocytic leukemia
   B. Hairy cell leukemia
   C. Mantle cell lymphoma
   D. Marginal zone lymphoma
   E. Myelofibrosis

5. A *littoral cell angioma* is a/an:
   A. Capillary hemangioma involving red pulp in a diffuse pattern
   B. Incidentally discovered splenic hamartoma
   C. Low-grade angiosarcoma
   D. Lymphangioma occurring as part of systemic lymphangiomatosis
   E. Sinuslike channels with endothelium-lined papillary projections

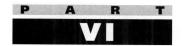

HEAD AND NECK

THE JAWS AND ORAL CAVITY

1. A nodular lesion is excised from the lower gingiva of a 30-year-old female patient. Histologically, it consists of vascular stroma containing numerous osteoclast-like giant cells and hemosiderin deposits. This is most consistent with:
   A. Granular cell tumor
   B. Masson hemangioma
   C. Peripheral giant cell granuloma
   D. Pyogenic granuloma
   E. Verruciform xanthoma

2. With respect to risk factors, the great majority of cases of squamous cell carcinoma of the mouth are associated with:
   A. Chronic trauma
   B. Iron deficiency
   C. Lifestyle
   D. Occupation
   E. Viruses

3. Which of the following is the most appropriate definition of *leukoplakia*?
   A. Carcinoma *in situ*
   B. Dysplastic lesion of the oral epithelium
   C. Intraepithelial neoplasia
   D. Lichen planus of the oral cavity
   E. White plaque greater than 5 mm that cannot be removed by rubbing

4. In which of the following oral lesions would you most probably find a squamous cell carcinoma on histological examination?
   A. Erythroplakia
   B. Hairy leukoplakia
   C. Leukoplakia
   D. Oral papilloma
   E. Tongue ulceration with eosinophilia

5. Of the histopathological parameters listed below, which one is the most significant predictor of regional lymph node metastasis in oral SCC?
   A. Desmoplastic reaction
   B. Grading
   C. Host inflammatory response
   D. Lymph node reaction pattern
   E. Pattern of tumor growth and invasion

6. An elderly patient presents with a large fungating mass growing from the lower lip and invading contiguous soft tissues and the mandible. Grossly, the lesion appears as a papillary neoplasm with white and red areas. Histologically, it consists of well-differentiated squamous epithelium with a frondlike pattern and a pushing margin. These characteristics are most consistent with:
   A. Adenosquamous cell carcinoma
   B. Basaloid squamous cell carcinoma
   C. Lymphoepithelioma-like carcinoma
   D. Spindle cell carcinoma
   E. Verrucous carcinoma

7. X-rays performed during a routine dental examination on a 30-year-old woman reveal a cystic lesion in the jaw. Which of the following is the most frequent cyst of the jaw?
   A. Dentigerous cyst
   B. Epidermoid and dermoid cysts
   C. Eruption cyst
   D. Fissural cyst
   E. Gingival cyst
   F. Keratocyst
   G. Lateral periodontal cyst
   H. Paradental
   I. Periapical cyst
   J. Primordial cyst
   K. Residual cyst

8. Dentigerous cysts are lesions most commonly associated with:
   A. Dental caries
   B. Gorlin syndrome
   C. McCune-Albright syndrome
   D. Traumatic injury
   E. Unerupted teeth

9. A multicystic tumor is resected from the jaw of a 40-year-old patient. It consists of epithelial islands resembling ameloblastic epithelium, in which peripheral cells exhibit prominent palisading of their nuclei, whereas central regions have a loose, stellate texture. Mitotic figures are inconspicuous, and nuclear atypia is minimal. The fibrous stroma between epithelial islands is paucicellular and without

apparent mitotic activity. Which of the following is the most likely diagnosis?
  A. Ameloblastic carcinoma
  B. Ameloblastic fibroma
  C. Ameloblastoid hyperplasia in dentigerous cyst
  D. Ameloblastoma
  E. Complex odontoma

10. Calcified parts of teeth are identifiable in which of the following odontogenic tumors?
  A. Adenomatoid odontogenic tumor
  B. Ameloblastic fibroma
  C. Ameloblastoma
  D. Odontoma
  E. Squamous odontogenic tumor

SALIVARY GLANDS

1. Which of the following is the most common location of heterotopic salivary gland tissue?
   A. Ear
   B. Lymph nodes
   C. Palatine tonsil
   D. Right sternomastoid muscle
   E. Thyroid gland

2. A 46-year-old male presents with an ulcer of the hard palate. A biopsy reveals necrosis, chronic inflammation, and squamous foci. The lesion exhibits a prominent lobular architecture. Which of the following is the most probable diagnosis?
   A. Leukoplakia
   B. Mucocele
   C. Necrotizing sialometaplasia
   D. Oral submucosal fibrosis
   E. Squamous cell carcinoma

3. Which of the following salivary gland tumors has the highest prevalence in males and is bilateral/multifocal in 10% of cases?
   A. Acinic cell tumor
   B. Adenoid cystic carcinoma
   C. Mucoepidermoid carcinoma
   D. Pleomorphic adenoma
   E. Warthin tumor

4. A well-demarcated slowly growing 4-cm tumor is resected from the left parotid gland of a 45-year-old female patient. Its cut surface is variegated, with myxoid and blue-gray areas. Histologic examination shows a tumor composed of epithelial elements organized in strands and acini, as well as a mesenchymal component including myxoid and chondroid areas. Which of the following is a recognized risk factor for this type of tumor?
   A. Epstein-Barr virus (EBV) infection
   B. HIV infection
   C. Radiation
   D. Sjögren syndrome
   E. Smoking

5. A well-circumscribed tumor of the parotid is composed by nests of uniform epithelial cells within a mesenchymal background. The nests show prominent peripheral palisading and contain scattered deposits of PAS-positive basement membrane–like material. No mitoses are identified. There is no perineurial or vascular invasion. Which of the following is the most likely diagnosis?
   A. Adenoid cystic carcinoma
   B. Basal cell adenocarcinoma
   C. Basal cell adenoma
   D. Myoepithelioma
   E. Warthin tumor

6. Which of the following is the most common malignant tumor of the salivary glands?
   A. Acinic cell carcinoma
   B. Adenoid cystic carcinoma
   C. Lymphoepithelioma-like carcinoma
   D. Malignant mixed tumor
   E. Mucoepidermoid carcinoma

7. Which of the following is a prominent feature of adenoid cystic carcinoma?
   A. Association with Mikulicz syndrome
   B. Cytoplasm packed with mitochondria
   C. Good long-term prognosis
   D. Most frequent in parotid gland
   E. Perineurial invasion is common

8. Histologic examination of a 2-cm parotid gland tumor demonstrates a predominantly solid growth composed of cells resembling normal serous cells of the salivary gland. The cells have abundant, slightly basophilic, granular cytoplasm, with a centrally placed small nucleus. Which of the following is the most likely diagnosis?
   A. Acinic cell carcinoma
   B. Adenoid cystic carcinoma
   C. Basal cell adenoma
   D. Mucoepidermoid carcinoma
   E. Myoepithelioma

9. A mass removed from the right parotid gland of a 23-year-old man reveals a multilocular cyst lined by squamous epithelium. The tissue between cysts contains a florid lymphocytic infiltrate with a germinal center formation. Immunostains demonstrate a mixed population of B and T lymphocytes. This lesion is frequently associated with:
   A. Coxsackievirus
   B. Epstein-Barr virus
   C. Human immunodeficiency virus

D. Human papillomavirus

E. Paramyxovirus

10. A 40-year-old woman presents with enlargement of the left parotid gland and dryness of the eyes and mouth. A biopsy of the parotid and minor salivary glands shows prominent periductal and perivascular lymphocytic infiltration with a germinal center formation. Scattered nests of myoepithelial cells are also noted. Laboratory studies reveal high titers of circulating antibodies to ribonucleo-proteins (RNP), including SS-A (Ro) and SS-B (La). Besides the increased risk of developing lymphoma, which of the following manifestations may be observed in this condition?

A. Esophageal fibrosis

B. Fibrinous serositis

C. Glomerulonephritis

D. Inflammatory myopathy

E. Tubulointerstitial nephritis

THE NOSE, PARANASAL SINUSES, AND NASOPHARYNX

1. A biopsy of a polypoid lesion in the nasal cavity reveals mixed inflammatory reaction containing thick-walled globular microcysts. Each cyst measures up to 200 μm in diameter and contains innumerable spores. Which of the following is the most likely diagnosis?
   - A. Actinomycosis
   - B. Aspergillosis
   - C. Mucormycosis
   - D. Myospherulosis
   - E. Rhinosporidiosis

2. A 40-year-old man presents with destructive ulcerative lesions of the nasal and nasopharyngeal cavities. Biopsies show extensive chronic inflammatory infiltrates, mostly consisting of foamy macrophages and plasma cells. PAS and Steiner stains identify small bacilli within macrophages. Which of the following is the most likely diagnosis?
   - A. Leprosy
   - B. Rhinoscleroma
   - C. Sinus histiocytosis with massive lymphadenopathy
   - D. Tuberculosis
   - E. Wegener granulomatosis

3. Which of the following statements best characterizes *lethal midline granuloma (LMG)*?
   - A. Angiotropic lymphoma involving the nasal cavity
   - B. Complication of chronic cocaine abuse
   - C. Destructive lesion due to large cell lymphoma
   - D. Syndrome encompassing different pathologic conditions
   - E. Synonym of aggressive cases of Wegener granulomatosis

4. A 35-year-old male undergoes resection of a nasal polyp. From an epidemiological standpoint, which of the following clinical or pathologic features is most likely to be associated with such a polyp?
   - A. Asthmatic attacks on aspirin ingestion
   - B. Cystic fibrosis
   - C. Epstein-Barr virus (EBV)
   - D. Occupational risk
   - E. Origin from the maxillary antrum

5. Which of the following statements applies to sinonasal papillomas?
   - A. Associated with human papillomavirus (HPV) in most instances
   - B. Often associated with cystic fibrosis (CF)
   - C. Schneiderian type usually has nonkeratinizing squamous epithelium
   - D. Those located in the lateral wall are of the fungiform type
   - E. Those located in the nasal septum are of the inverted type

6. Which of the following occupational groups are at increased risk of developing a squamous cell carcinoma of the nose or paranasal cavities?
   - A. Battery and ammunition workers
   - B. Coal workers
   - C. Grinders and diamond polishers
   - D. Nickel refiners
   - E. Wood workers

7. Which of the following tumors shows the strongest association with Epstein-Barr virus?
   - A. Keratinizing nasopharyngeal carcinoma
   - B. Lethal midline granuloma
   - C. Nonkeratinizing nasopharyngeal carcinoma
   - D. Olfactory neuroblastoma
   - E. Sinonasal carcinoma

8. A biopsy of a mass located in the left ethmoid sinus reveals a carcinoma characterized by a glandular architecture. Knowing that the patient is a 65-year-old retired woodworker, which of the following is the most likely diagnosis?
   - A. Adenoid cystic carcinoma
   - B. Intestinal-type adenocarcinoma
   - C. Low-grade sinonasal adenocarcinoma
   - D. Mucoepidermoid carcinoma
   - E. Undifferentiated nasopharyngeal carcinoma

9. A 40-year-old man presents with an intranasal polypoid mass arising from the roof of the nasal fossa. The mass is red and soft. Microscopic examination reveals clusters of small cells with high nucleocytoplasmic ratio forming occasional

Homer-Wright rosettes. Marked capillary proliferation in a lobular pattern is also present. These features are most consistent with a lesion arising from:

    A. Erectile-like fibrovascular tissue

    B. Lymphoid tissue

    C. Melanocytes

    D. Olfactory neuroepithelium

    E. Squamous epithelium of the nasal fossa

10. An 18-year-old male with a history of recurrent nasal epistaxis undergoes the resection of a mass located in the posterolateral wall of the roof of the nasal fossa. Histologically, the lesion consists of a bundle of vascular structures within a stroma rich in stellate cells and mast cells. Which of the following hormones is thought to play a role in the pathogenesis of this lesion?

    A. Estradiol

    B. Growth hormone

    C. Progesterone

    D. Serotonin

    E. Testosterone

22

PATHOLOGY OF THE LARYNX

1. A vocal cord nodule is removed from a 45-year-old attorney who presented with chronic hoarseness. Histologically, it is composed of hyalinized stroma containing dilated blood vessels with perivascular fibrinous exudate. Which of the following is the most likely diagnosis?
   A. Angioma
   B. Laryngeal nodule (singer's nodule)
   C. Laryngeal papilloma
   D. Localized amyloidosis
   E. Pyogenic granuloma

2. A 22-year-old patient has undergone multiple resections of laryngeal papillomas since the age of 16. The lesions appear composed of well-differentiated squamous epithelium with a papillary architecture. Mild nuclear atypia with koilocytotic changes are observed. Which of the following is the most likely etiology of these lesions?
   A. Exposure to alcohol
   B. Exposure to cigarette smoking
   C. Inherited mutations of epidermal growth factor receptor gene
   D. Viral infection
   E. Voice overuse

3. Compared to juvenile papillomas, laryngeal papillomas arising in adults are:
   A. Associated with human papillomavirus (HPV)
   B. More commonly associated with dysplasia
   C. More prone to recurrence
   D. Usually multiple
   E. All of the above

4. A transglottic cancer of the larynx is a tumor that:
   A. Arises from the true cord
   B. Arises in the pyriform sinus
   C. Crosses the ventricle vertically
   D. Involves the false cord
   E. Lies below the true cord

5. Which of the following laryngeal tumors has the lowest metastatic potential?
   A. Basaloid squamous carcinoma
   B. Carcinomas with neuroendocrine differentiation
   C. Salivary glandlike tumors
   D. Squamous cell carcinoma
   E. Verrucous carcinoma

23

THE EAR

1. A small painful nodule excised from the upper right helix of a 28-year-old male shows an ulcer demarcated by acanthotic epidermis. Chronic inflammatory infiltration is present at the bottom of the ulcer, extending to the perichondrium. These features are most consistent with:
   A. Chondrodermatitis nodularis helicis chronica
   B. Gout
   C. Ochronosis
   D. Malakoplakia
   E. Spectacle frame acanthoma

2. A mass is removed from the middle ear of a 48-year-old woman. This photomicrograph shows its histopathological features. Which of the following is the most likely diagnosis?

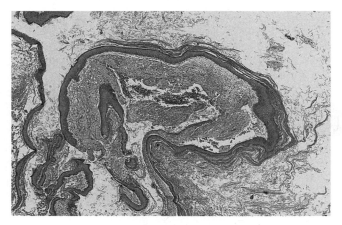

QUESTION 23.2

A. Adenoma of the middle ear
B. Cholesteatoma

C. Cholesterol granuloma
D. Dermoid cyst
E. Squamous cell carcinoma

3. The most common form of malignancy affecting the external ear is:
   A. Adenocarcinoma
   B. Adenoid cystic carcinoma
   C. Basal cell carcinoma
   D. Mucoepidermoid carcinoma
   E. Squamous cell carcinoma

4. A total stapedectomy is performed for treatment of otosclerosis in a 45-year-old male. Which of the following histologic changes is most likely to be present?
   A. Extensive osteolysis of the footplate
   B. New woven bone formation in the crura
   C. New woven bone formation in the footplate
   D. Spongiosis and formation of large marrow cavities
   E. No changes: Pathologic changes are limited to otic capsule

5. A 30-year-old female patient presents with progressive hearing loss and pain in the right ear. MRI reveals a middle ear mass, which is resected. Histologically, the tumor is composed of nests of cells, which are immunoreactive for synaptophysin but negative for keratin and epithelial membrane antigen (EMA). S100 and glial fibrillary acidic protein (GFAP) immunohistochemistry is negative, except for a few scattered cells. This tumor is most likely a/an:
   A. Adenoma of the middle ear
   B. Choristoma
   C. Meningioma
   D. Paraganglioma
   E. Schwannoma

THE EYE AND OCULAR ADNEXA

1. The designation of *phthisis bulbi* refers to:
   A. Atrophic disorganized eye with ossification
   B. Chronically inflamed eye
   C. Excised globe due to severe trauma
   D. Glaucomatous eye
   E. Globe with heavy deposition of iron or copper

2. Which of the following types of corneal dystrophies is most frequently observed in corneal specimens submitted to the pathologist in the United States?
   A. Fuch's endothelial dystrophy
   B. Granular dystrophy
   C. Lattice dystrophy
   D. Macular dystrophy
   E. Meesmann juvenile epithelial dystrophy

3. A conjunctival biopsy is performed in a 50-year-old female with a history of chronic interstitial lung disease. The biopsy reveals nonnecrotizing granulomas, but stains for microorganisms are negative. Which of the following is the most probable cause?
   A. Cat-scratch fever
   B. Rheumatoid arthritis
   C. Sarcoidosis
   D. Treponema pallidum
   E. Tularemia

4. The microscopic appearance of an intraocular tumor is shown in this picture. Which of the following features is most significant in the prognosis of this neoplasm?
   A. Extent of necrosis
   B. Extent of optic nerve invasion
   C. Immunohistochemical features
   D. Mitotic activity
   E. Presence of calcification

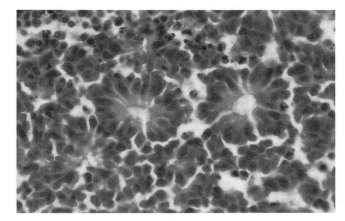

QUESTION 24.4

5. Enucleation of the right eyeball is performed on a 42-year-old male because of a clinical diagnosis of intraocular melanoma. Gross examination reveals a mushroom-shaped mass arising from the choroid. Histologic examination and immunohistochemical stains confirm the clinical diagnosis of melanoma. The cellular features associated with the worst prognosis include:
   A. Epithelioid morphology, prominent nucleoli, high mitotic rate
   B. Spindle shape, inconspicuous nucleoli, indistinct cell borders
   C. Spindle shape, plump nuclei, and distinct nucleoli
   D. Intermediate features between spindle and epithelioid morphology
   E. Combination of the above

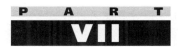

INTRATHORACIC ORGANS
AND BLOOD VESSELS

NONNEOPLASTIC PULMONARY DISEASE

1. A 48-year-old woman presents with slowly progressive respiratory insufficiency. Chest X-rays show a diffuse infiltrative process most prominent at the lung base. An open lung biopsy shows extensive fibrosis of the interalveolar septa, dilatation of alveolar ducts, and chronic inflammatory infiltration of the septa. Histopathologic changes are patchy, with areas of advanced fibrosis alternating with areas of active inflammation and new collagen deposition. These findings are most consistent with:

A. Desquamative interstitial pneumonia
B. Giant cell interstitial pneumonia
C. Lymphocytic interstitial pneumonia
D. Nonspecific interstitial pneumonia
E. Usual interstitial pneumonia

2. Which of the following is true about asbestos bodies?
A. Best demonstrated by routine histologic techniques
B. Best examined by special biophysical methods

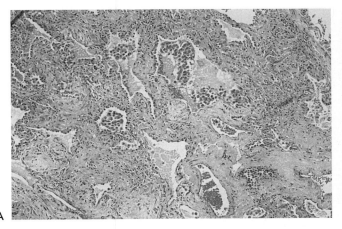

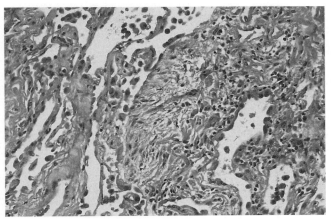

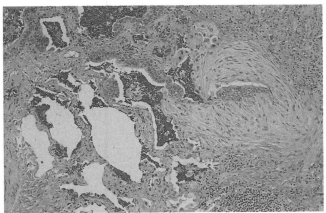

QUESTION 25.1

C. Present preferentially in mesotheliomas

D. Synonymous of ferruginous bodies

E. Not found in hilar lymph nodes

3. A 38-year-old woman with a history of heavy smoking presents with slowly progressive respiratory insufficiency. Chest x-rays show a bilateral ground-glass interstitial infiltrate involving the lung base. An open lung biopsy reveals the following histopathologic changes: alveolar spaces filled with histiocytes; hyperplasia of alveolar type II cells; lymphomonocytic, plasma cell, and neutrophilic interstitial infiltrate. These changes are relatively homogeneous. The most likely diagnosis is:

A. Centriacinar emphysema with chronic bronchitis

B. Desquamative interstitial pneumonia

C. Nonspecific interstitial pneumonia

D. Respiratory bronchiolitis

E. Usual interstitial pneumonia

4. Extrinsic allergic alveolitis (also called hypersensitivity pneumonitis) is a reaction to long-term exposure to various antigens of animal or plant origin. The inflammatory infiltrate present in the lung is predominantly composed of:

A. Cytotoxic T lymphocytes and plasma cells

B. Eosinophils and neutrophils

C. Helper T lymphocytes and plasma cells

D. Histiocytes and multinucleated giant cells

E. Lymphocytes and histiocytes

5. Pulmonary conditions such as Löffler syndrome, tropical eosinophilia, allergic bronchopulmonary aspergillosis, and bronchocentric granulomatosis usually result from hypersensitivity reactions to:

A. Allergens of plant origin

B. Bacterial organisms

C. Fungi, parasites, and drugs

D. Nitrogen dioxide (NO_2)

E. Viruses

6. An adult patient presents with a chest X-ray picture of bilateral areas of diffuse consolidation. Biopsies of involved areas demonstrate multiple necrotizing granulomas in close proximity to small bronchi. Bronchial spaces are filled with mucus, neutrophils, and eosinophils. No histologic evidence of arteritis is seen. Peripheral eosinophilia is mild, and antineutrophil cytoplasmic antibodies (ANCA) are undetectable. Which of the following is the most likely diagnosis?

A. Allergic bronchopulmonary aspergillosis (ABPA)

B. Allergic granulomatosis (Churg-Strauss syndrome)

C. Bronchiolitis obliterans–organizing pneumonia

D. Bronchocentric granulomatosis

E. Wegener granulomatosis limited to the lungs

7. Which of the following histopathologic findings is considered most characteristic of bronchiolitis obliterans–organizing pneumonia?

A. Hyaline membranes

B. Interstitial fibrosis

C. Intrabronchiolar fibroblastic plugs

D. Macrophages within alveolar spaces

E. Peribronchial granulomas

8. A lymphoma originating from BALT (bronchial-associated lymphoid tissue) is usually:

A. An aggressive high-grade lymphoma

B. Associated with lymphatic tracking

C. Composed of T lymphocytes, similar to lymphocytic interstitial pneumonia (LIP)

D. Not associated with lymphoepithelial lesions

E. Seen in young patients

9. The entity known as lymphomatoid granulomatosis is a/an:

A. Infectious condition due to mycobacteria

B. Leukemic infiltration

C. Malignant lymphoid proliferation

D. Process akin to mycobacterial pseudotumor

E. Reactive lymphoid process

10. A 20-year-old man undergoes surgery for resection of a well-circumscribed mass in the right lung. Histologically, it is composed of spindle cells arranged in fascicles variably admixed with a plasma cell population. The spindle cells react with antibodies to vimentin and actin and are negative for CD68. The plasma cell component is polyclonal as evaluated by light chain immunohistochemistry. The diagnosis most compatible with these features is:

A. Bronchiolitis obliterans–organizing pneumonia

B. Lymphomatoid granulomatosis

C. Mycobacterial pseudotumor

D. Plasma cell granuloma

E. Pulmonary hyalinizing granuloma

11. A 13-year-old child presents with recurrent hemoptysis and iron-deficiency anemia. Granular perihilar infiltrates are present on chest x-rays. Which of the following histologic findings supports a diagnosis of idiopathic hemosiderosis instead of Goodpasture syndrome?

A. Absence of IgG deposition along basement membranes

B. Accumulation of hemosiderin-laden macrophages

C. Hyperplasia of alveolar cells

D. Presence of interstitial fibrosis

E. Presence of interstitial lymphocytic infiltration

12. A 35-year-old woman manifests increasingly severe respiratory distress and chest pain. Cardiac catheterization leads to a clinical diagnosis of pulmonary hypertension of unknown origin. In the earliest stages of this condition, an open lung biopsy would reveal predominantly:

A. Fibrin thrombi

B. Intimal hyperplasia

C. Medial thickening

D. Plexogenic lesions

E. Reduplication of elastic lamina

13. The condition known as *lymphangiomyomatosis* is seen exclusively in:
    A. Children
    B. Young men
    C. Women of childbearing age
    D. Postmenopausal women
    E. Elderly persons

14. Which of the following pulmonary conditions is due to the accumulation of surfactant apoprotein within alveoli?
    A. Alveolar proteinosis
    B. Amyloidosis, diffuse alveolar septal type
    C. Goodpasture syndrome
    D. Idiopathic hemosiderosis
    E. Pulmonary alveolar microlithiasis

26

PULMONARY NEOPLASMS

1. Which of the following clinical *or* pathological features is most commonly associated with squamous cell carcinoma of the lung?
   A. Development in close proximity to lung scars
   B. Diffuse pneumonia-like infiltrate on chest X-rays
   C. Lambert-Eaton syndrome
   D. Origin from a major bronchus
   E. Presence of HPV in close to 100% of cases

2. The most typical ultrastructural feature of small cell carcinoma is:
   A. Abundant mitochondria and smooth endoplasmic reticulum
   B. Dense-core membrane bound granules (100 to 200 nm)
   C. Dense secretory granules (300 to 400 nm) and intranuclear tubular inclusions
   D. Long slender microvilli
   E. Osmiophilic lamellar bodies

3. A peripheral lung tumor shows the following microscopic features: small cells with a high nucleocytoplasmic ratio, granular "salt-and-pepper" chromatin, arrangement in trabecular and solid nests, and neurosecretory granules. Which of the following favors a diagnosis of small cell carcinoma over that of carcinoid tumor?
   A. Areas of spindly tumor cells
   B. Diffuse immunoreactivity for chromogranin
   C. High mitotic activity [more than 20/10 high power fields (HPF)]
   D. Neurosecretory granules of large size
   E. Peripheral location

4. Which of the following subtypes of lung cancer is thought to arise most commonly from neoplastic transformation of Clara cells?
   A. Clear cell carcinoma
   B. Mucinous type of bronchioloalveolar carcinoma
   C. Nonmucinous type of bronchioloalveolar carcinoma
   D. Small cell carcinoma of the classic type
   E. Undifferentiated large cell carcinoma

5. Which of the following pulmonary tumors is characterized by tubular glands and stroma with a pattern resembling fetal lung in the third month of gestation?
   A. Blastoma
   B. Carcinosarcoma
   C. Fetal adenocarcinoma
   D. Hamartoma
   E. Lymphangiomyomatosis

6. Which of the following is true about bronchial carcinoids?
   A. Atypical variant is characterized by monotonous cells
   B. Central variant is composed of spindle-shaped cells
   C. Most cases are endocrinologically inactive
   D. Occur most commonly in the peripheral lung parenchyma
   E. Represent approximately one-third of all lung tumors

7. The most common salivary gland–like tumors arising in the lungs is:
   A. Acinic cell carcinoma
   B. Adenoid cystic carcinoma
   C. Mucoepidermoid carcinoma
   D. Oncocytoma
   E. Pleomorphic adenoma

8. Which of the following immunohistochemical stains is diffusely positive on clear cell tumor (sugar tumor) of the lungs?
   A. Factor VIII—related antigen
   B. HMB-45
   C. Keratin
   D. Leukocyte common antigen (CD45)
   E. Smooth muscle actin

9. A lobectomy is submitted for intraoperative consultation. It contains a well-circumscribed tumor with a tan, bulging cut surface. It can be easily shelled out. A specimen taken from the periphery shows papillary structures with cellular atypia. Which of the following frozen section diagnoses should be given?
   A. Adenocarcinoma
   B. Bronchioloalveolar carcinoma
   C. Pulmonary blastoma
   D. Sclerosing hemangioma
   E. Sugar tumor

10. A 3-cm, round, subpleural nodule is found on CT scan in the left lung of a 14-year-old boy. A biopsy demonstrates

fascicles of spindly cells separated by collagen bundles and admixed with a plasma cell–rich chronic inflammatory infiltrate. Focally, vascular proliferation is pronounced. The spindle cell component is immunoreactive for vimentin and CD68, but not for keratin, CD34, smooth muscle actin, or synaptophysin. No microorganism is identified on special stains. Which of the following is the most likely diagnosis?

A. Carcinoid
B. Hamartoma
C. Hemangiopericytoma
D. Inflammatory pseudotumor
E. Plasmacytoma

11. A 2-cm coin lesion with a "popcorn" pattern of calcification on a chest X-ray is excised. Histologically, it consists of islands of cartilage admixed with adipose and smooth muscle tissue, with occasional epithelium-lined clefts. Which of the following is the most likely pathogenesis of this lesion?

A. Acquired lesion resulting from overgrowth of mesenchymal tissue
B. Congenital lesion resulting from developmental anomalies
C. Congenital lesion resulting from separation of lung parenchyma from the bronchial tree
D. Inflammatory proliferation of mesenchymal elements
E. Neoplastic transformation of bronchial cartilage

12. Which of the following markers is recognized by an antibody that reacts with virtually all cases of small cell carcinoma and neuroblastoma?

A. ACTH
B. Chromogranin
C. Neural cell adhesion molecule (N-CAM)
D. Neuron-specific enolase (NSE)
E. Vimentin

13. Antibodies to surfactant apoprotein are useful in identifying which of the following pulmonary cells or their neoplastic counterparts?

A. Clara cells ⟶ α₁AT
B. Goblet cells
C. Kulchitsky cells
D. Squamous cells
E. Type II alveolar epithelial cells

27

THE PLEURA

1. Subserosal fibroblast-like cells are responsible for regeneration of the mesothelial lining after various insults. Immunohistochemically, such cells are characterized by expression of vimentin, actin, and:
   A. CD34
   B. CD99
   C. CEA
   D. Keratin
   E. S100 protein

2. A well-circumscribed 5-cm nodule is excised from the visceral pleura of a 40-year-old presenting with chest pain and hypoglycemia. Histologically, it is composed of a meshwork of fibroblast-like cells within a dense fibrous background. Scattered areas have a hemangiopericytoma-like quality, whereas others are hypercellular. Occasional clusters of cells forming papillae are found. Most cells are immunoreactive for vimentin and CD34, but negative for keratin. Which of the following is the most likely diagnosis?

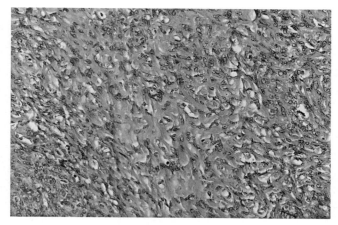

QUESTION 27.2

   A. Fibrosarcoma
   B. Hemangiopericytoma
   C. Mesothelioma
   D. Schwannoma
   E. Solitary fibrous tumor

3. A biopsy of a pleural tumor reveals papillary and acinar formations within a dense fibrous stroma. Which of the following findings is most consistent with a diagnosis of mesothelioma and rules out adenocarcinoma?
   A. Alcian blue positivity not removed by hyaluronidase pretreatment
   B. Cytokeratin immunoreactivity
   C. Mucicarmine positivity
   D. PAS-positive, diastase-resistant cytoplasmic staining
   E. Slender long microvilli without glycocalyx on electron microscopy

4. A tumor in a pleural decortication specimen is diagnosed

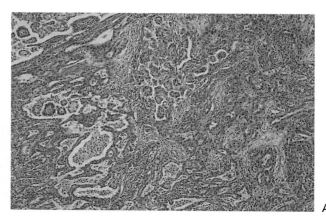

A

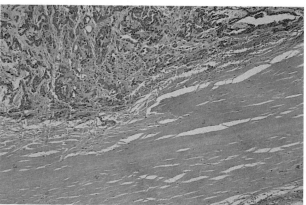

B

QUESTION 27.3

as a well-differentiated epithelial type mesothelioma. Which of the following entities should be considered in the differential diagnosis?

A. Adenocarcinoma of the lung
B. Epithelioid hemangioendothelioma
C. Metastatic carcinoma
D. Reactive mesothelial hyperplasia
E. All of the above

5. Which of the following morphologic features is most helpful in differentiating fibrous mesothelioma from fibromatosis?

A. Abundant collagen
B. Actin expression
C. Bland cytologic features
D. Keratin expression
E. Storiform pattern

28

THE MEDIASTINUM

1. A patient comes to medical attention with signs and symptoms of superior vena cava syndrome. Lymphoma is the most common cause of this syndrome in adults. Which of the following is the second most common cause?
   A. Acute leukemia
   B. Fibrosing mediastinitis
   C. Metastatic bronchogenic carcinoma
   D. Pericardial cysts
   E. Thymic carcinoma

2. Multilocular *thymic cysts*:
   A. Account for 80% of all mediastinal lesions
   B. Derive from a reactive inflammatory process
   C. Represent thymic cystic lymphangiomas
   D. Result from cystic degeneration of thymomas
   E. Result from malformation of the third branchial pouch

3. A mediastinal cyst is incidentally discovered in a 25-year-old man. It is unilocular, located in the superior mediastinum, and focally calcified. The excised cyst contains slightly turbid fluid, and the wall consists of ciliated columnar epithelium with foci of mature cartilage. Which of the following is the most likely diagnosis?
   A. Bronchogenic cyst
   B. Cystic hygroma
   C. Enteric cyst
   D. Pericardial cyst
   E. Unilocular thymic cyst

4. A diagnosis of *immature* teratoma of the mediastinum principally rests on microscopic demonstration of immature:
   A. Bone or cartilage-forming mesenchyme
   B. Neuroepithelium
   C. Squamous epithelium
   D. Striated muscle
   E. Vascular structures

5. A 40-year-old patient undergoes surgery for resection of a mediastinal mass. The tumor is surrounded by a thick, focally calcific capsule. Histologically, the mass consists of epithelial cells admixed with an abundant lymphoid cell population (Q 28.5A). The most significant histologic features include the following: lobulation with angular-shaped lobules, lymphocyte-rich perivascular serum lakes (Q 28.5B), rosette-like formations without lumina, and whorling nests of squamous cells. The nuclei of epithelial cells are vesicular with inconspicuous nucleoli, whereas lymphocytes exhibit variable degrees of activation. These features are most consistent with:
   A. Hodgkin disease
   B. Large cell lymphoma
   C. Lymphoblastic lymphoma
   D. Seminoma
   E. Thymic carcinoid
   F. Thymoma

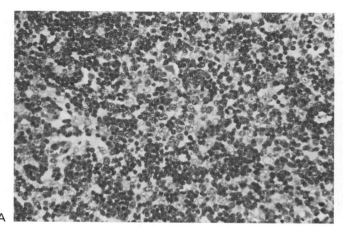
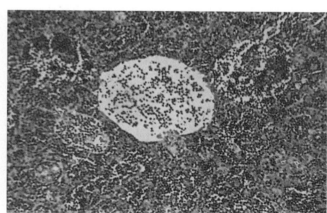

A   B

QUESTION 28.5

6. Various histologic classifications of lymphoma have been proposed, which are usually based on morphologic features of epithelial neoplastic cells (spindle vs. plump shape) and prevalence of lymphoid versus epithelial cells. The following table lists several types of thymomas that differ in these histologic parameters. Which of these cases is associated with the best prognosis?

Epithelial Cell Component	Lymphocytic Component
A. Predominantly spindly	Variable
B. Predominantly plump	Prevalent over epithelial component
C. Predominantly plump	Approximately equal to epithelial component
D. Predominantly plump	Minor compared to epithelial component
E. Marked atypia	Variable

7. Lymphoid hyperplasia of the thymus is most likely to be associated with:
   A. Castleman disease
   B. DiGeorge syndrome
   C. Germinoma
   D. Hodgkin disease
   E. Myasthenia gravis

8. A 33-year-old woman with myasthenia gravis undergoes resection of an enlarged thymic gland. Which of the following features favors lymphocyte-predominant thymoma over thymic hyperplasia?
   A. Effacement of thymic architecture
   B. Foci of medullary differentiation
   C. Keratin immunoreactivity in an arborizing pattern
   D. Serum lakes in perivascular location
   E. All of the above

9. A mediastinal lesion comes to the pathologist's attention. The patient has a fever, anemia, weight loss, and hypergammaglobulinemia. Histologically, the specimen consists of lymphoid tissue containing prominent follicular aggregates and numerous small-caliber vessels with hyalinized walls. Lymphocytes are often arranged in an <u>onionskin pattern around small vessels</u>. Thymic architecture is not identifiable. Which of the following is the most likely diagnosis?
   A. Castleman disease
   B. Lymphocyte-predominant thymoma
   C. Lymphoid hyperplasia
   D. Normal thymus
   E. Thymic carcinoma

10. A 33-year-old man presents with a thymic mass and an elevated white blood cell count. A thymic resection shows histologic features highly suggestive of lymphocyte-predominant thymoma (LPT), but lymphoblastic lymphoma (LBL) cannot be entirely ruled out. The immunostain that may be most helpful in this differential diagnosis is:

   A. CD3
   B. CD43
   C. CD99 (MIC-2)
   D. Cytokeratin
   E. Terminal deoxynucleotidyl transferase

11. Predominantly epithelial, spindle cell thymomas (type A according to the WHO classification) may have a morphologic pattern most commonly resembling:
   A. Atypical carcinoid
   B. Castleman disease
   C. Hemangiopericytoma — *Ck~, vimet tu*
   D. Lipoma
   E. Schwannoma (neurilemmoma)

12. A characteristic feature of mediastinal schwannomas is:
   A. Early clinical manifestations
   B. Lack of well-defined capsule
   C. Large size and prominent regressive changes
   D. Poorer prognosis compared to retroperitoneal schwannomas
   E. Presence of clusters of well-differentiated ganglion cells

13. A nonencapsulated thymic mass shows the histologic features of anaplasia. Focal necrosis and intravascular invasion are seen. Neoplastic cells are plump, with eosinophilic cytoplasm, vesicular nuclei, and prominent nucleoli. Occasional squamous pearls are noted. Which of the following types of thymic carcinoma is the most likely diagnosis?
   A. Adenosquamous
   B. Clear cell
   C. Keratinizing squamous cell
   D. Lymphoepithelioma-like
   E. Nonkeratinizing squamous cell

14. An adult patient presents with Cushing syndrome. Radiologic investigations lead to identification of a mediastinal tumor, which is excised. The tumor is solid and composed of ribbons of uniform cells forming scattered well-formed rosettes with central lumina. Which of the following ultrastructural features is most likely to be found?

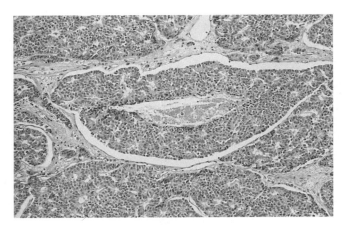

QUESTION 28.14

A. Complex desmosomes and tonofilaments

B. Dense-core granules and perinuclear masses of microfilaments

C. Glycogen-rich cytoplasm and prominent nucleoli

D. Nuclear blebs and absence of epithelial features

E. Synaptic junctionlike structures

15. A mediastinal tumor with a prominent "zellballen" architecture on histologic examination is most likely a:

A. Melanoma

B. Mesothelioma

C. Neuroblastoma

D. Paraganglioma

E. Thymic carcinoma, lymphoepithelioma-like

16. An adolescent male presents with a cervical tumor around the thyroid. Histologic examination of the tumor reveals a biphasic pattern similar to synovial sarcoma, with a mesenchymal highly cellular spindle cell component containing scattered mucin-secreting glandular structures. Which of the following is the most likely diagnosis?

A. Carcinoma with thymuslike elements (CASTLE)

B. Ectopic cervical thymoma

C. Ectopic hamartomatous thymoma

D. Spindle epithelial tumor with thymuslike elements (SETTLE)

E. Synovial sarcoma

17. A well-encapsulated thymoma is excised from an adult patient. Histologically, it is composed of a mixture of epithelial cells and lymphocytes, with a predominant spindle cell population. Which of the following is the single most important prognostic parameter?

A. Extracapsular invasion

B. Predominance of plump epithelial cells

C. Predominance of spindle epithelial cells

D. Presence of abortive Hassall's corpuscles

E. Proportion between epithelial and lymphoid cells

29

THE HEART

1. A 24-year-old male suffers from congestive heart failure. He has no history of therapeutic or illicit drug use, valvular disease, or systemic disorder. A myocardial biopsy shows myofibers arranged as in the picture. Occasional fibers contain basophilic granules. These morphologic features are most consistent with:

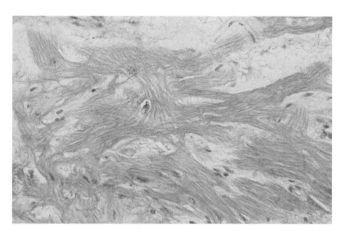

QUESTION 29.1

A. Amyloidosis
B. Dilated cardiomyopathy
C. Hypertrophic cardiomyopathy
D. Infiltrative cardiomyopathy
E. Myocarditis

2. An endomyocardial biopsy shows numerous myocytes with basophilic cytoplasm and complete loss of cross-striations. Inflammatory infiltration is not noted. EM studies reveal disintegration of myofilaments. Which of the following is the most plausible explanation for these findings?

A. Acute rejection of moderate degree
B. Acute viral myocarditis
C. Dilated cardiomyopathy
D. Toxicity due to adriamycin
E. Toxicity due to cyclophosphamide

3. In order to make a morphologic diagnosis of definite myocarditis, which of the following changes is required?

A. Eosinophilic infiltration
B. Giant cells
C. Inflammatory infiltration
D. Inflammatory infiltration and fibrosis
E. Inflammatory infiltration and myocyte necrosis

4. Aschoff bodies in an endomyocardial biopsy indicate a diagnosis of:

A. Chagas disease
B. Lyme disease
C. Rheumatic heart disease
D. Rocky Mountain spotted fever (RMSF)
E. Toxoplasma myocarditis

5. An endomyocardial biopsy performed 2 weeks after cardiac transplantation shows a single well-demarcated focus of endocardial lymphocytic infiltrate composed of B and T lymphocytes, macrophages, and plasma cells. This change is probably a consequence of:

A. Acute rejection
B. Cyclosporin A toxicity
C. EBV infection
D. Prior biopsy
E. None of the above

6. Although graft vasculopathy remains the long-term limitation of cardiac transplantation, acute rejection is of significance because of its treatability and immediate short-term consequences. It is diagnosed on cardiac biopsy. An endomyocardial biopsy with multifocal aggressive infiltrate and/or myocyte damage is correctly graded as:

A. 1b
B. 3a
C. 3b
D. 4
E. No rejection

7. A surgically resected mitral valve has a "fish-mouth" shape due to commissural fusion. These changes are most likely the result of:

A. Infective endocarditis
B. Left ventricular enlargement
C. Myxomatous degeneration
D. Papillary muscle rupture
E. Rheumatic heart disease

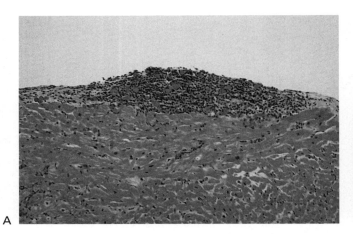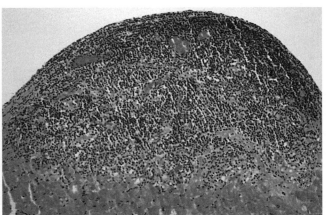

QUESTION 29.5

8. Echocardiography reveals a solid mass filling the left atrium in a 44-year-old female with signs and symptoms of mitral valve obstruction. Which of the following neoplasms is most likely to result in this picture?

    A. Fibroelastoma

    B. Mesothelial/monocytic incidental cardiac excrescences (MICE)

    C. Metastatic melanoma

    D. Myxoma

    E. Rhabdomyoma

BLOOD VESSELS

1. In a pathologic examination of endarterectomy specimens, it is essential to:
   A. Define the plane of surgical dissection through arterial wall
   B. Identify presence and extent of inflammatory infiltration
   C. Look for changes suggestive of cystic medial degeneration
   D. Photograph gross specimen for medicolegal reasons
   E. Submit parts of the specimen for culture

2. A false aneurysm (pseudoaneurysm) is most likely to develop in which of the following settings?
   A. Developmental defects in arterial media
   B. Gunshot or stab wound
   C. Hypertension, diabetes, smoking
   D. Infective endocarditis, drug abuse
   E. Marfan syndrome

3. An aneurysm developing in the abdominal aorta is most commonly associated with:
   A. Atherosclerosis
   B. Cystic medial degeneration

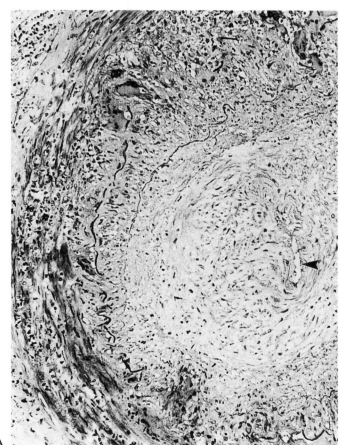

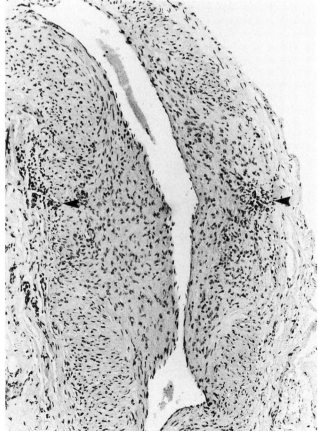

A   B

QUESTION 30.4

C. Infection

D. Malformation

E. Trauma

4. A 70-year-old patient with an acute onset of temporal headache, fever of unknown origin, and a high erythrosedimentation rate undergoes a temporal artery biopsy. This reveals chronic inflammatory infiltration of the vessel wall with Langhans and foreign body–type giant cells. Elastic stain demonstrates fragments of elastin within histiocytes and giant cells. This condition may lead to:

A. Blindness

B. Degos disease

C. Hepatitis B

D. Loss of radial pulse

E. Polymyalgia rheumatica

5. A renal biopsy reveals fibrinoid necrosis of medium-sized arteries, with accompanying obliterating thrombosis and focal ectasias. Vascular lesions appear at different stages. Laboratory tests indicate a recent hepatitis B infection; antineutrophil cytoplasmic antibodies (ANCAs) are negative. These features are most consistent with:

A. Churg-Strauss syndrome

B. Giant cell arteritis

C. Leukocytoclastic cutaneous arteritis

D. Polyarteritis nodosa

E. Wegener granulomatosis

6. A 20-year-old male develops purpura, fever, and hematuria after penicillin treatment for a streptococcal infection. Skin and renal biopsies show vasculitis involving arterioles and venules. Multifocal microscopic hemorrhages and glomerular necrosis are also noted. Antineutrophil cytoplasmic antibodies of the perinuclear type (p-ANCA) are present. No immune deposits are identified in skin or kidney biopsies. These clinical, laboratory, and pathologic features are most consistent with:

A. Henoch-Schönlein purpura

B. Microscopic polyangiitis

C. Polyarteritis nodosa

D. Rheumatic disease

E. Wegener granulomatosis

7. Which of the following is the most common pattern of so-called *renal artery dysplasia*?

A. Intimal fibroplasia—hyperplasia of intima

B. Medial fibroplasia—fibrosis of media alternating with aneurysms

C. Medial hyperplasia—fibrosis of media without aneurysms

D. Periarterial fibroplasia—adventitial and periadventitial fibrosis

E. Perimedial fibroplasia—hyperplasia of smooth muscle layer

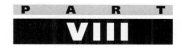

P A R T

VIII

ALIMENTARY CANAL AND ASSOCIATED ORGANS

ESOPHAGUS

1. A patient undergoes endoscopic examination for evaluation of gastroesophageal reflux. The mucosa of the lower esophageal segment is severely hyperemic. Biopsies from this area reveal epithelial hyperplasia, increased thickness of the lamina propria, and inflammatory infiltration. Which of the following histologic parameters is *diagnostic* of gastroesophageal reflux esophagitis (GERD)?
   A. Ballooned squamous cells
   B. Dilatation of venules in lamina propria
   C. Epithelial hyperplasia
   D. Erosion/ulceration
   E. Intraepithelial eosinophils
   F. Intraepithelial lymphocytes
   G. Intraepithelial neutrophils
   H. None of the above

2. An esophageal biopsy from a 25-year-old man with retrosternal pain shows the histopathological changes in this picture. This form of esophagitis is due to:

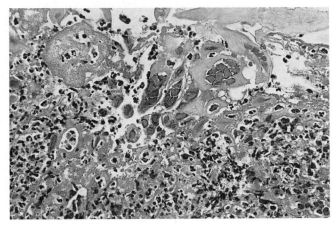

QUESTION 31.2

   A. Cytomegalovirus
   B. Herpes simplex virus (HSV)
   C. Measles
   D. *Tropheryma whippelii*
   E. Varicella-zoster virus

3. A histologic change that definitively supports a diagnosis of *Barrett esophagus* within an esophageal biopsy is:
   A. Cardiac-type glands
   B. Columnar cells with PAS-positive secretion
   C. Endocrine cells
   D. Goblet cells with acid mucin
   E. Villous surface of the mucosa

4. An esophageal biopsy is taken from a patient followed because of gastroesophageal reflux. A representative picture shows the most significant histopathological changes. These changes are most likely associated with:

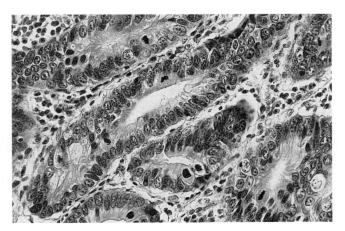

QUESTION 31.4

   A. Barrett esophagus of the atrophic fundal type
   B. Barrett esophagus of the junctional type
   C. Barrett esophagus of the specialized columnar type
   D. Reflux esophagitis with *H. pylori*
   E. Reflux esophagitis with reactive hyperplasia

5. Superficial squamous cell carcinoma of the esophagus is a carcinoma characterized by:
   A. Circumferential involvement of the esophagus
   B. Distal invasion of the gastric wall
   C. Growth confined to submucosa, regardless of nodal status
   D. Infiltration limited to lamina propria
   E. Invasion limited to mucosa and submucosa, with negative nodes

6. One of the following histopathologic types of esophageal cancer has an extremely aggressive behavior and may be confused with adenoid cystic carcinoma. Which one is it?
   A. Adenosquamous carcinoma
   B. Basaloid carcinoma
   C. Lymphoepithelioma-like carcinoma
   D. Small cell carcinoma
   E. Verrucous carcinoma

7. Which of the following statements applies to esophageal adenocarcinoma?
   A. The "inlet patch" is the most frequent location
   B. Has a better prognosis than squamous cell carcinoma
   C. Incidence is steadily decreasing in the United States
   D. Majority of cases develop from Barrett esophagus
   E. Minority of cases arise from the gastroesophageal junction

THE STOMACH

1. A gastric biopsy of the antral/pyloric region shows replacement of the normal gastric epithelium by intestinal-type epithelium. Gastric columnar cells are replaced by absorptive cells and goblet cells producing acid sulfomucin. These findings are consistent with:
   A. Intestinal metaplasia, large bowel type, complete
   B. Intestinal metaplasia, large bowel type, incomplete
   C. Intestinal metaplasia, small bowel type, complete
   D. Intestinal metaplasia, small bowel type, incomplete
   E. Pyloric metaplasia

2. Gastric biopsies from a patient with dyspeptic symptoms reveal inflammatory infiltration in the foveolar areas, consisting mostly of lymphocytes with few neutrophils and eosinophils. Glandular atrophy is insignificant, but there is a decrease is cytoplasmic mucin. Which of the following diagnoses is most consistent with these histologic features?
   A. Acute gastritis
   B. Atrophic gastritis
   C. Eosinophilic gastroenteritis
   D. Gastric atrophy
   E. Superficial gastritis

3. Which of the following histopathologic changes of the antral mucosa is most frequently associated with *Helicobacter pylori* gastritis?
   A. Erosions
   B. Lymphoid follicles with germinal centers of deep mucosa
   C. Neutrophilic infiltration of surface epithelium
   D. Pit abscesses
   E. Severe atrophic gastritis

4. Endoscopic and biopsy studies performed in a patient with gastric hypochlorhydria reveal chronic atrophic gastritis involving the fundus and sparing the antral region. Which of the following pathogenetic mechanisms is prevalent in this form of gastritis?
   A. Alcohol abuse
   B. Autoimmune
   C. Duodenal reflux
   D. *H pylori* infection
   E. Tobacco abuse

5. A gastric biopsy shows the alterations demonstrated in this photomicrograph. Which of the following is the most likely diagnosis?

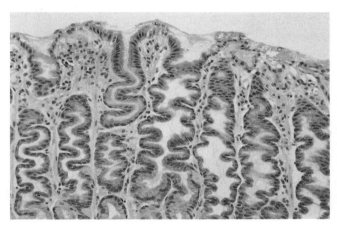

QUESTION 32.5

   A. Eosinophilic gastritis
   B. Granulomatous gastritis
   C. Helicobacter gastritis
   D. Lymphocytic gastritis
   E. Reactive gastropathy

6. The most frequent type of gastric polyp is:
   A. Adenoma
   B. Fundic gland polyp
   C. Hamartomatous polyp
   D. Hyperplastic polyp
   E. Inflammatory fibroid polyp

7. The gross appearance of gastric mucosa in Zollinger-Ellison syndrome is often strikingly similar to:
   A. Fundic gland polyps
   B. Gardner syndrome
   C. Hyperplastic polyps
   D. Inflammatory fibroid polyps
   E. Ménétrier disease

8. There is a definite, although weak association between the form of gastric adenocarcinoma shown in this picture and which of the following forms of metaplasia?

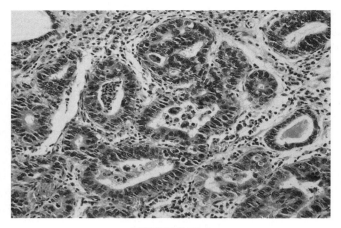

QUESTION 32.8

   A. Intestinal metaplasia, large bowel type, complete
   B. Intestinal metaplasia, large bowel type, incomplete
   C. Intestinal metaplasia, small bowel type, complete
   D. Intestinal metaplasia, small bowel type, incomplete
   E. Pyloric metaplasia

9. Which of the following is the most important prognostic factor in gastric adenocarcinoma?
   A. CA19-9 levels
   B. CEA level
   C. Pathologic stage
   D. Patient age
   E. Tumor histologic type

10. Which of the following is true about superficial spreading ("early") gastric carcinoma?
   A. Adenocarcinoma that has not penetrated the basement membrane
   B. Carcinoma associated with a 50% 5-year survival rate
   C. Carcinoma limited to mucosa/submucosa without node metastasis
   D. Carcinoma limited to mucosa/submucosa with or without node metastasis
   E. Well-differentiated carcinoma limited to the mucosa

11. The type of gastric endocrine tumor that develops in the fundus in association with achlorhydria and hypergastrinemia will most likely secrete or contain:
   A. ACTH
   B. Enterochromaffin-like (ECL) cells

   C. Histamine
   D. Serotonin
   E. Somatostatin

12. A 55-year-old man presents with vague dyspeptic symptoms. Endoscopy reveals prominent accentuation of mucosal rugae in a cerebriform pattern. Gastric biopsies show a diffuse infiltrate of small lymphocytes and centrocyte-like cells forming structures such as the one in this photomicrograph. There are scattered lymphoid follicles. Many cells show features of plasmacytoid differentiation, and some contain PAS-positive intranuclear inclusions. Which of the following is the most likely diagnosis?

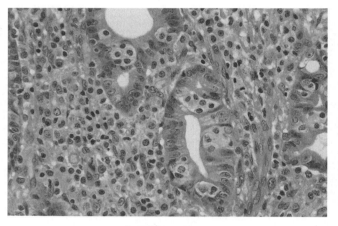

QUESTION 32.12

   A. Large cell lymphoma
   B. Lymphoplasmacytoid lymphoma
   C. MALT-related lymphoma
   D. Plasma cell granuloma
   E. Pseudolymphoma

13. A patient undergoes surgery for resection of a gastric neoplasm previously diagnosed as gastrointestinal stromal tumor (GIST) on biopsy. This class of tumors is presumably derived from:
   A. Interstitial cells of Cajal
   B. Myofibroblasts
   C. Schwann cells
   D. Smooth muscle cells
   E. Undifferentiated mesenchymal cells

NONNEOPLASTIC INTESTINAL DISEASES

1. Which of the following macroscopic mucosal patterns is usually seen in jejunal biopsies from patients with celiac sprue?
   A. Cerebroid
   B. Flat
   C. Leaflike
   D. Mosaic
   E. Villouslike

2. A 35-year-old HIV-negative man presents with malabsorption syndrome and lymphadenopathy. A jejunal biopsy shows numerous macrophages in the lamina propria, which are stuffed with PAS-positive granules. Electron microscopy reveals rodlike structures in their cytoplasm. Which of the following is the most likely pathogen in this condition?
   A. *Bartonella henselae*
   B. *Mycobacterium avium-intracellulare*
   C. *Salmonella*
   D. *Tropheryma whippelii*
   E. *Yersinia*

3. A duodenal biopsy from a patient suffering from intermittent diarrhea and malabsorption is shown in this high-power photomicrograph of a trichrome-stained section. Which of the following is the most likely diagnosis?
   A. Capillariasis
   B. Cryptosporidiosis
   C. Giardiasis
   D. Microsporidiosis
   E. Strongyloidiasis

4. Which of the following microscopic features is most characteristic of the quiescent stage of ulcerative colitis (UC in remission)?
   A. Crypt abscesses and decreased mucin content
   B. Diffuse mucosal and submucosal inflammatory infiltration
   C. Entirely normal mucosa
   D. Mucosal atrophy and distortion of gland architecture
   E. Regenerative activity of glandular epithelium

5. A colonic biopsy shows the histological changes highlighted in this picture, which is from a patient with UC.

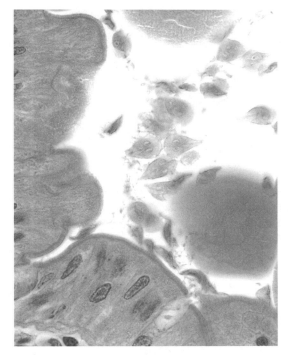

QUESTION 33.3

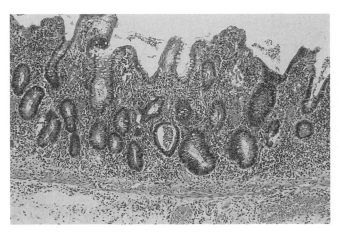

QUESTION 33.5

Which of the following features favors a diagnosis of Crohn disease over ulcerative colitis?

    A. Colonic involvement
    B. Crypt abscesses
    C. Nonnecrotizing granulomas
    D. Pseudopolyps
    E. Ulcers

6. A 59-year-old woman presents with intractable watery diarrhea of unknown etiology. All of the clinical and radiologic investigations are normal. Endoscopically, the colonic mucosa appears unremarkable. A colon biopsy shows increased inflammatory cells in the lamina propria and a thick hyaline membrane underneath the epithelial layer. Which of the following is the most likely diagnosis?

    A. Bacterial colitis
    B. Collagenous colitis
    C. Eosinophilic colitis
    D. Lymphocytic colitis
    E. Pseudomembranous colitis

7. A 32-year-old male presents with constipation and rectal bleeding. Clinical differential diagnosis includes Crohn disease, villous adenoma, and adenocarcinoma. Rectal biopsies reveal round pools of mucin lined by a single-cell epithelial layer. Desmoplastic reaction is absent. These features are most consistent with:

    A. Mucinous adenocarcinoma
    B. Mucosal prolapse syndrome
    C. Pneumatosis cystoides intestinalis
    D. Ulcerative colitis
    E. Villous adenoma

8. A patient with AIDS develops intractable watery diarrhea. A jejunal biopsy shows round faintly basophilic 3-μm bodies attached to the luminal surface, as illustrated by this high-power picture. Which of the following H&E changes would be expected in the bowel mucosa?

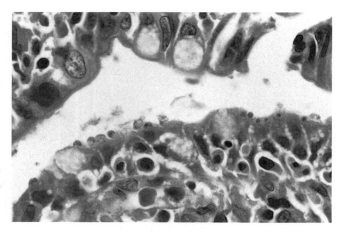

QUESTION 33.8

    A. Crypt abscesses
    B. Eosinophilic infiltration
    C. Extensive lymphocytic infiltration
    D. Granulomas
    E. Minimal nonspecific changes

9. An AIDS patient with intractable diarrhea undergoes a GI biopsy. On high power, clusters of small dotlike structures are seen in a paranuclear location within epithelial cells of intestinal villi. These are gram-positive but AFB-negative. The most likely pathogen is:

    A. Cryptosporidia
    B. Cytomegalovirus
    C. *Giardia lamblia*
    D. Microsporidia
    E. Spirochetes

10. A colonic biopsy from an area of stricture located in the splenic flexure is examined histologically. Which of the following microscopic changes favors a diagnosis of ischemic bowel disease over inflammatory bowel disease?

    A. Crypt abscesses
    B. Fibrosis of the lamina propria
    C. Individual cell necrosis in crypts
    D. Linear deep fissures
    E. Volcano-like masses of fibrin and neutrophils

11. A previously healthy 70-year-old woman undergoes a barium enema and colonoscopy for evaluation of chronic lower intestinal bleeding. Imaging studies are negative, but a source of bleeding is identified in the cecum. Which of the following is the most likely cause of this patient's bleeding?

    A. Angiodysplasia (vascular ectasias)
    B. Angiosarcoma
    C. Cavernous hemangioma
    D. Diverticular disease
    E. Varices

12. Which of the following changes is most likely to be present in a suction mucosal/submucosal biopsy of the aganglionic segment from a patient with Hirschprung disease?

    A. Absence of ganglion cells in the intramural plexus
    B. Absence of ganglion cells in the submucosal plexus
    C. Decreased acetylcholinesterase reaction
    D. Reduced number of nerve fibers
    E. Reduced number of satellite cells

13. An intravenous pyelography reveals prominent displacement of the ureters toward the midline. Which of the following retroperitoneal processes is most likely to produce such a finding?

    A. Idiopathic retroperitoneal fibrosis
    B. Leiomyosarcoma
    C. Liposarcoma
    D. Malignant fibrous histiocytoma
    E. Malignant lymphoma

34

INTESTINAL NEOPLASMS

1. Which of the following features is most characteristic of hyperplastic colorectal polyps?
   A. Decreased mucin content
   B. Inconspicuous basement membrane
   C. Increased mitoses at the base of glands
   D. Increased mitoses at the tips of glands
   E. Mild-to-moderate cellular atypia

2. Histologic examination of a tangentially cut colonic biopsy reveals tightly clustered crypts as shown in this low-power photomicrograph. Which of the following is the most likely diagnosis?

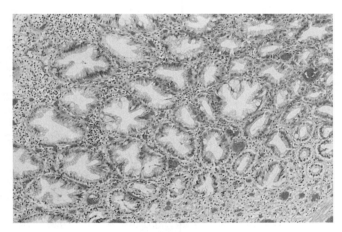

QUESTION 34.2

   A. Adenomatous polyp
   B. Hyperplastic polyp
   C. Juvenile polyp
   D. Normal colonic mucosa
   E. Serrated adenoma

3. A polyp is resected from the proximal portion of the jejunum. Histologically, it consists of glands containing both absorptive and goblet cells supported by a stalk. Within the stalk, there are smooth muscle bundles continuous with the underlying muscularis mucosae. Which of the following additional features is most likely to be observed in this patient?
   A. Innumerable adenomatous polyps of the colon
   B. Malignant brain tumors
   C. Osteomas of the mandible and long bones
   D. Perioral and perianal pigmentation
   E. Soft tissue tumors

4. The presence of conspicuous cystic spaces within the head of a benign rectal polyp suggests a diagnosis of:
   A. Adenomatous polyp
   B. Hamartomatous polyp
   C. Inflammatory polyp
   D. Inflammatory fibroid polyp
   E. Juvenile polyp

5. Which of the following types of colonic polyps is associated with familial polyposis and found in up to one-third of adult individuals at autopsy?
   A. Hamartomatous polyp
   B. Hyperplastic polyp
   C. Juvenile polyp
   D. Tubular adenoma (adenomatous polyp)
   E. Villous adenoma (villous papilloma)

6. Most villous adenomas have which of the following clinical-pathologic characteristics?
   A. Centrally ulcerated mass in the sigmoid
   B. Composed of normal glands and crypts
   C. Found usually in young patients
   D. Low propensity for malignant degeneration
   E. Sessile soft mass in the rectum

7. The definition of *intramucosal neoplasia/carcinoma* should be reserved for adenomas with:
   A. Epithelial misplacement
   B. Height less than two times that of normal mucosa
   C. High-grade dysplasia
   D. Malignant glands invading through muscularis mucosae
   E. Small malignant glands infiltrating the lamina propria

8. A colectomy specimen from a 28-year-old man shows innumerable tubular adenomas carpeting the entire mucosal surface of the colon. Which of the following is the approximate incidence rate of colon adenocarcinoma in patients with this condition?
   A. Less than 5%
   B. 10% to 20%
   C. 30% to 50%
   D. 50% to 80%
   E. 100%

9. Adenocarcinomas of the small bowel:
   A. Are half as frequent as colonic adenocarcinomas
   B. Are most frequent in the ileum
   C. Are never seen in association with Crohn disease
   D. Develop most commonly in the duodenum
   E. Usually arise from Brunner gland nodules

10. This high-power photomicrograph shows a histologic type of colorectal carcinoma. Which of the following is it?

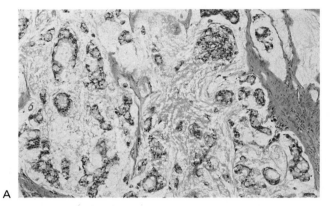

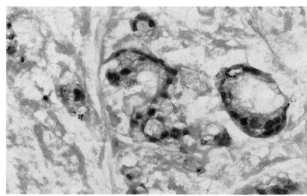

QUESTION 34.10

   A. Adenocarcinoma
   B. Adenosquamous carcinoma
   C. Mucinous adenocarcinoma
   D. Signet ring cell carcinoma
   E. Small cell cancer
   F. Squamous cell carcinoma
   G. Undifferentiated (medullary) carcinoma

11. A 65-year-old man undergoes a partial colectomy for resection of adenocarcinoma. The tumor infiltrates the muscularis propria without reaching the serosa. Which of the following molecular/morphologic features is associated with a better prognosis?
   A. Crohn-like inflammatory reaction
   B. Endocrine cells expressing chromogranin
   C. K-*ras* mutations
   D. Microacinar pattern
   E. Multiplicity of tumor

12. A brain metastasis of unknown primary carcinoma is examined histologically. Which of the following immunohistochemical features favors a diagnosis of metastatic colorectal carcinoma?
   A. Dotlike perinuclear positivity for keratin-20
   B. Positive glial fibrillary acidic protein (GFAP)
   C. Positive keratin-7 and negative keratin-20
   D. Positive keratin-20 and negative CEA
   E. Positive keratin-20 and negative keratin-7

13. Which of the following is true about carcinoid of the appendix?
   A. Adenocarcinoid is by definition malignant
   B. Frequently associated with carcinoid syndrome
   C. Goblet cell type is consistently negative for chromogranin
   D. Insular type is associated with a poor prognosis
   E. Represents an incidental finding in about 1 of 300 appendices

14. Which of the following features is characteristic of rectal carcinoids?
   A. Frequently associated with carcinoid syndrome
   B. Frequently immunoreactive for prostatic specific antigen
   C. Insular or nesting arrangement is the usual microscopic pattern
   D. Multicentric when associated with inflammatory bowel disease
   E. Never give rise to lymph node metastases

15. Intestinal lymphomas account for 17% of primary tumors of the small bowel and less than 5% of colorectal tumors. Which of the following is the most frequent type in Western countries?
   A. B-cell lymphoma of MALT type
   B. Burkitt lymphoma
   C. Enteropathy-associated lymphoma
   D. Follicular lymphoma
   E. Immunoproliferative small intestinal disease

16. Which of the following is a small bowel lymphoma encountered in Third World countries and associated with monoclonal production of IgA heavy chains?
   A. B-cell lymphoma of MALT type
   B. Burkitt lymphoma
   C. Enteropathy-associated lymphoma
   D. Follicular lymphoma
   E. Immunoproliferative small intestinal disease

17. A patient with celiac sprue (gluten-sensitive enteropathy) is prone to developing which of the following types of small intestinal lymphomas?
   A. Histiocytic lymphoma
   B. Hodgkin disease
   C. Immunoproliferative small intestinal disease
   D. MALT-associated lymphoma
   E. T-cell lymphoma

18. A small tumor is removed from the second duodenal segment. It is characterized by a heterogeneous population

of cells arranged in a nesting pattern. A high-power view is shown in the picture. Which of the following is the most likely diagnosis?

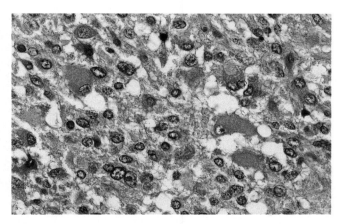

QUESTION 34.18

A. Carcinoid tumor
B. Gangliocytic paraganglioma
C. Gastrointestinal autonomic nerve tumor (GANT)
D. Gastrointestinal stromal tumor (GIST)
E. Schwannoma

PANCREAS

1. The pancreas of a 50-year-old patient shows extensive hemorrhagic and fat necrosis. Chalky-white deposits are observed in the omentum. Besides alcoholism, the most common etiologic factor associated with this condition is:
   A. Acute ischemia
   B. Bile stones
   C. Drugs
   D. Hyperlipoproteinemia
   E. Infections

2. In industrialized countries, the most important cause of chronic pancreatitis is:
   A. Alcoholism
   B. Cholelithiasis
   C. Hereditary conditions
   D. Hyperparathyroidism
   E. Protein malnutrition

3. A subtotal pancreatic resection is performed in a patient with malabsorption. The histopathologic changes include atrophy of the exocrine component, dense intralobular and perilobular fibrosis, calcific deposits in the ducts, and dilated ducts containing an inspissated secretion. There is apparent hyperplasia of the islets of Langerhans. Which of the following is the most common complication of this condition?
   A. Ductal adenocarcinoma
   B. Islet cell carcinoma
   C. Migratory thrombophlebitis
   D. Obstructive jaundice
   E. Pancreatic pseudocyst

4. In the differential diagnosis between pancreatic adenocarcinoma and chronic pancreatitis, which of the following changes favors adenocarcinoma?
   A. Chronic inflammation
   B. Ductal dilatation
   C. Fibrosis
   D. Loss of lobular architecture
   E. Parenchymal atrophy

5. On histologic examination, a pancreatic tumor shows a mixture of different neoplastic components including areas that appear as in this low-power picture and other areas of glandular differentiation. There are bizarre osteoclast-like cells and atypical mitotic figures. Which of the following features is characteristic of this neoplasm?

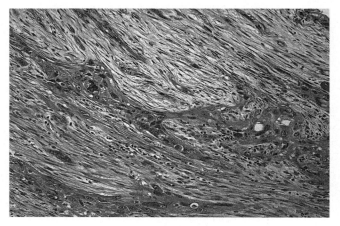

QUESTION 35.5

   A. Butyrate esterase reaction
   B. Evidence of neuroendocrine differentiation
   C. Female predilection
   D. Keratin expression
   E. Origin from acinar cells

6. A pancreatic tumor is found at the postmortem examination of a 75-year-old woman who died of a myocardial infarction. On the cut surface, the tumor shows small cysts filled with serous fluid. Histologically, the septa between cysts are lined by cuboidal cells with clear cytoplasm and contain scattered islets of Langerhans. Which of the following is the most likely diagnosis?
   A. Acinar cell carcinoma
   B. Chronic pancreatitis
   C. Microcystic cystadenoma
   D. Mucinous cystadenoma
   E. Polycystic disease

7. A 4-year-old boy presents with jaundice and an abdominal mass. There is a family history of adenomatous polyposis coli. He undergoes resection of a pancreatic tumor. Histologically, the neoplasm appears as in this photomicrograph. Which of the following is the most likely diagnosis?
   A. Acinar cell carcinoma
   B. Ductal adenocarcinoma
   C. Islet cell tumor

D. Pancreatoblastoma
E. Solid cystic-papillary epithelial neoplasm

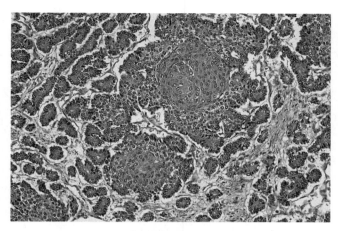

QUESTION 35.7

8. A pancreatic neoplasm resected from a 18-year-old woman is characterized by a pseudopapillary architecture and shows the histological features demonstrated in this picture. Which of the following additional features are characteristic of this tumor?

A. Butyrate esterase positivity
B. Innumerable mitochondria
C. Osteoclast-like giant cells
D. PAS-positive globules
E. Squamoid corpuscles

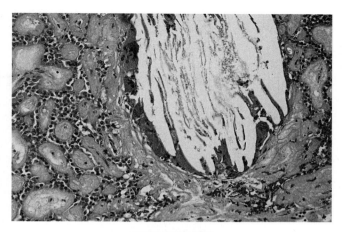

QUESTION 35.8

9. The most frequent islet cell tumor is also the least frequently malignant. Which one is it?

A. Gastrinoma
B. Glucagonoma
C. Insulinoma
D. Somatostatinoma
E. VIPoma

10. Which of the following pancreatic conditions is described by the designation of *nesidioblastosis*?

A. Atypical changes of islet cells
B. Extensive pancreatic heterotopia
C. Islet hyperplasia in chronic pancreatitis
D. Islets in connection with ductules
E. Squamous metaplasia of interlobular ducts

36

NONNEOPLASTIC LIVER DISEASE

1. Following a 3-hour-long exploratory laparotomy, a surgeon performs a wedge liver biopsy in an immunocompetent patient with hepatomegaly and jaundice. This shows a lobular neutrophilic exudate with hepatocellular necrosis, predominantly found in a subcapsular location. Which of the following is the most likely diagnosis?
   A. Alcoholic hepatitis
   B. Drug-induced damage
   C. Infection
   D. Sepsis
   E. Surgical hepatitis

2. A liver biopsy from a 2-month-old infant with cholestatic jaundice reveals prominent small bile duct proliferation, bile plugs, portal edema, and scattered hepatic giant cells. The lobular architecture is preserved. Which of the following is the most likely cause of these changes?
   A. Alpha-1-antitrypsin deficiency
   B. Extrahepatic biliary atresia
   C. Galactosemia
   D. Hereditary fructose intolerance
   E. Infection

3. Extrahepatic biliary atresia (EBA) is:
   A. Caused by congenital absence of bile ducts
   B. Commonly associated with patency of ducts at porta hepatis
   C. Due to postnatal bile duct destruction
   D. Usually limited to hepatic bile ducts
   E. Usually limited to the common bile duct

4. A diagnosis of *intrahepatic biliary atresia* is primarily based on the finding of:
   A. Ductular proliferation and portal edema
   B. Fibrosis and inflammation of portal tracts
   C. Giant cell transformation and extramedullary hematopoiesis
   D. Loss of ductules
   E. Loss of interlobular ducts

5. The most characteristic morphologic change in the liver of patients with alpha-1-antitrypsin deficiency is:
   A. Bile duct destruction
   B. Cytoplasmic keratin inclusions
   C. Iron accumulation
   D. Microvesicular steatosis
   E. PAS-positive cytoplasmic globules

6. A 20-year-old male with chronic liver disease, increased copper in the urine, and Kayser-Fleisher rings on slit-lamp examination will most likely have which of the following associated alterations?
   A. Antinuclear, anti–smooth muscle and antimitochondrial antibodies
   B. Degeneration of putamen in the brain
   C. Glucose intolerance
   D. Increased serum levels of ceruloplasmin
   E. Panacinar emphysema

7. A 25-year-old male undergoes clinical and pathologic investigations because of progressive jaundice and elevated liver enzymes. Endoscopic retrograde cholangiopancreatography demonstrates alternating segments of stenosis and dilatation of extrahepatic biliary tree. A liver biopsy shows changes similar to those seen in this picture. Which of the following conditions is most commonly associated with this liver disease?
   A. Crohn disease
   B. Progressive systemic fibrosis

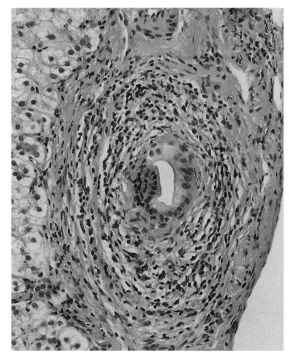

QUESTION 36.7

C. Retroperitoneal fibrosis

D. Riedel thyroiditis

E. Ulcerative colitis

8. A 50-year-old woman undergoes a liver biopsy because of persistent pruritus, jaundice, and elevated liver enzymes. The biopsy shows chronic hepatitis characterized by lymphohistiocytic infiltration around small bile ducts, with concomitant degeneration of ductules. Piecemeal necrosis is also present. Rhodamine staining demonstrates marked copper accumulation. Which of the following is the finding most likely associated with this condition?

A. Antihepatitis C virus antibodies

B. Antimitochondrial autoantibodies

C. Homozygosis for PiZZ genotype of alpha-1-antitrypsin

D. Iron accumulation in pancreas and myocardium

E. Mitochondrial crystalline inclusions and "fish-mouth" canaliculi on EM

9. A patient with laboratory evidence of liver dysfunction has a history of chronic intake of anabolic steroids. Which of the following patterns of liver injury would be expected?

A. Cholestasis

B. Granulomatous inflammation

C. Hepatocyte necrosis

D. Macrovesicular steatosis

E. Microvesicular steatosis

10. An autopsy is performed on a patient that has died of fulminant hepatic failure (FHF). The liver weighs 900 g. Histologic examination shows large areas of acute hepatocyte necrosis with scattered neutrophils. Which of the following is the most common virus causing this condition?

A. Hepatitis A virus

B. Hepatitis B virus

C. Hepatitis C virus

D. Hepatitis D virus

E. Hepatitis E virus

11. A patient with a history of hemophilia A and repeated blood transfusions develops chronic hepatitis. Which of the following viruses is the most common cause of chronic hepatitis in this clinical setting?

A. Hepatitis A virus

B. Hepatitis B virus

C. Hepatitis C virus

D. Hepatitis D virus

E. Hepatitis E virus

12. According to the grading/staging system proposed by Scheuer, a liver biopsy showing bridging fibrosis with architectural disarray but no cirrhosis is classified as:

A. Grade 0

B. Grade 1

C. Grade 2

D. Grade 3

E. Grade 4

13. A young woman with chronic liver dysfunction undergoes a liver biopsy. This shows mild-to-moderate periportal inflammation, single-hepatocyte necrosis, and periportal fibrosis. There is a mixed portal infiltrate containing plasma cells. Laboratory investigations have also demonstrated circulating anti–smooth muscle antibodies and hypergammaglobulinemia. Enzyme immunoassay for anti-HCV antibodies is positive, but a recombinant immunoblot assay (RIBA) fails to detect anti-HCV antibodies. Which of the following is the most likely diagnosis?

A. Alcoholic hepatitis

B. Autoimmune (lupoid) hepatitis

C. Chronic hepatitis C infection

D. Drug-induced hepatitis

E. Primary biliary cirrhosis

14. Which of the following statements best characterizes hyperacute (humoral) rejection of a liver allograft?

A. Characterized by loss of bile ducts in portal spaces

B. Characterized by lymphocytic infiltration of portal spaces

C. Characterized by subendothelial lymphocytes in portal veins

D. Occurs within 24 hours following transplantation

E. Occurs from 5 to 30 days following transplantation

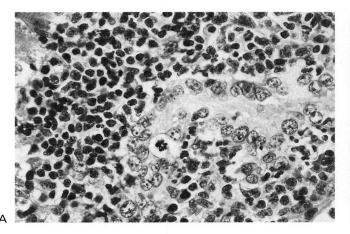

A

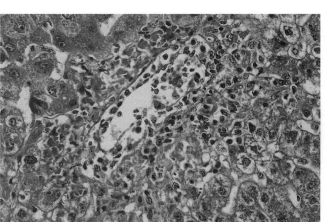

B

QUESTION 36.15

15. These photomicrographs show the main histological changes of a liver biopsy obtained 14 days after orthotopic liver transplantation. This histologic picture is most consistent with:
    A. Acute (cellular) rejection
    B. Chronic (ductopenic) rejection
    C. Humoral rejection
    D. Portal vein thrombosis
    E. Preservation injury

16. Six months following liver transplantation, a liver biopsy reveals changes similar to those present in this photomicrograph. Such changes would be most likely associated with:

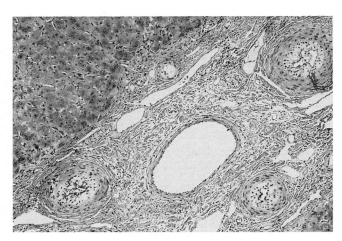

QUESTION 36.16

A. Bile duct proliferation
B. Endothelialitis
C. Loss of bile ducts
D. Marked inflammation
E. Platelet and fibrin microthrombi

17. A liver biopsy is performed because of a clinical diagnosis of chronic hepatitis. The presence of "ground-glass" hepatocytes would favor a diagnosis of:
    A. Hepatitis A
    B. Hepatitis B
    C. Hepatitis C
    D. Primary biliary cirrhosis
    E. Steatohepatitis

MASSES OF THE LIVER

1. Aspiration of a cystic lesion in the right hepatic lobe yields odorless, orange, pasty material. Microscopic examination of this material shows necrotic debris, with no neutrophils. Occasional histiocyte-like round cells with a small round nucleus with a karyosome are identified. Which of the following is the most likely diagnosis?
   A. Amebiasis
   B. Biliary cystadenoma
   C. Echinococcosis
   D. Pyogenic abscess
   E. Solitary unilocular cyst

2. The autopsy of a 40-year-old woman reveals hemoperitoneum and a subcapsular hemorrhagic mass in the right hepatic lobe. The mass is partially encapsulated, and the adjacent liver parenchyma appears compressed. Histologically, the lesion is composed of cords of well-differentiated hepatocytes with abundant glycogen content. Conspicuous thick-walled vessels are scattered throughout the lesion, but there are no identifiable central veins or portal tracts. Which of the following is the most important predisposing factor for this lesion?
   A. Aflatoxin exposure
   B. *Bartonella henselae* infection
   C. Hepatitis B virus infection
   D. Oral contraceptives use
   E. Thorotrast exposure

3. A well-demarcated subcapsular nodule is identified by MRI in the right hepatic lobe of a 35-year-old woman with abdominal discomfort. The lesion is removed. Its cut section is shown in this macroscopic photograph. Microscopic examination shows liver lobules with fatty changes separated by thick fibrous bands. The central scar contains thick-walled arteries. These gross and microscopic features are consistent with:
   A. Early cirrhosis
   B. Focal nodular hyperplasia
   C. Hepatoblastoma
   D. Liver adenoma
   E. Nodular regenerative hyperplasia

4. A 50-year-old woman with rheumatoid arthritis presents with signs and symptoms of portal hypertension. An abdominal MRI is suggestive of liver cirrhosis. A needle biopsy

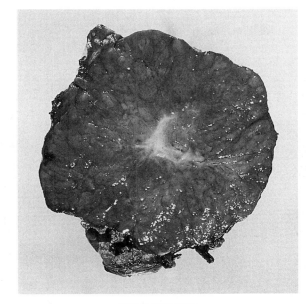

QUESTION 37.3

reveals areas of congestion alternating with areas of expanded lobules. Central veins are not seen. Which of the following mechanisms plays a crucial role in the pathogenesis of this disorder?
   A. Drug-induced injury to hepatocytes
   B. Drug-induced injury to sinusoids
   C. Extrahepatic biliary injury
   D. Hepatitis B virus infection
   E. Microvascular alterations

5. The following is a list of factors or conditions that predispose to the development of hepatocellular carcinoma (HCC). In which of them does HCC occur constantly in noncirrhotic livers?
   A. Alcohol abuse
   B. Hepatitis B virus
   C. Hepatitis C virus
   D. Hereditary hemochromatosis
   E. Hypercitrillunemia

6. Which of the following morphological or immunohistochemical features is most significant in making a diagnosis of hepatocellular carcinoma?

A. Bile formation
B. CAM 5.2 immunoreactivity
C. Cytoplasmic CEA immunoreactivity
D. Sinusoidal pattern
E. Tubular architecture

7. A patient undergoes partial hepatectomy for a neoplasm. The tumor consists of nodules of large cells with prominent nucleoli, separated by broad fibrohyaline bands. Which of the following is the most likely clinical setting associated with this tumor type?

A. Markedly elevated serum alpha-fetoprotein
B. 20-year-old patient with chronic hepatitis B
C. 30-year-old patient with normal liver
D. 50-year-old patient with alcoholic cirrhosis
E. Elderly patient with hemochromatosis

8. The patient is a 16-month-old baby with a hepatic tumor. On histological examination, the tumor is characterized by a "light/dark" pattern shown on this low-power picture. This tumor is most likely a:

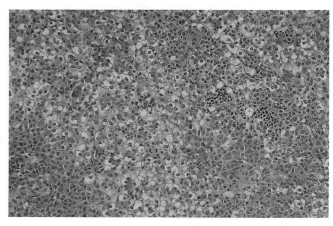

QUESTION 37.8

A. Bile duct hamartoma
B. Hemangioblastoma
C. Hepatoblastoma
D. Malignant mesenchymoma
E. Mesenchymal hamartoma

9. The cut surface of a liver removed at autopsy shows scattered white nodules in the liver parenchyma. Histologically, they consist of disorderly clusters of bile ductules lined by bland epithelial cells without an identifiable connection with the bile system. These features are most consistent with:

A. Bile duct adenoma
B. Bile duct carcinoma
C. Bile duct hamartoma
D. Mesenchymal hamartoma
E. Metastatic carcinoma

10. Multiple tan-white masses are found at autopsy in the liver of a 65-year-old man. The intervening hepatic parenchyma is normal. The neoplasm consists of small tubular structures within a dense fibrotic stroma. Neoplastic cells vary markedly in size and shape within the same tubule. Mucin production is demonstrated by mucicarmine stain, but no bile is detected. Perineural invasion is seen. The cytoplasm of tumor cells is labeled by CAM 5.2, keratin AE1-antibody, and anti-CEA antibodies. These features are most consistent with:

A. Angiosarcoma
B. Bile duct carcinoma
C. Bile duct hamartoma (von Meyenburg complex)
D. Hepatocellular carcinoma
E. Metastatic carcinoma

11. Which of the following factors is known to increase the risk of developing angiosarcoma of the liver, but not that of bile duct carcinoma or hepatocellular carcinoma?

A. Anabolic steroid treatment
B. Cirrhosis of any etiology
C. Clonorchis parasite infestation
D. Occupational exposure to vinyl chloride
E. Thorotrast exposure

12. A 34-year-old woman who takes oral contraceptives undergoes surgery for resection of multiple intrahepatic tumors. Histologically, the lesions consist of plump cells with acidophilic and vacuolated cytoplasm. Neoplastic cells infiltrate vascular channels. Immunoreactivity for factor VIII–related antigen is detected. Ultrastructural studies reveal Weibel-Palade bodies. Which of the following is the most likely diagnosis?

A. Angiosarcoma
B. Epithelioid hemangioendothelioma
C. Focal nodular hyperplasia
D. Hemangioma
E. Liver cell adenoma

38

GALLBLADDER, EXTRAHEPATIC BILIARY TREE, AND AMPULLA

1. *Acalculous* acute cholecystitis may develop most frequently in patients with:
   A. Acquired immunodeficiency disease (AIDS)
   B. Chronic hemolytic diseases
   C. Infections with *Ascaris lumbricoides*
   D. Infections with *Escherichia coli*
   E. Infections with liver flukes

2. Most cases of carcinoma of the gallbladder are associated with:
   A. Cholelithiasis
   B. Gardner syndrome
   C. Porcelain gallbladder
   D. Sclerosing cholangitis
   E. Ulcerative colitis

3. A 10-year-old female presents with signs and symptoms of cholestatic jaundice. A lesion involving the common bile duct is resected. The surgical specimen is shown in this gross photograph. The diagnosis is:
   A. Biliary atresia
   B. Caroli disease

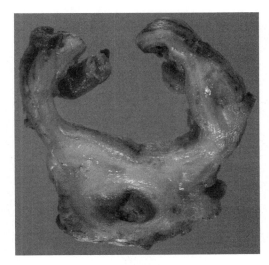

QUESTION 38.3

   C. Choledochal cyst
   D. Phrygian cap
   E. Sclerosing cholangitis

39

ANUS AND PERIANAL AREA

1. Which of the following histologic patterns is most suggestive of the basaloid variant of anal carcinoma?
    A. Extensive mucin production
    B. Spindle cell tumor
    C. Tumor nests with peripheral palisading
    D. Villous architecture
    E. Well-differentiated squamous epithelium with minimal atypia

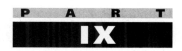

URINARY TRACT AND MALE GENITAL SYSTEM

40

DEVELOPMENTAL ABNORMALITIES OF THE KIDNEY

1. Which of the following developmental anomalies has been linked to maternal use of angiotensin-converting enzyme (ACE) inhibitors and maternal cocaine abuse?
   A. Congenital hydronephrosis
   B. Renal dysplasia
   C. Renal hypoplasia
   D. Renal segmental atrophy
   E. Renal tubular dysgenesis

2. The condition known as renal segmental atrophy (or Ask-Upmark kidney) is most likely due to:
   A. Autosomal dominant genetic defect
   B. Autosomal recessive genetic defect
   C. Congenital anomaly of ureteral muscle
   D. Segmental hypoplasia
   E. Vesicoureteral reflux

3. A 9-month-old infant comes to clinical attention because of renal insufficiency and enlarged kidneys. Radiologic and sonographic studies show large and hyperechoic kidneys. A renal biopsy shows the changes depicted in the photomicrograph. These findings are consistent with autosomal recessive polycystic kidney disease (AR-PKD). Which of the following pathologic lesions is most likely to be associated with this kidney condition?
   A. Angiomas in the retina and cerebellum
   B. Angiomyolipoma
   C. Cardiac rhabdomyoma
   D. Hepatic fibrosis
   E. Pancreatic cysts

4. Which of the following features is not characteristic of renal pathology in autosomal dominant polycystic kidney disease (AD-PKD)?

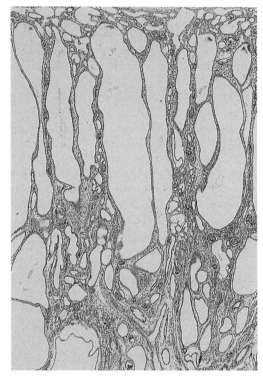

QUESTION 40.3

A. Lithiasis and infection are rare in renal cysts
B. Renal cysts are lined by hyperplastic epithelium with papillary formations
C. Renal parenchyma between cysts is dysplastic
D. Renal pathology is usually associated with pyelocaliceal occlusion
E. Virtually all nephrons are affected by cystic dilatation

ADULT RENAL DISEASES

1. Electron microscopy on a renal biopsy from a 9-year-old boy with nephritic syndrome and elevated antistreptococcal antibody titers reveals subepithelial electron-dense dome-shaped "humps." The morphologic pattern most probably demonstrable on light microscopic examination is:
    A. Diffuse extracapillary proliferative glomerulonephritis
    B. Diffuse intracapillary proliferative glomerulonephritis
    C. Focal glomerulonephritis
    D. Membranous glomerulopathy
    E. Normal glomerular morphology

2. A 12-year-old boy has nephrotic syndrome and low complement levels. The main findings on renal biopsy are as follows: diffuse mesangial hypercellularity, pronounced accentuation of glomerular lobules, a double-contour ("tram-track") appearance of glomerular basement membrane on PAS/silver stains, and mesangial deposition of C3 and IgG. Which of the following is the most likely diagnosis?
    A. Membranoproliferative (mesangiocapillary) glomerulonephritis, type I
    B. Membranoproliferative (mesangiocapillary) glomerulonephritis, type II
    C. Membranous glomerulopathy
    D. Minimal change glomerulopathy
    E. Postinfectious glomerulonephritis

3. *Dense deposit disease* (DDD) is an alternative designation of which of the following glomerulopathies?
    A. Light chain disease
    B. Membranoproliferative (mesangiocapillary) glomerulonephritis, type I
    C. Membranoproliferative (mesangiocapillary) glomerulonephritis, type II
    D. Membranous glomerulopathy
    E. Minimal change glomerulopathy

4. Which of the following is true about *rapidly progressive (crescentic) glomerulonephritis (RPGN)*?
    A. Crescents consist exclusively of parietal cells of Bowman capsule
    B. Finding 20% of glomeruli with crescents supports the diagnosis

C. Most cases are associated with a known underlying condition
D. Most cases are associated with linear deposition of anti-GBM IgG
E. Prognosis depends on extent of crescent formation and IF pattern

5. A 4-year-old child presents with nephrotic syndrome, and a renal biopsy shows no light microscopic changes. Ultrastructural changes are shown here. Which of the following immunofluorescence findings would most likely be present?
    A. Absence of C3 and immunoglobulin deposits
    B. Continuous granular C3 deposition along capillary wall
    C. Granular IgG/C3 deposits along GBM
    D. Linear IgG deposition along GBM
    E. Mesangial IgA deposits

6. A clinical evaluation of a young adult with generalized edema shows heavy proteinuria (4.5 g/day). The past medical history is unremarkable. In the United States, which of the following is the most common glomerular disease accounting for this presentation?
    A. Diabetic nephropathy
    B. Focal segmental glomerulosclerosis
    C. IgA nephropathy (Berger disease)
    D. Membranous glomerulonephritis
    E. Minimal change disease

7. Focal segmental glomerulosclerosis (FSGS) is the usual morphological pattern of HIV-associated nephropathy (HIVAN). Which of the following light microscopic changes is most characteristic of HIVAN?
    A. Argyrophilic spikes on the basement membrane
    B. Crescent formation
    C. Glomerular collapse and interstitial fibrosis
    D. Obsolescent glomeruli
    E. None of the above

8. A renal biopsy is performed on a 34-year-old man for the evaluation of proteinuria in the nephrotic range. A representative silver-stained section is shown in the photomicrograph. IF demonstrates finely granular deposits of IgG and C3 along the capillary wall. EM shows effacement of foot

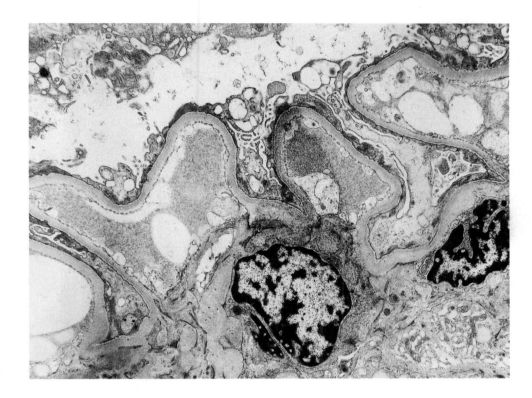

QUESTION 41.5

processes, associated with numerous subepithelial electron-dense deposits, which are separated from each other by extensions of the basement membrane. Which of the following is the most likely diagnosis?

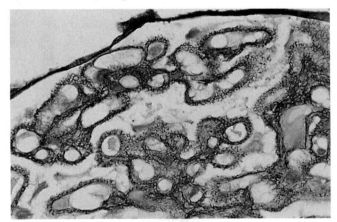

QUESTION 41.8

A. Focal segmental glomerulosclerosis
B. Membranoproliferative glomerulonephritis, type I
C. Membranoproliferative glomerulonephritis, type II
D. Membranous glomerulonephritis
E. Minimal change glomerulopathy

9. A 55-year-old woman with a 15-year history of type II diabetes mellitus is found to have microalbuminuria. All other renal function tests are normal. At this early stage, the most likely glomerular change of diabetic nephropathy is:

A. Expansion of the mesangial matrix
B. Fibroepithelial crescents
C. Insudative lesions such as fibrin caps and capsular drops
D. Mesangial intercapillary nodules (of Kimmelstiel-Wilson)
E. Thickening of the basement membrane

10. Which of the following is the most common form of glomerulonephritis worldwide and manifests with recurrent gross or microhematuria?

A. Alport syndrome
B. IgA nephropathy (Berger disease)
C. Pauci-immune crescentic glomerulonephritis
D. Postinfectious glomerulonephritis
E. Thin membrane disease

11. Microscopic hematuria is discovered in an otherwise healthy 20-year-old man. There is a family history of similar abnormality. A renal biopsy appears normal on light microscopy, but the glomerular basement membrane is less than 200 nm thick on EM. Which of the following extrarenal abnormalities is most likely associated with this condition?

A. Deafness
B. Hypoplasia of patella
C. Lens dislocation
D. Nail dysplasia
E. None of the above

12. A hereditary form of glomerulopathy caused by defective collagen synthesis and associated with sensorineural deafness and ocular abnormalities is:

A. Alport syndrome
B. Berger disease
C. Fabry disease
D. Onychoosteodysplasia
E. Thin membrane disease

13. A 35-year-old man presents with nephritic syndrome. Several years prior to this, he suffered from an episode of generalized purpura due to cryoglobulinemia. Which of the following ultrastructural changes is most characteristic of glomerular disease secondary to cryoglobulinemia?

    A. Diffuse vacuolization of glomerular endothelial cells
    B. Laminated intraepithelial inclusions called "zebra bodies"
    C. Subendothelial deposits with a fingerprint-like pattern
    D. Subepithelial electron-dense "humps"
    E. Tubulovesicular inclusions in endothelial cells

14. A 60-year-old woman with a long history of rheumatoid arthritis comes to medical attention because of heavy proteinuria. Which of the following alterations is most likely to be identified on a renal biopsy?

    A. Amyloid deposition
    B. IgA mesangial deposition
    C. Immune complex deposition
    D. Light chain mesangial deposition
    E. Urate crystal deposition within tubules

15. A 30-year-old woman with systemic lupus erythematosus (SLE) undergoes a renal biopsy because of proteinuria and microhematuria. The biopsy shows glomerular changes consistent with class IV lupus nephritis according to the WHO classification. Which of the following glomerular changes is present in this renal biopsy?

    I   A. No light microscopic changes identifiable
    II B. Mild mesangial expansion *(mesangial lupus G. N.)*
    III C. Focal segmental necrotizing glomerulonephritis
    IV D. Diffuse proliferative glomerulonephritis
    V   E. Membranous glomerulonephritis
    VI F. Global and segmental glomerular sclerosis

16. A 65-year-old man with heavy proteinuria and hypertension undergoes a renal biopsy. There is no clinical/laboratory evidence of diabetes mellitus. The main biopsy finding consists of diffuse and nodular mesangial accumulation of PAS-positive material. Which of the following changes may explain these findings?

    A. Amyloid deposition
    B. IgA deposition
    C. Immune complex formation
    D. Immunoglobulin light chain deposition
    E. Thickening of basement membrane

17. The following microscopic changes are observed in an autopsy kidney: periglomerular fibrosis, atrophic and dilated tubules, and interstitial fibrosis. This histopathological picture is most likely due to:

    A. Acute pyelonephritis

B. Allergic tubulointerstitial nephritis
C. Chronic pyelonephritis
D. Malakoplakia
E. Xanthogranulomatous pyelonephritis

18. In the United States, the most common cause of end-stage renal disease (ESRD) among Caucasians is diabetic nephropathy. In African-Americans, the most common cause is:

    A. Autosomal dominant polycystic kidney disease (AD-PKD)
    B. Chronic interstitial nephritis
    C. Diabetic nephropathy
    D. Glomerulonephritides
    E. Hypertension

19. Hyperacute rejection of renal allograft is:

    A. Characterized by emperipolesis of tubular epithelium
    B. Characterized by swelling and detachment of endothelium
    C. Mediated principally by cytotoxic lymphocytes
    D. Preventable by cyclosporine treatment
    E. Preventable by routine pretransplant cross-matching

20. Acute *cellular* rejection of renal allografts is:

    A. Characterized by fibrointimal thickening of vessels
    B. Characterized by prominent endothelial damage
    C. Highly responsive to immunosuppressive treatment
    D. Most common cause of long-term failure of renal transplantation
    E. Virtually irreversible once it manifests

21. Acute *humoral* rejection of renal allografts is:

    A. Characterized by emperipolesis of tubular epithelium
    B. Entirely preventable by cross-matching techniques
    C. Histologically similar to arteriolonephrosclerosis
    D. Mediated predominantly by endothelial cell damage
    E. Responsive to immunosuppressive treatment

22. A patient presents with progressive decline in renal function and hypertension 4 years after receiving allograft renal transplantation. Which of the following changes is the most likely underlying cause of this presentation?

    A. Destruction of tubules
    B. Endothelial swelling
    C. Fibrointimal thickening of vessels
    D. Interstitial lymphomonocytic infiltration
    E. Mesangial prominence with "tram-tracking" of GBM

23. Which of the following toxic effects of cyclosporine closely mimics hemolytic-uremic syndrome and is reversible upon drug withdrawal?

    A. Functional toxicity
    B. Tubular toxicity
    C. Vascular interstitial toxicity, acute
    D. Vascular interstitial toxicity, chronic
    E. None of the above

ADULT RENAL TUMORS

1. In addition to nucleoli and nuclear shape, which of the following elements should be assessed according to the Fuhrman system in grading renal cell carcinoma (RCC)?
   A. Cytoplasmic features (clear vs. granular)
   B. Growth pattern (solid vs. acinar)
   C. Mitotic figures
   D. Nuclear size
   E. Nucleocytoplasmic ratio

2. Cytogenetic studies performed on a renal tumor demonstrate the presence of terminal deletion of the short arm of chromosome 3. Which of the following is the most likely neoplasm?
   A. Collecting duct carcinoma
   B. Oncocytoma
   C. Renal cell carcinoma, chromophobe type
   D. Renal cell carcinoma, clear cell type
   E. Renal cell carcinoma, papillary type

3. A biopsy of a renal mass shows an epithelial tumor composed predominantly of cells with abundant granular cytoplasm. This feature can be found in:
   A. Chromophobe carcinoma
   B. Conventional (clear cell) carcinoma
   C. Oncocytoma
   D. Papillary carcinoma
   E. All of the above

4. The microscopic features of a 5-cm cortical renal tumor are shown in the picture. Fibrovascular cores contain abundant foamy macrophages, and hemosiderin is present in many cells. Cytogenetic studies reveal various chromosomal abnormalities, including trisomies 7, 16, and 17. This type of renal cell tumor arises from:
   A. Cells from distal convoluted tubule
   B. Cells of proximal convoluted tubule

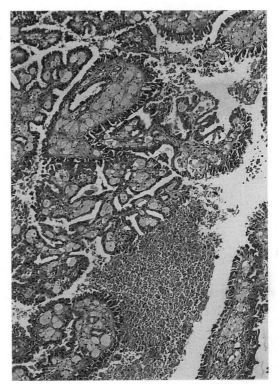

QUESTION 42.4

   C. Collecting ducts of renal medulla
   D. Intercalated cells of renal cortex
   E. Urothelial cells of the pelvis

5. Features of the renal tumor depicted in this photomicrograph include all of the following, *except:*
   A. Extremely good prognosis
   B. Perinuclear clearing
   C. Negative colloidal iron staining

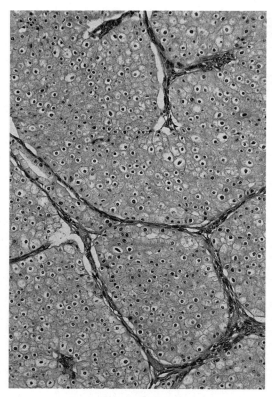

QUESTION 42.5

D. Numerous cytoplasmic vesicles on EM
E. Presumed origin from intercalated cells

6. A feature of chromophobe renal cell carcinoma is:
   A. Association with tuberous sclerosis
   B. Good prognosis
   C. High prevalence of 3p deletion
   D. Mean age at diagnosis of 25 years
   E. Tendency for renal vein invasion

7. On gross examination, a renal tumor appears as a well-demarcated, mahogany-brown, 6.5-cm mass with a central stellate scar. Which of the following microscopic features will most likely be associated with such gross appearance?
   A. Neoplastic ducts and tubules in a desmoplastic stroma
   B. Nests and tubules of malignant cells with prominent nucleoli
   C. Oncocytic cells with eosinophilic cytoplasm and round nuclei
   D. Papillary architecture lined by hemosiderin-laden epithelial cells
   E. Solid sheets of cells with sharp borders and perinuclear clearing

8. A 20-year-old African-American male with sickle cell trait undergoes removal of a renal tumor. Histologically, this tumor is most likely to be:
   A. Chromophobe cell carcinoma
   B. Clear cell (classic) renal cell carcinoma
   C. Collecting duct carcinoma
   D. Medullary carcinoma
   E. Oncocytoma

9. Metanephric adenomas are frequent tumors found in approximately 15% to 20% of adult autopsies. They are characterized by which of the following features?
   A. Associated more frequently with tuberous sclerosis
   B. Contain foamy histiocytes
   C. Histologically similar to papillary carcinoma
   D. Located most frequently in the medulla
   E. Presence of deletion of short arm of chromosome 3

10. A renal tumor composed of a mixture of adipose tissue, vessels, and HMB-45–reactive smooth muscle cells is frequently associated with:
    A. Beckwith-Wiedemann syndrome
    B. Neurofibromatosis
    C. Sickle cell trait
    D. Tuberous sclerosis
    E. von Hippel-Lindau syndrome

43

RENAL NEOPLASMS OF CHILDHOOD

1. A nephrectomy specimen is received for staging of a previously diagnosed Wilms tumor. The tumor appears confined within the kidney and completely resected. In distinguishing between stage I and stage II, which of the following anatomical structures should be examined?
   - A. Lymph nodes
   - B. Peritoneum
   - C. Renal sinus
   - D. Renal vein
   - E. Resection margins

2. A 3-year-old child undergoes surgery for resection of a large abdominal mass centered in the right kidney. The tumor is composed of various histologic elements, including an undifferentiated small cell component, a fibroblastic stroma, and scattered epithelial structures. The latter consist of tubules and abortive glomerular formations. Areas of skeletal muscle differentiation are seen in the stromal component. Which of the following is the most important prognostic factor?
   - A. Age
   - B. Extent of epithelial differentiation
   - C. Muscle differentiation
   - D. Size
   - E. Stage

3. The renal tumor known as *mesoblastic nephroma* is characterized by:
   - A. Development in fetal life
   - B. Highly aggressive behavior
   - C. Mesenchymal and epithelial elements
   - D. Multiple cysts lined by tubular epithelium
   - E. Small round cell morphology

4. A nephrectomy specimen from a 2-year-old boy shows a well-circumscribed homogeneous tumor in the medullary region. Its histological features are shown in this medium-power picture. Mitoses are frequent. Only vimentin immunoreactivity is demonstrated in tumor cells. The child has metastases in the skull and the brain. Which of the following is the most likely diagnosis?

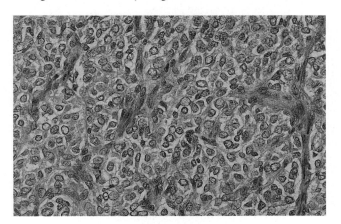

QUESTION 43.4

   - A. Clear cell sarcoma
   - B. Medullary fibroma
   - C. Mesoblastic nephroma
   - D. Multicystic nephroma
   - E. Wilms tumor

44

THE UROTHELIAL TRACT: RENAL PELVIS, URETER, URINARY BLADDER, AND URETHRA

1. Histologic examination of a bladder specimen reveals glandular structures and cystic spaces within the bladder wall, as shown in this photomicrograph. This finding is most consistent with:

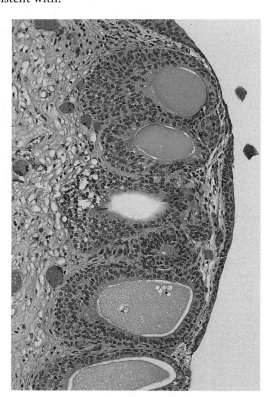

QUESTION 44.1

    A. BCG treatment
    B. Follicular cystitis
    C. Invasive adenocarcinoma
    D. Mesonephroid metaplasia
    E. Reactive change

2. A middle-aged woman has a 3-month history of supra-pubic discomfort, dysuria, and frequency. Urine cultures are negative. The finding of mucosal fissures on cystoscopy and mucosal/submucosal chronic inflammation with mast cells on biopsy are most consistent with:

    A. Cystitis glandularis
    B. Follicular cystitis
    C. Interstitial cystitis
    D. Malakoplakia
    E. Ulcerative cystitis

3. A 68-year-old woman undergoes excision of a polypoid, easily bleeding mass protruding through the urethral meatus. Histologically, it is composed of vascular tissue with chronic inflammatory cells and islands of squamous epithelium. The most likely diagnosis is:

    A. Crohn disease
    B. Fibroepithelial polyp
    C. Mesonephric adenoma
    D. Urethral carcinoma
    E. Urethral caruncle

4. A plaque of the urinary bladder mucosa is biopsied. The biopsy shows a mixed inflammatory infiltrate predominantly located within the lamina propria, consisting of nodules of histiocytes surrounded by lymphoid aggregates. As shown by the arrow in this picture, there are round laminated

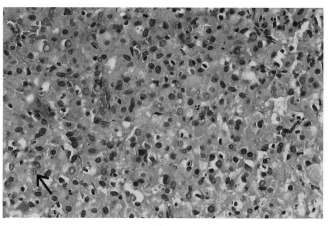

QUESTION 44.4

inclusions. Which of the following mechanisms is related to this lesion?

A. Autoimmune response
B. Defects in phagocytic function
C. Drug toxicity
D. Metaplastic change
E. Response to radiation

5. Which of the following factors is the most important predisposing condition for the development of bladder cancer in the United States?

A. Arylamine exposure
B. Cigarette smoking
C. Cyclophosphamide treatment
D. Human papillomavirus infection
E. *Schistosoma hematobium* infection

6. Pathologic staging of transitional cell carcinoma (TCC) of the bladder shows the poorest interobserver reliability in evaluating the depth of invasion into:

A. Lamina propria
B. Muscularis mucosa
C. Pelvic wall
D. Perivesical fat
E. Prostate

7. Biopsies of a 2.0-cm exophytic tumor in the bladder trigone of a 57-year-old man show papillary structures lined by more than ten layers of epithelial cells. Nuclear atypia is moderate, mitoses are rare, and there are foci of necrosis. The neoplasm infiltrates the underlying muscularis mucosa. Which of the following is the most important parameter influencing the prognosis?

A. Cell layers
B. Infiltration of the muscularis
C. Mitoses
D. Necrosis
E. Nuclear atypia

8. A 66-year-old man presents with dysuria, urgency, and microhematuria. Following cytologic studies and cystoscopy, biopsies reveal the presence of the lesion shown in this picture. Which of the following is true about this lesion?

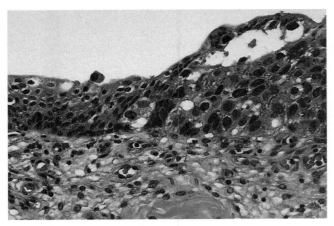

QUESTION 44.8

A. Characterized by full-thickness cellular atypia
B. Found usually in association with papillary or invasive tumors
C. High nuclear-cytoplasmic ratio is always present
D. Manifests usually with dysuria and hematuria
E. Umbrella cells are always absent

9. A biopsy of a mass in the trigone area of the urinary bladder shows a malignant tumor with microscopic features similar to those in the picture. This type of urinary bladder cancer is most frequent in association with:

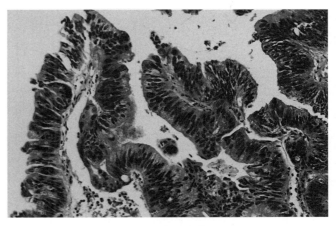

QUESTION 44.9

A. Bladder exstrophy
B. Cigarette smoking
C. Cystitis glandularis/cystica
D. Mesonephric rests in the bladder mucosa
E. Schistosoma hematobium infection

10. Cystoscopic studies reveal a large polypoid mass in the urinary bladder of a 6-year-old child. Histologically, the tumor is composed of a mucinous matrix with sheets of small blue cells. It exhibits a conspicuous "cambium layer," consisting of an accumulation of neoplastic cells beneath the mucosa. Which of the following is the most likely diagnosis?

A. Adenocarcinoma
B. Leiomyosarcoma
C. Lymphoma
D. Rhabdomyosarcoma
E. Sarcomatoid carcinoma

11. Four weeks following transurethral resection of the prostate, a 60-year-old man undergoes follow-up cystoscopic examination, which reveals a small nodule in the bladder neck. A biopsy of this lesion shows a spindle cell growth with a high mitotic rate. The cells are arranged in interweaving fascicles and display immunoreactivity for keratin and actin. Which of the following is the most likely diagnosis?

A. Inflammatory pseudotumor
B. Leiomyosarcoma
C. Mesonephroid metaplasia
D. Postoperative granuloma
E. Postoperative spindle cell nodule

45

THE PROSTATE AND SEMINAL VESICLES

1. Which of the following histopathologic features in a prostatic biopsy favors a diagnosis of adenocarcinoma over that of prostatic hyperplasia?
   A. Conspicuous nucleoli
   B. Cystic dilatation of glands
   C. Lymphocytic infiltration
   D. Prominent papillary infoldings
   E. Squamous metaplasia

2. Besides age, which of the following is a well-recognized factor that influences the incidence of prostatic carcinoma?
   A. Exposure to environmental toxins
   B. Fat consumption
   C. Nodular hyperplasia
   D. Race
   E. Vitamin A intake

3. In regard to prostate cancer screening, which of the following is true?
   A. Complex form of prostate-specific antigen (PSA) is released predominantly by hyperplastic prostate
   B. False-negative rate of core biopsies is approximately 25%
   C. Free form of PSA is released predominantly by prostate cancer
   D. Transrectal ultrasonography (TRUS) has a 95% sensitivity
   E. Tumor seeding after perineal needle biopsy is a common event

4. A prostatic carcinoma is detected by a biopsy. Both its dominant grade and secondary grade appear as illustrated in this picture. Which of the following is the corresponding Gleason score?
   A. 0
   B. 3
   C. 6
   D. 9
   E. 12

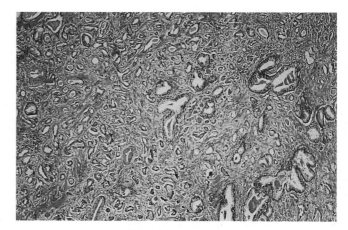

QUESTION 45.4

5. A prostatic needle biopsy from a patient with an elevated serum PSA is submitted for histopathological evaluation. Most of the tissue in the biopsy consists of normal glands and stroma, but there is a small focus of crowded small glands suspicious for malignancy. In this context, which of the following parameters is most helpful in making a diagnosis of cancer?
   A. Amphophilic cytoplasm
   B. Blue-tinged mucinous secretions
   C. Intraluminal crystalloids
   D. Mitoses
   E. Nuclear hyperchromasia/enlargement
   F. Prominent nucleoli
   G. Sharp luminal borders
   H. All of the above

6. In transurethral prostate resection (TUR) specimens, which of the following parameters is most helpful in the differential diagnosis between prostatic adenosis and low-grade adenocarcinoma?
   A. Architectural features
   B. Back-to-back glands

C. Intraluminal crystalloids
D. Medium-sized nucleoli
E. Minimal infiltrative behavior

7. Besides perineural infiltration and glomerulations, which of the following features is by itself diagnostic of prostatic cancer?

A. Back-to-back glands
B. Intraluminal crystalloids
C. Mucinous fibroplasia
D. Prominent nucleoli
E. Small crowded glands

8. This photomicrograph shows the most significant finding

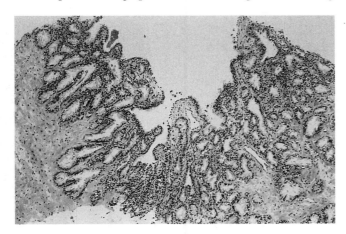

QUESTION 45.8

in a prostatic needle biopsy of a 60-year-old man with a slightly elevated serum PSA. Which of the following is the most likely diagnosis?

A. Atrophic glands
B. Colonic mucosa
C. Cowper glands
D. Seminal vesicles
E. Verumontanum hyperplasia

9. Which of the following features will differentiate low-grade from high-grade prostatic intraepithelial neoplasia (PIN)?

A. Absence of immunolabelling for basal cell–specific markers
B. Architectural features
C. Macronucleoli
D. Mitotic figures
E. Nuclear enlargement

10. A patient undergoes radical prostatectomy because of a palpable (stage II) carcinoma. Which of the following is correct regarding the pathological staging of this cancer?

A. Capsular invasion is seldom detected
B. Extracapsular extension usually occurs anteriorly
C. Microscopic extraprostatic extension is found in 50% of cases
D. Perineural infiltration has prognostic significance
E. Tumor is usually difficult to detect on gross examination

NONNEOPLASTIC DISEASES OF THE TESTIS

1. Persons undergoing vasectomy are particularly prone to developing which of the following conditions?
   A. Fibrosarcoma
   B. Lipoma
   C. Proliferative funiculitis
   D. Testicular infarction
   E. Vasitis nodosum

2. A 55-year-old man presents with unilateral painless enlargement of the testis. A biopsy discloses granulomatous inflammation within the stroma without evidence of neoplasm. Numerous neutrophils and plasma cells are also present. Special stains for fungi or acid-fast bacilli are negative. Michaelis-Gutmann bodies are not seen. Which of the following is the prevalent etiologic/pathogenetic factor in this condition?
   A. Autoimmune
   B. Infectious
   C. Sarcoidosis
   D. Treponema
   E. None of the above

TESTICULAR AND PARATESTICULAR TUMORS

1. The lesion shown in this photomicrograph is considered a precursor of all germ cell tumors, *except:*

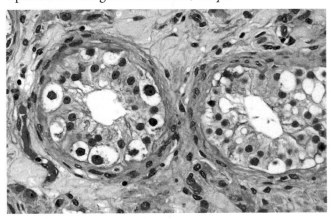

QUESTION 47.1

A. Choriocarcinoma
B. Classic seminoma
C. Embryonal carcinoma
D. Spermatocytic seminoma
E. Teratoma

2. A testicular biopsy in a 40-year-old patient shows a neoplasm consisting of cells with conspicuous nucleoli and clear cytoplasm arranged in a nesting pattern. Fibrous septae between neoplastic nests contain numerous lymphocytes. Mitotic figures are rare. Tumor cells are immunoreactive for placental alkaline phosphatase (PLAP). Which of the following is the most likely diagnosis?

A. Anaplastic seminoma
B. Embryonal cell carcinoma
C. Lymphoma
D. Seminoma
E. Spermatocytic seminoma

3. A 70-year-old man undergoes orchiectomy for a testicular tumor. Histologically, the tumor reveals a 3-cell population, including small round cells, intermediate cells, and multinucleated giant cells. Nucleoli are evident in the intermediate and giant cells. Mitotic activity is present. Which of the following features is typical of this tumor?

A. Associated with cryptorchidism
B. PLAP immunoreactivity is usually detected
C. May occur in extratesticular sites
D. Metastatic spread is rare
E. Orchiectomy and radiation is the recommended treatment

4. A testicular tumor from a 30-year-old man consists of highly anaplastic epithelial cells with poorly defined borders in a glandular arrangement. Multifocal coagulative necrosis is noted. Neoplastic cells express keratin, specifically CK8 and 18. Which of the following is true about this tumor?

A. In its pure form accounts for 30% of testicular neoplasms
B. Mitotic activity is low or absent
C. Most commonly associated with yolk sac or trophoblastic components
D. Most frequent in children under 3 years
E. Uniformly positive for placental alkaline phosphatase (PLAP)

5. The most common testicular neoplasm in children less than 3 years of age is characterized by a spongy texture on the cut surface. Microscopically, its most typical pattern is characterized by fibrovascular cores "festooned" by tumor cells, as shown in this picture. Which of the following is it?

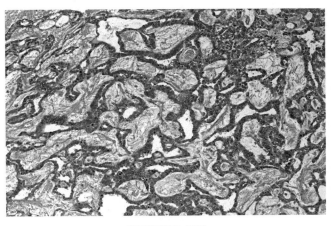

QUESTION 47.5

A. Choriocarcinoma
B. Embryonal carcinoma
C. Seminoma
D. Teratoma
E. Yolk sac tumor

6. A testicular teratoma:
   A. Behaves as a malignant tumor in children and as a benign tumor in adults
   B. Consists of a cyst filled with keratin and hair
   C. In adults, is usually associated with other germ cell tumors
   D. In prepubertal age, is usually immature
   E. Occurs more frequently in pure form in adult patients

7. An 18-year-old male is evaluated for the acute onset of right hemiplegia. A CT scan shows a well-demarcated hemorrhagic mass in the left frontal lobe. Further investigations lead to the discovery of a testicular tumor. Which of the following is the most likely tumor in this context?
   A. Choriocarcinoma
   B. Embryonal carcinoma
   C. Seminoma
   D. Teratoma
   E. Yolk sac tumor

8. Histologic examination of a 2-cm testicular tumor from a 40-year-old man with gynecomastia shows sheets of polygonal cells with eosinophilic cytoplasm. Electron microscopy reveals intracytoplasmic elongated crystalloids. Which of the following is the most likely diagnosis?
   A. Adrenogenital syndrome
   B. Choriocarcinoma
   C. Leydig cell hyperplasia
   D. Leydig cell tumor
   E. Sertoli cell tumor

9. Which of the following histologic patterns is most characteristic of *Sertoli cell tumors*?
   A. Glandular arrangement
   B. Mixture of cytotrophoblast and syncytiotrophoblast

C. Round nests between lymphocyte-rich septa
D. Stromal fibrovascular core surrounded by double-cell layer
E. Tubules reminiscent of immature seminiferous tubules

10. Which of the following is the most common testicular neoplasm in patients over the age of 60 years?
   A. Classic seminoma
   B. Embryonal carcinoma
   C. Lymphoma
   D. Mixed germ cell tumor
   E. Spermatocytic seminoma

11. A tumor attached to the epididymis is resected. Its histological appearance is shown in this picture. Which of the following is the most likely diagnosis?

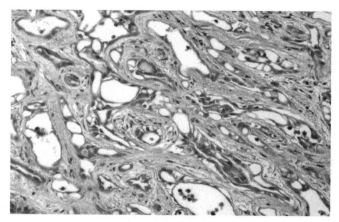

QUESTION 47.11

A. Adenomatoid tumor
B. Lipoma
C. Melanotic neuroectodermal tumor
D. Papillary cystadenoma
E. Rhabdomyosarcoma

48

THE PENIS

1. Which of the following is the cause of *Fournier gangrene?*
   A. Excessive sexual activity
   B. Implantation of foreign material
   C. Penile torsion
   D. Staphylococci and streptococci
   E. Syphilis

2. A 25-year-old male presents with an ulcerated painless perianal mass, clinically diagnosed as carcinoma. Biopsy of the lesion shows extensive lymphohistiocytic and plasmacellular infiltration. Scrapings of the lesions stained with Wright stain demonstrates large histiocytic cells containing microcysts filled with deeply stained bodies. Which of the following is the etiologic agent?

   A. *Bartonella henselae*
   B. *Calymmatobacterium donovanii*
   C. *Chlamydia trachomatis*
   D. *Haemophilus ducreyi*
   E. *Treponema pallidum*

3. Erythroplasia of Queyrat and Bowen disease refer to conditions histologically characterized by:
   A. Acanthosis with spotty proliferation of atypical cells
   B. Carcinoma *in situ*
   C. Prominent koilocytotic atypia
   D. Squamous hyperplasia with papillomatosis
   E. Superficial spreading squamous cell carcinoma

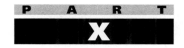
FEMALE REPRODUCTIVE SYSTEM AND PERITONEUM

GESTATIONAL TROPHOBLASTIC DISEASE

1. Upon gross examination, the abortus from a 14-week gestation consists of a mass of vesicles. These are of varying sizes, from 0.1 to 3.0 cm. Microscopically, all trophoblastic villi are swollen and devoid of central vessels. The lining trophoblastic cells are variably hyperplastic. No fetal parts are identified. This condition is characterized by:

    A. Diploidy (46,XX or 46,XY)
    B. Normal volume of uterus
    C. No significant risk of choriocarcinoma
    D. Parthenogenetic origin
    E. Triploidy (69,XXX or 69,XXY)

2. *An exaggerated placental site* is found in up to 2% of first-trimester abortions. This benign lesion is characterized by an increased number of:

    A. Cytotrophoblastic cells
    B. Intermediate trophoblastic cells
    C. Smooth muscle cells
    D. Syncytiotrophoblastic cells
    E. All of the above

3. Which of the following comments is true about gestational choriocarcinoma:

    A. Develops most frequently from ectopic pregnancy
    B. Most cases follow partial mole
    C. Poorly responsive to chemotherapy
    D. Rarely metastasizes to the brain
    E. Risk is influenced by blood group

4. One year after a term pregnancy, a 40-year-old woman undergoes hysterectomy because of a neoplasm infiltrating the uterine fundus to the serosa. Its histological appearance is shown in this photomicrograph. Cells are immunoreactive for keratin, human placental lactogen (hPL), and inhibin-alpha, but negative for hCG. Which of the following is the most likely diagnosis?

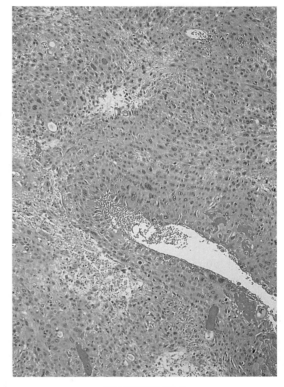

QUESTION 49.4

    A. Choriocarcinoma
    B. Epithelioid trophoblastic tumor
    C. Exaggerated placental site
    D. Placental site nodule
    E. Placental site trophoblastic tumor

50

THE PLACENTA

1. The umbilical cord of a placenta from a preterm delivery is narrow and wrinkled. A 10-cm segment adjacent to the placental disc is flattened. Which of the following conditions is most likely associated with these changes?
   A. Abruptio placentae
   B. Ectopic implantation
   C. Infection
   D. Maternal history of cocaine abuse
   E. Oligohydramnios

2. A placenta is submitted for gross and histologic evaluation in a case of clinically diagnosed abruptio placentae. Which of the following microscopic findings is most compatible with this diagnosis?
   A. Intravillous and intervillous hemorrhage
   B. Meconium-laden macrophages in amniotic membrane
   C. Neutrophil-rich infiltration of membranes
   D. Myocytes and hemorrhage in the maternal plate
   E. Thrombi in fetal blood vessels

3. A 30-year-old woman has a spontaneous abortion at 30-week gestation. On histological examination of the placenta, the maternal floor contains an extensive perivillous deposition of eosinophilic fibrinoid material with numerous intermediate X cells. A histopathological diagnosis of maternal floor infarction is made. This condition is associated with an increased risk of:
   A. Abruptio placentae
   B. Ectopic pregnancies
   C. Fetal hydrops
   D. Postmaturity
   E. Recurrent reproductive failure

4. A 35-year-old pregnant woman presented with fever, uterine tenderness, and leukocytosis. She delivered a male baby at 30-week gestation. Histological examination of the placenta and amniotic sac reveals a mild chorioamnionitis, with occasional foci of villitis. Which of the following is the most likely infectious agent in this situation?
   A. *Bacteroides fragilis*
   B. *Chlamydia trachomatis*
   C. *Escherichia coli*
   D. Fusobacterium
   E. Group B streptococci

5. The cause of villitis of unknown etiology (VUE) is most likely:
   A. Chronic hypoxia
   B. Immunological reaction
   C. Infectious agents
   D. Malformative process
   E. None of the above

6. A tan-green discoloration of a placenta and its membranes is noticed on gross examination. Histologically, numerous meconium-laden macrophages are found in the superficial plate, extraplacental amniotic membrane, and in the Wharton jelly of the umbilical cord. There is focal necrosis of umbilical arteries. These changes are compatible with an antenatal meconium exposure of at least:
   A. Few minutes
   B. 1 hour
   C. 3 hours
   D. 12 hours
   E. 24 to 48 hours

7. In this photomicrograph, chorionic villi display a change that may be produced by chronic fetal placental hypoxia. Which of the following is it?

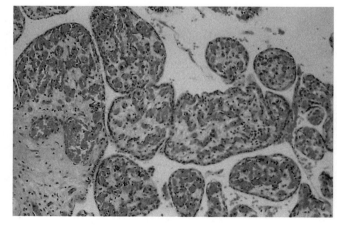

QUESTION 50.7

   A. Chorangiosis
   B. Chorioamnionitis
   C. Intravillous hemorrhage
   D. Villitis of unknown origin
   E. Villous dysmaturity

THE VULVA AND VAGINA

1. Which of the following is the most common type of vulvar cyst in the adult?
   A. Bartholin duct
   B. Epidermoid
   C. Hymenal
   D. Pilonidal
   E. Skene duct

2. The lesion known as *condyloma latum* is due to which of the following infectious agents?
   A. *Calymmatobacterium granulomatis*
   B. *Chlamydia trachomatis*
   C. *Haemophilus ducreyi*
   D. Human papillomavirus
   E. *Treponema pallidum*

3. A 28-year-old woman presents with a large polypoid vulvar mass, which is excised. At low magnification, the lesion appears as in this photomicrograph. There is no nuclear atypia nor mitotic activity. The most probable diagnosis is:

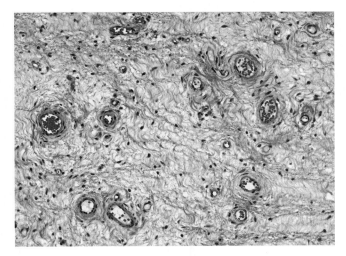

QUESTION 51.3

   A. Aggressive angiomyxoma
   B. Angiomyofibroblastoma
   C. Fibroepithelial polyp
   D. Hemangioma
   E. Leiomyoma with myxoid features

4. Which of the following vulvar lesions is a high-risk cancer precursor and is associated with HPV?
   A. Bowenoid papulosis
   B. Kraurosis
   C. Lichen planus
   D. Lichen sclerosus et atrophicus
   E. Squamous cell hyperplasia

5. A biopsy of a vulvar lesion shows a keratinizing neoplasm such as that in the picture. Which of the following is true about this neoplasm?

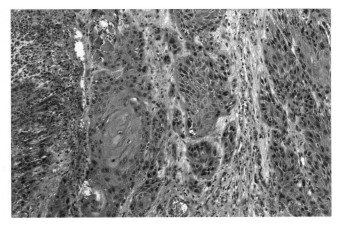

QUESTION 51.5

   A. Characterized by a papillary surface
   B. Frequently found in association with squamous hyperplasia
   C. Most commonly occurs in young women
   D. Often associated with bowenoid-type VIN
   E. Usually associated with HPV type 16 or 33

6. Which of the following features distinguishes Paget disease of the vulva from Paget disease of the breast?
   A. Association with an underlying carcinoma
   B. Immunoreactivity for apocrine marker (GCDFP-15)
   C. Immunoreactivity for epithelial markers
   D. Immunoreactivity for HMB-45
   E. Presence of pruritic crusted erythema

7. Hidradenoma papilliferum was diagnosed histologically in an ulcerated vulvar nodule. Which of the following breast lesions is morphologically similar to this tumor?
   A. Adenomyoepithelioma
   B. Fibroadenoma
   C. Intraductal papilloma
   D. Myoepithelioma
   E. Paget disease

8. A true statement concerning vaginal adenosis is:
   A. Inapparent on gross inspection
   B. May be associated with microglandular hyperplasia
   C. Progresses to adenocarcinoma in a high proportion of cases
   D. Related to bacterial vaginosis
   E. Usually manifests in prepubertal age

9. A vaginal polypoid mass is excised from a 43-year-old woman. Histologically, it is composed of large strap cells with cross-striations in a fascicular arrangement. No cambium layer is present underneath the epithelial layer. Which of the following is the most likely diagnosis?
   A. Aggressive angiomyxoma
   B. Mixed tumor of vagina
   C. Rhabdomyoma
   D. Rhabdomyosarcoma
   E. Stromal polyp

10. The most common malignant tumor of the vagina is strongly associated with HPV infection, and its most important risk factor is previous cervical carcinoma. Which of the following is it?

   A. Clear cell adenocarcinoma
   B. Embryonal rhabdomyosarcoma
   C. Endometrioid adenocarcinoma
   D. Mesonephric (wolffian) adenocarcinoma
   E. Squamous cell carcinoma

11. This photomicrograph shows the histological features of a vaginal tumor that occurs in children and adolescents. Which of the following is a risk factor for development of this tumor?

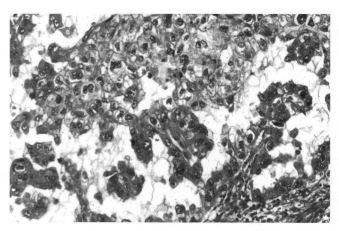

QUESTION 51.11

   A. Bacterial vaginosis
   B. HPV infection
   C. Postnatal exposure to estrogens
   D. Prenatal exposure to diethylstilbestrol (DES)
   E. Vaginal endometriosis

52

THE CERVIX

1. Which of the following histopathologic changes are associated with *Chlamydia trachomatis* cervicitis?
   A. Follicular cervicitis
   B. Granulomatous inflammation
   C. Multinucleated cells with intranuclear inclusions
   D. Neutrophilic infiltration
   E. Ulcers

2. Which of the following comments is correct about invasive squamous cell carcinomas of the cervix?
   A. Associated with good prognosis if of the basaloid type
   B. Consistently euploid or polyploid
   C. Express keratin, but not CEA or progesterone receptors
   D. Most often associated with HPV types 6 and 11
   E. Most often associated with HPV types 16 and 18

3. A cervical biopsy discloses the changes shown in this picture. There are no atypical mitotic figures. These changes should be reported as:

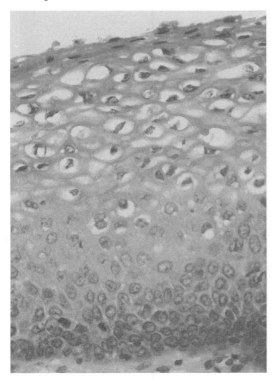

QUESTION 52.3

A. Condyloma, no evidence of SIL
B. High-grade SIL
C. Low-grade SIL
D. Reactive epithelial changes, nonspecific
E. Vaginal papillomatosis

4. A cervical biopsy reveals the changes shown in this picture. Which of the following is the diagnosis?

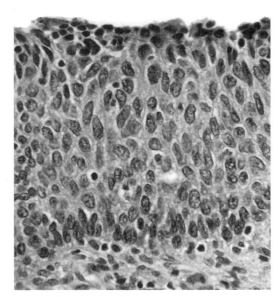

QUESTION 52.4

A. Adenoid basal carcinoma
B. Curettage-related changes
C. High-grade SIL
D. Low-grade SIL
E. Marked atrophy
F. Reactive epithelial changes

5. A cervical biopsy from a small polypoid lesion discloses collections of histiocytic cells in the stroma. The patient did not have previous surgery or biopsy procedures. This finding should be interpreted as:
   A. Decidual reaction
   B. Necrobiotic granuloma
   C. Normal finding
   D. Placental implantation site
   E. Squamous cell carcinoma

6. Which of the following is probably the condition most frequently mistaken for microinvasive squamous cell carcinoma?
  A. Decidual reaction
  B. Granulomas
  C. High-grade squamous intraepithelial lesion
  D. Placental implantation site
  E. Sheets of epithelioid histiocytes

7. Which of the following nonneoplastic lesions of the uterine cervix is strongly associated with oral contraceptive use?
  A. Arias-Stella reaction
  B. Endocervical polyp
  C. Microglandular hyperplasia
  D. Nabothian cysts
  E. Tunnel clusters

8. This photomicrograph shows a lesion detected in a cervical biopsy from a 40-year-old woman. Which of the following is true about this lesion?
  A. Arises from reserve cells at the squamocolumnar junction
  B. Associated with HPV in the majority of cases
  C. Often associated with squamous intraepithelial lesion
  D. Usually seen next to invasive adenocarcinoma
  E. All of the above

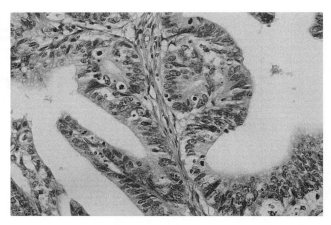

QUESTION 52.8

9. Of the following morphologic variants of cervical adenocarcinoma, one is characterized by extremely well differentiated architectural and cytological features and may be difficult to differentiate from normal glands. Which one is it?
  A. Adenoma malignum
  B. Adenosquamous carcinoma
  C. Clear cell carcinoma
  D. Glassy cell carcinoma
  E. Villoglandular papillary adenocarcinoma

53

THE UTERINE CORPUS

1. Compared to dilation and curettage (D and C), an endometrial biopsy (EMB) is:
   A. As effective in detecting malignancy
   B. Better suited to removing endometrial polyps
   C. Less accepted by patients
   D. More expensive
   E. More likely to cause postoperative adhesions

2. An endometrial biopsy reveals endometrial glands lined by cells with pleomorphic large nuclei and abundant clear cytoplasm, as shown in the picture. Mitotic figures are not seen. This histologic appearance may be found in all of the following conditions, *except:*

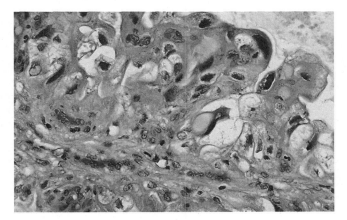

QUESTION 53.2

   A. Ectopic pregnancy
   B. Exogenous hormonal administration
   C. Gestational trophoblastic disease
   D. Postmenopause
   E. Uterine pregnancy

3. An endometrial biopsy from a patient with an intrauterine device (IUD) is evaluated for assessment of possible chronic endometritis. This diagnosis would be confirmed by finding:
   A. Granulomas
   B. Lymphocytic infiltration
   C. Neutrophilic infiltration
   D. Plasmacellular infiltration
   E. Viral inclusions

4. In which of the following forms of dysfunctional uterine bleeding (DUB) is endometrial hyperplasia most likely to develop?
   A. Anovulatory cycle
   B. Inadequate proliferative phase
   C. Inadequate secretory phase
   D. Irregular shedding
   E. Membranous dysmenorrhea

5. A 48-year-old woman undergoes an endometrial biopsy for the evaluation of abnormal uterine bleeding. The main histologic findings are illustrated on low power in this photomicrograph. There are mitoses in the glandular epithelium, but no cytologic atypia. Foci of ciliated cell metaplasia are seen. Which of the following is the most likely diagnosis?

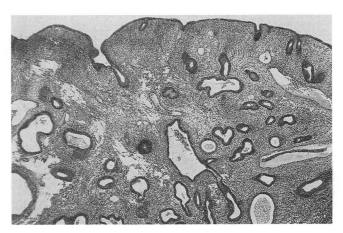

QUESTION 53.5

   A. Complex hyperplasia without atypia
   B. Disordered proliferative endometrium
   C. Endometrial atrophy with ciliated cell metaplasia
   D. Inactive (weakly proliferative) endometrium
   E. Simple hyperplasia without atypia

6. Which of the following statements applies to endometrial hyperplasia?
   A. Associated with inadequate corpus luteum function
   B. Cystically dilated glands are more frequent in severe hyperplasia

C. Cytologic atypia is the best predictor for subsequent cancer

D. Mild hyperplasia progresses to carcinoma in 30% of cases

E. Squamous metaplasia increases the risk of malignant degeneration

7. The majority of endometrial polyps have which of the following features?

A. Contain dilated thick-walled blood vessels

B. Decidual changes are frequent

C. Do not contain hyperplastic glands

D. Often show foci of adenocarcinoma

E. Stroma is composed of mitotically active cells

8. The International Federation of Gynecology and Obstetrics (FIGO) grading system of endometrioid adenocarcinoma is based mostly on which of the following parameters?

A. Architectural features

B. Hormone receptor status

C. Mitotic rate

D. Nuclear atypia

E. Nuclear atypia and architectural features

9. So-called *morules* are typically found in which of the following forms of endometrial metaplasia?

A. Clear cell metaplasia

B. Eosinophilic metaplasia

C. Papillary metaplasia

D. Squamous metaplasia

E. Tubal (ciliated) metaplasia

10. This high-power picture shows a type of endometrial carcinoma that does not develop in association with hyperestrinism and is characterized by extremely aggressive behavior. Which of the following is it?

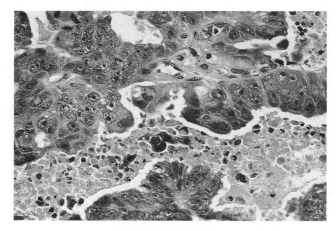

QUESTION 53.10

A. Adenosquamous

B. Clear cell

C. Mucinous

D. Papillary serous

E. Small cell

11. Which of the following is a uterine tumor histologically similar to fibroadenoma of the breast and composed of glandular and stromal elements?

A. Adenofibroma

B. Benign leiomyoblastoma

C. Endolymphatic stromal myosis

D. Mixed müllerian tumor

E. Symplasmic leiomyoma

12. A hysterectomy specimen from a 70-year-old woman reveals a large polypoid mass consisting of an epithelial glandular component admixed with a sarcoma-like component. The latter includes cellular anaplastic elements resembling the normal endometrial stroma as well as neoplastic cells with cross-striations and myoglobin immunoreactivity. Which of the following is true about this cancer?

A. Better prognosis than endometrial adenocarcinoma

B. Carcinomatous component has the highest metastatic potential

C. Neoplastic components often include skin and thyroid

D. Histologically reminiscent of phylloides tumors

E. Usually occurs in women of reproductive age

13. The main morphologic feature differentiating low-grade from high-grade stromal sarcomas of the endometrium is:

A. Immunohistochemical profile

B. Lymphatic/vascular invasion

C. Mitotic count

D. Type of margin (pushing vs. infiltrative)

E. Vascularity

14. Which of the following applies to uterine leiomyosarcomas?

A. Arise from malignant transformation of leiomyomas

B. Consist usually of clear cells with sharp outlines

C. Differentiation from leiomyomas is based mostly on mitotic count

D. Invade locally but rarely metastasize to distant organs

E. Occur exclusively in women of postmenopausal age

54

OVARIAN SURFACE EPITHELIAL-STROMAL TUMORS

1. All of the following statements about ovarian tumors are correct, *except:*
    A. Approximately one-eighth of tumors in patients younger than 45 are malignant
    B. Approximately one-third of tumors in patients older than 50 are malignant
    C. Borderline surface epithelial tumors are extremely rare in young women
    D. Mature cystic teratoma is the most common ovarian tumor
    E. Primitive germ cell tumors are extremely rare in women older than 50

2. Ovarian serous tumors are composed of an epithelium that microscopically and ultrastructurally resembles:
    A. Endocervical epithelium
    B. Endometrial epithelium
    C. Intestinal epithelium
    D. Transitional epithelium
    E. Tubal epithelium

3. Ovarian mucinous tumors are composed of an epithelium that microscopically and ultrastructurally resembles:
    A. Endocervical epithelium
    B. Endometrial epithelium
    C. Intestinal epithelium
    D. Transitional epithelium
    E. Tubal epithelium

4. A large cystic sac containing thick mucinous fluid is present in the left ovary of a 40-year-old woman. Microscopically, the wall consists of nonciliated columnar cells arranged mostly in a single layer and papillary projections. There is a focus of increased cytologic atypia and stratification, as shown in this picture. Stromal invasion is absent. These features are most consistent with:

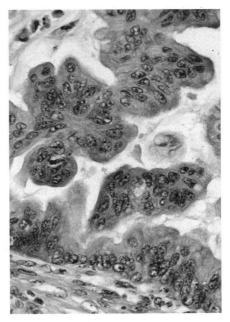

QUESTION 54.4

    A. Borderline mucinous tumor
    B. Mucinous cystadenocarcinoma
    C. Mucinous cystadenoma
    D. Serous cystadenocarcinoma
    E. Serous cystadenoma

5. This photomicrograph shows an ovarian lesion. Which of the following is the most likely diagnosis?
    A. Adenofibroma
    B. Endometrioid carcinoma
    C. Endometriosis
    D. Granulosa cell tumor
    E. Sertoli cell tumor

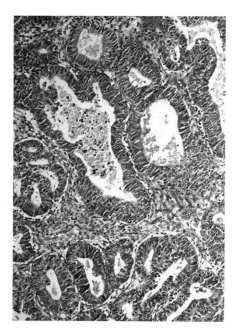

QUESTION 54.5

6. Which of the following ovarian tumors is most frequently associated with ovarian/pelvic endometriosis?
    A. Clear cell carcinoma
    B. Endometrioid carcinoma
    C. Endometrioid stromal sarcoma
    D. Malignant mesodermal mixed tumors
    E. Mucinous tumors
    F. Serous tumors
    G. Squamous cell carcinoma

7. A solid ovarian tumor histologically shows nests of transitional-like epithelium separated by fibroblastic stroma. Scattered small microcystic spaces are present. The cells have clearly outlined borders and frequent nuclear grooving. The patient is a 40-year-old woman with signs of hyperestrinism. Which of the following is the tissue of origin of this neoplasm?
    A. Germ cells
    B. Stromal cells
    C. Surface epithelium
    D. Urothelium
    E. Walthard nests

SEX CORD–STROMAL, STEROID CELL, AND GERM CELL TUMORS OF THE OVARY

1. This photograph shows a high-power view of an ovarian tumor from a 30-year-old woman who presented with abnormal uterine bleeding and abdominal pain. Neoplastic cells were immunoreactive for inhibin. Which of the following is the most likely diagnosis?

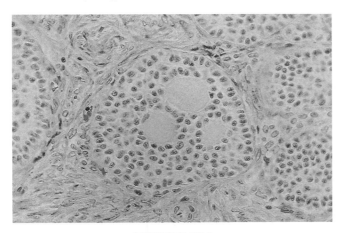

QUESTION 55.1

A. Adult-type granulosa cell tumor
B. Embryonal carcinoma
C. Juvenile-type granulosa cell tumor
D. Sertoli-Leydig cell tumor
E. Thecoma

2. A syndrome characterized by an ovarian tumor, ascites, and right pleural effusion is typically associated with:

A. Fibroma
B. Granulosa cell tumor
C. Leydig cell tumor
D. Sclerosing stromal tumor
E. Thecoma

3. This photomicrograph demonstrates the most significant histopathological findings in a 4-cm tumor located in the ovarian hilus and associated with clinical signs of virilization. Which of the following is the most likely diagnosis?

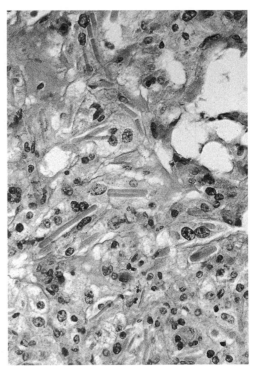

QUESTION 55.3

A. Leydig cell tumor
B. Luteinized thecoma
C. Sertoli cell tumor
D. Steroid cell tumor, NOS
E. Stromal luteoma

4. An ovarian dysgerminoma contains scattered isolated foci of glandlike structures immunoreactive for alpha-fetoprotein (AFP) and keratin. This immunohistochemical pattern is evidence of differentiation toward:

A. Early carcinomatous differentiation
B. Embryonal carcinoma
C. Choriocarcinoma

D. Yolk sac tumor

E. None of the above

5. An ovarian neoplasm composed of interlacing cords of cuboidal cells, pseudopapillary formations around a central vessel (Schiller-Duval bodies), and intra- and extracellular PAS-positive droplets will exhibit immunoreactivity for:

A. Alpha-fetoprotein (AFP)

B. Human chorionic gonadotropin (hCG)

C. Human placental lactogen (HPL)

D. Placental alkaline phosphatase (PLAP)

E. Synaptophysin

6. Histologic examination of multifocal peritoneal nodules in a 12-year-old girl shows neoplastic glial tissue immunoreactive with antibodies to glial fibrillary acidic protein (GFAP). Which of the following accounts for this condition?

A. Carcinoid tumor of the ovary

B. Development from autocthonous neural tissue

C. Ectopic neural tissue

D. Immature teratoma of the ovary

E. Metastasis of glioblastoma multiforme

7. An ovarian tumor that occurs predominantly in sexually abnormal patients (e.g., gonadal dysgenesis) is:

A. Gonadoblastoma

B. Lipid cell tumor

C. Sertoli-Leydig cell tumor

D. Sex cord tumor with annular tubules

E. Teratoma

MISCELLANEOUS PRIMARY TUMORS, SECONDARY TUMORS, AND NONNEOPLASTIC LESIONS OF THE OVARY

1. Small cell carcinomas of the ovary have histopathologic features that may resemble which of the following ovarian neoplasms?
   A. Brenner tumor
   B. Dysgerminoma
   C. Embryonal carcinoma
   D. Gonadoblastoma
   E. Granulosa cell tumor

2. Which of the following macroscopic or microscopic features favors a primary ovarian neoplasm over metastasis?
   A. Expansile growth pattern
   B. Microscopic surface mucin
   C. Multinodular invasive growth
   D. Prominent vascular invasion
   E. Single cell invasion

3. The ovaries of a 50-year-old patient show a multinodular appearance. Histologically, the lesions are composed of scattered single cells within a spindle cell stroma, as shown in this picture. Which of the following is the most likely origin of this tumor?
   A. Appendix
   B. Colon
   C. Ovary itself
   D. Stomach
   E. Uterus

4. The majority of ovarian infections in the United States are secondary to:
   A. Acute appendicitis
   B. Malakoplakia
   C. Pelvic inflammatory disease (PID)
   D. Pelvic tuberculosis
   E. Use of an intrauterine device (IUD)

5. Which of the following is the pathologic substrate of an ovarian condition known as *hyperreactio luteinalis*?
   A. Bilateral luteinized follicle cysts
   B. Decidual reaction of ovarian stroma

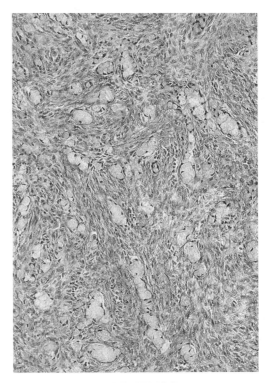

QUESTION 56.3

   C. Massive ovarian edema
   D. Stromal hyperplasia and hyperthekosis
   E. Unilateral luteoma

6. Which of the following features is typically absent in ovaries associated with *polycystic ovarian disease* (Stein-Leventhal syndrome)?
   A. Corpora lutea
   B. Cystic follicles
   C. Follicle cysts
   D. Luteinization of theca interna
   E. Stromal hyperplasia/hyperthekosis

THE FALLOPIAN TUBE AND
BROAD LIGAMENT

1. A postmortem examination of a woman with a history of sterility reveals bilateral nodular enlargement of the isthmic segment of the fallopian tubes. Microscopically, the enlargements consist of glandlike spaces of varying size and shape surrounded by a rim of thick smooth muscle. The most likely pathogenesis of this condition is:

A. Analogous to adenomyosis
B. Analogous to endometriosis
C. Infectious
D. Metaplastic
E. Related to previous sterilization procedure

2. The usual microscopic appearance of tubal adenocarcinoma is extremely similar to that of:

A. Endometrioid adenocarcinoma
B. Mesothelioma
C. Mucinous adenocarcinoma
D. Ovarian papillary serous carcinoma
E. Transitional cell carcinoma

3. A tumor localized in the broad ligament appears as a well-circumscribed, solid, bosselated mass with yellow-white cut surfaces. Its histological appearance is shown in this picture. Cells are immunoreactive for keratin, but not for EMA, S100 protein, CEA, or B72.3. Which of the following is the most likely diagnosis?

A. Adenomatoid tumor
B. Endometrioid adenocarcinoma
C. Ependymoma

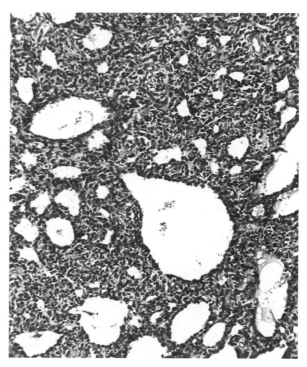

QUESTION 57.3

D. Female adnexal tumor of probable wolffian origin
E. Sertoli cell tumor

THE PERITONEUM

1. Scattered white miliary-like nodules are found in the visceral peritoneum during an exploratory laparotomy in a patient who underwent a previous abdominal surgery. On microscopic examination, the nodules consist of granulomas with PAS-positive birefringent granules within histiocytes and giant cells. These granules display a Maltese-cross pattern under polarized light. This material is most likely:

    A. Barium
    B. Cellulose
    C. Paraffin
    D. Starch
    E. Talc

2. During an exploratory laparotomy on a 40-year-old woman, multiple gray-white nodules are incidentally discovered within the pelvic peritoneum. The histological appearance of these nodules is shown in this picture. Which of the following is the most likely diagnosis?

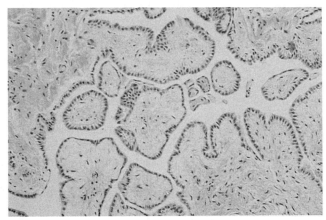

QUESTION 58.2

    A. Adenomatoid tumor
    B. Gliomatosis peritonei
    C. Localized fibrous tumor
    D. Müllerian metaplasia
    E. Well-differentiated mesothelioma

3. A 24-year-old male presents with ascites. Imaging studies reveal a multinodular tumor in the pelvic cavity, which is resected. On histologic examination, a small cell tumor organized in nests within a fibroblastic stroma is found. Neoplastic cells show diffuse cytoplasmic immunoreactivity for keratin and punctate reactivity for desmin. Further studies show the presence of t(11;22) involving the Ewing sarcoma (EWS) and Wilms tumor (WT1) genes. Which of the following is the diagnosis?

    A. Ewing sarcoma
    B. Intraabdominal desmoplastic small cell tumor
    C. Lymphoma
    D. Neuroblastoma
    E. Wilms tumor

4. Paracentesis on a patient with ascites leads to the demonstration of mucinous fluid with fragments of atypical glandular epithelium. Which of the following is the most usual source of this condition?

    A. Adenocarcinoid of the appendix
    B. Adenocarcinoma of the colon
    C. Cystadenocarcinoma of the ovary
    D. Mucinous tumor of the appendix
    E. Signet-ring carcinoma of the bowel

5. This photomicrograph demonstrates the histological appearance of a red-brown peritoneal lesion removed from a woman with cyclic abdominal pains. At the time of surgery, the patient would be most likely in which of the following hormonal status?

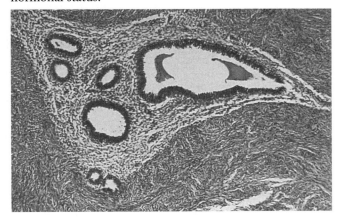

QUESTION 58.5

    A. Estrogen replacement therapy
    B. Postmenopause
    C. Pregnancy
    D. Proliferative phase of menstrual cycle
    E. Secretory phase of menstrual cycle

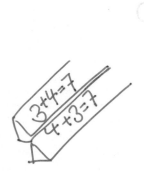

ANSWERS AND EXPLANATIONS

CHAPTER 1

1. Correct choice: C
SPONGIOTIC DERMATITIS (p. 6)—Spongiotic dermatitis describes a nonspecific histopathologic pattern whose clinical counterpart is known as *eczematous dermatitis*. This is a common response to pathogenic stimuli, either exogenous (e.g., allergic and irritant contact dermatitis) or endogenous (e.g., nummular eczema and related conditions). Intraepidermal edema (i.e., *spongiosis*) is a defining microscopic feature, but morphological changes vary according to the stage. Spongiosis predominates in the acute stage, whereas papillomatosis and acanthosis become progressively more important in subacute/chronic stages.

2. Correct choice: A
CONTACT DERMATITIS, ALLERGIC VERSUS IRRITANT (p. 7)—Contact dermatitis manifests with a similar picture of eczematous/spongiotic dermatitis, regardless of its etiopathogenesis. The *allergic* form results from prior sensitization to specific allergens and is accompanied by prominent tissue eosinophilia. The *nonallergic* form is a nonimmune mediated response to irritants such as soaps and detergents. Spongiosis is common to allergic and nonallergic contact dermatitis, as well as the *endogenous* forms of dermatitis.

3. Correct choice: D
NUMMULAR ECZEMA AND RELATED FORMS (p. 7)—Nummular eczema manifests with itchy coin-shaped lesions covered by a scaly crust. It affects adults without apparent predisposing conditions. In contrast to fungal infections, nummular eczema does not show central clearing nor hyphae or spores on KOH-treated scrapings. This category of eczematous disorders is known as the *endogenous eczema group*. Besides nummular eczema, it includes atopic dermatitis, dyshidrosis, and seborrheic dermatitis, all conditions apparently unrelated to any known exogenous agent.

4. Correct choice: B
SUBACUTE SPONGIOTIC DERMATITIS AND T-CELL LYMPHOMA (p. 7)—Distinguishing between subacute spongiotic dermatitis and the patch stage of T-cell lymphoma is a common problem. Lymphoma is associated with *epidermotropism*, that is, atypical lymphocytes within the epidermis. Spongiotic dermatitis is characterized by *exocytosis*, that is, intraepidermal lymphocytes without nuclear atypia. Acanthosis and papillomatosis are typical of subacute/chronic stages of spongiotic dermatitis, whereas spongiosis (intraepidermal edema) is most characteristic of acute spongiotic dermatitis. When nuclear atypia of intraepidermal lymphocytes is hard to assess, the presence of spongiosis should favor a diagnosis of spongiotic dermatitis over lymphoma.

5. Correct choice: D
PITYRIASIS ROSEA AND SECONDARY SYPHILIS (pp. 7 and 14)—Secondary syphilis of the skin can be roughly classified as macular or papular. Macular lesions are nonspecific, but the papular lesions of later stages show distinctive features, for example, swelling/hyperplasia of endothelial cells in dermal vessels and a plasma cell-rich perivascular infiltrate. Bandlike lymphocytic infiltration resembling lichen planus, acanthosis, and parakeratosis mimicking psoriasis, and noncaseating granulomas may be seen, but they are not specific of syphilis. *Moth-eaten alopecia* is also characteristic of secondary syphilis. The histopathology of pityriasis rosea is that of a spongiotic dermatitis (*endogenous form*), with focal papillary hemorrhages.

6. Correct choice: A
DERMATOPHYTOSIS (p. 8)—Fungal infection of the skin may manifest with spongiotic dermatitis. If fungal organisms (hyphae or spores) are not readily apparent on hematoxylin and eosin (H&E) stain, an infectious etiology should be suspected when neutrophils are seen in the epidermis, especially in the stratum corneum. Periodic acid-Schiff (PAS) staining may then be used to identify the organism. Short and thick hyphae are associated with *Pityrosporum* infection, and pseudohyphae and budding yeasts with *Candida*. *Dermatophytes* are characterized by slender, septate or nonseptate hyphae.

7. Correct choice: D
PSORIASIS (p. 9)—In its classic presentation, psoriasis is rarely biopsied. However, variants of this condition may create some diagnostic uncertainty and undergo biopsy examination. Pustular psoriasis is characterized by sterile pustules that develop by confluence of *Munro microabscesses*, focal collections of neutrophils within the parakeratotic scale. Salient features of psoriasis include confluent parakeratosis, regular acanthosis with suprapapillary thinning, and the absence of a granular layer. Perivascular lymphocytic infiltration and focal hemorrhages are present in the upper dermis.

8. Correct choice: C
INTERFACE DERMATITIS, LICHENOID PATTERN (p. 9)—Inflammatory conditions of the skin manifesting with a bandlike lymphocytic infiltrate along the dermal–epidermal junction are referred to as *interface dermatitis*. This pattern of inflammatory response is common to numerous skin disorders of heterogeneous pathogenesis. Interface dermatitis can be further classified into *lichenoid* and *vacuolar* patterns (see table that follows). The lichenoid pattern is characterized by disruption of the basement membrane and necrosis of keratinocytes in the basal layer (with resultant formation of colloid bodies), without appreciable vacuolar changes. Lichen planus is the prototypical example of this inflammatory pattern. Choice D names interface dermatitis conditions in which a vacuolar pattern is prevalent.

matitis herpetiformis, choice C with pemphigus vulgaris, choice D with bullous pemphigoid, and choice E with porphyria.

11. Correct choice: E
GRAFT VERSUS HOST DISEASE (p. 13)—Early stages of GVHD (weeks following transplantation) are characterized by the microscopic picture mentioned in this case. Later stages (months/years) are associated with diffuse dermal fibrosis without significant inflammation, mimicking *scleroderma*. In the initial stage, the degree of chronic inflammation correlates with prognosis. The most significant changes of actinic keratosis include interfollicular parakeratosis, disorderly maturation of keratinocytes, chronic inflammation, and basophilic degeneration of the upper dermis. Late radiation dermatitis shows bizarre, stellate-shaped fibroblasts in the dermis with modest inflammatory changes.

LICHENOID AND VACUOLAR INTERFACE DERMATITIS: TWO MAJOR INFLAMMATORY PATTERNS INVOLVING THE DERMAL–EPIDERMAL JUNCTION

	Lichenoid	Vacuolar
Morphologic changes	Dense lymphocytic infiltrate along dermal–epidermal junction	Inflammatory infiltrate along dermal–epidermal junction present or absent
	Necrosis of basal keratinocytes	Intracytoplasmic vacuoles within basal keratinocytes
	Colloid bodies	Disruption of basement membrane
	Disruption of basement membrane	Pigment incontinence
	Pigment incontinence	
Major conditions	Lichen planus	Lupus erythematosus
	Lichen nitidus	Dermatomyositis
	Lichenoid drug eruption	PLEVA and lymphomatoid papulosis
		Acute graft versus host disease

9. Correct choice: E
LICHEN PLANUS (p. 10)—Lichen planus is an inflammatory, usually self-limiting dermatosis characterized by "pruritic, purple, polygonal papules" symmetrically distributed on the flexor surfaces of elbows and wrists. Oral lesions are often present and consist of white reticulated mucosal changes. Histologically, it is characterized by a bandlike lymphocytic infiltrate obscuring the dermal–epidermal junction, hyperkeratosis, hypergranulosis, irregular acanthosis and Civatte bodies. The latter (also called *colloid bodies*) are apoptotic bodies usually seen close to the basement membrane. The morphological changes associated with lichen planus can be considered within the context of *lichenoid interface dermatitis*. Choice A is associated with psoriasis, choice B with lupus erythematosus, choice C with erythema nodosum, and choice D with lichen simplex chronicus.

10. Correct choice: B
LUPUS ERYTHEMATOSUS (p. 11)—Deposition of IgG, IgM, and C3 in a granular pattern along the dermal–epidermal junction is highly characteristic of lupus skin lesions, both systemic (SLE) and discoid (DLE). Morphologically, this pattern of inflammation is known as *vacuolar interface dermatitis* (as opposed to *lichenoid*), because the inflammatory activity at the dermal–epidermal junction is associated with vacuolar degeneration of the basal epidermis. This category includes pityriasis lichenoides et varioliformis acuta (PLEVA) and lymphomatoid papulosis. Dermatomyositis is histologically similar to SLE/DLE. Choice A is associated with der-

12. Correct choice: A
ERYTHEMA MULTIFORME (p. 15)—Erythema multiforme (EM) is an acute inflammatory disease characterized by concomitant development of macules, papules, bullae, and so on. The classic *target* lesion is a papule with a central bulla surrounded by erythema. Frequently involved is the skin of palms and soles as well as mucosae. The severity of EM varies. Up to 90% of cases of the milder form (*EM minor*) are secondary to herpes simplex infection. The most severe forms (*Stevens-Johnson syndrome* and *toxic epidermal necrolysis*) are caused by drugs, for example, sulfonamides. Microscopic changes are similar to those of *fixed drug eruption*: chronic inflammation of the upper dermis, vacuolar changes resulting in focal subepidermal bullae, and scattered dyskeratotic (i.e., necrotic) keratinocytes.

13. Correct choice: C
PEMPHIGUS FOLIACEUS (p. 18)—This condition leads to subcorneal bullae, in which the plane of cleavage is just below the stratum corneum. The roof of the bulla, therefore, is extremely thin (leaflike) and tends to separate easily from the underlying epidermal layers. Inflammatory cells are rare. In other conditions, subcorneal bullae are associated with a significant inflammatory infiltrate, eosinophilic in erythema toxicum neonatorum, neutrophilic in impetigo contagiosa and staphylococcal scalded-skin syndrome. Patients with pemphigus foliaceus often seek medical care when bullae have already converted into crusts. Choices A and E are closely related conditions caused by

Staphylococcus aureus and associated with subcorneal bullae filled with neutrophils.

14. Correct choice: E
PEMPHIGUS VULGARIS (p. 20)—The mechanism of bulla development in pemphigus vulgaris is acantholysis, that is, disruption of intercellular attachment, leading to intraepidermal bullae. Autoantibodies against epidermal desmosomal proteins such as *desmoglein-3* mediate the immune mechanism leading to destruction of the intercellular junction. Pemphigus vulgaris thus results in suprabasal bullae, in which the epidermal cells remaining attached to the basement membrane come to resemble a "row of tombstones." Depending on the level of intraepidermal cleavage, pemphigus can be superficial (*foliaceus* and *erythematosus*) or deep (*vulgaris* and *vegetans*).

15. Correct choice: B
KERATOSIS FOLLICULARIS (p. 21)—Also known as *Darier disease*, this hereditary, autosomal dominant condition is characterized by a lifelong eruption of crusted vesicular lesions on the neck and trunk. The lesions consist of suprabasal acantholytic vesicles

that contain characteristic *grains* (acantholytic cells) and dermal papillae (*villi*) lined by a single layer of keratinocytes. *Corps ronds* and *grains* are large dyskeratotic cells scattered within the superficial epidermal layers. Choice A, also known as *Hailey-Hailey disease*, is similar to pemphigus vulgaris but is autosomal dominant. Choice D, also known as *Grover disease*, is similar to Darier disease but related to heat and sweating. Choice E is morphologically indistinguishable from Darier disease, but occurs as a localized lesion on sun-exposed areas.

16. Correct choice: A
BULLOUS PEMPHIGOID AND SUBEPIDERMAL BULLAE (p. 22)—The level of cleavage within the epidermis is an important screening factor in the diagnosis of bullous diseases (see the table that follows). Skin conditions associated with subepidermal bullae may be further divided into those with inflammation and those without inflammation. *Bullous pemphigoid* is the prototype of subepidermal bullae with inflammation. Large bullae develop in the trunk, flexor surfaces, and intertriginous regions. The detachment of the epidermis from the underlying basement membrane is

MAJOR BULLOUS DISEASES CLASSIFIED BY LEVEL OF CLEAVAGE

Subcorneal/ Intracorneal	Without acantholysis	Subcorneal pustular dermatosis	Large unilocular bullae filled with neutrophils develop on trunk and body folds.
		Scabies	Itchy papule and characteristic burrows. Mites identifiable on biopsy.
	With acantholysis	Pemphigus foliaceus	Most superficial type of pemphigus. No or scanty inflammatory infiltrate and a few acantholytic cells.
		Bullous impetigo	Staphylococcal infection. Honey-colored crusts resulting from neutrophil-filled bullae (pustules).
Intraepidermal	Without acantholysis	Spongiotic dermatitis	Bullae result from confluence of spongiotic vacuoles in the context of acute and subacute spongiotic dermatitis.
		Erythema toxicum neonatorum	Asymptomatic pustular condition of neonates. Eosinophils are numerous within pustules.
		Dermatophytosis	Trichophyton most common agent.
	With acantholysis	Pemphigus group: vulgaris, vegetans, erythematous	*Vulgaris*: suprabasal bullae. *Vegetans*: intraepidermal abscesses and marked acanthosis. *Erythematous*: superficial bullae. Eosinophils present within epidermis and dermis.
		Familial benign pemphigus (Hailey-Hailey disease)	Autosomal dominant. Suprabasal bullae predominate, but acantholysis present throughout epidermis.
		Keratosis follicularis (Darier disease)	Suprabasal acantholytic vesicles with *grains* (acantholytic cells) and dermal papillae (*villi*) lined by a single layer of keratinocytes.
		Transient acantholytic dermatosis (Grover disease)	Similar to Darier disease, but results from heat and sweating.
		Herpes simplex/zoster infection	Diagnostic nuclear inclusions.
Subepidermal	With inflammation	Bullous pemphigoid	Detachment of the epidermis from the underlying basement membrane associated with a mixed inflammatory infiltrate in the upper dermis.
		Dermatitis herpetiformis	Papillary dermal microabscesses. Granular deposits of IgA identifiable by immunofluorescence.
	Without inflammation	Epidermolysis bullosa	Group of heterogeneous inherited disorders. Separation of epidermis from underlying dermis with no inflammation.
		Porphyria cutanea tarda	Sunlight exposure and trauma act as triggers. Characteristic dermal papillae protruding into bulla in a "festooned" pattern.

related to autoantibodies to desmosomal proteins. Epidermolysis bullosa and porphyria cutanea tarda manifest with subepidermal bullae without inflammation.

17. Correct choice: B

DERMATITIS HERPETIFORMIS (p. 23)—The most characteristic clinical manifestations are clusters of extremely pruritic vesicles and bullae on the back, often in association with gluten enteropathy. Hypersensitivity to *gliadin*, a protein of gluten, is thought to play a crucial pathogenetic role, and clinical manifestations resolve on a gluten-free diet. Microabscesses within the tips of dermal papillae and IgA/IgG deposition by direct immunofluorescence are diagnostic features.

18. Correct choice: A

LYME DISEASE AND OTHER FORMS OF GYRATE ERYTHEMAS (p. 26)—*Gyrate erythema* may manifest in different conditions. Erythema chronicum migrans is the pathognomonic lesion of the cutaneous stage of *Lyme disease*, caused by *B. burgdorferi* transmitted from rodents to humans by the bite of a deer tick. Nonspecific histologic changes include superficial and deep perivascular lymphoplasmacytic infiltration. Erythema chronicum migrans begins 2 to 3 weeks following the tick bite at the inoculation site: a red papule enlarges centrifugally, developing central clearing and reaching a large diameter (up to 25 cm). Choice B may be associated with *erythema gyratum repens*, and choice C with rheumatic fever with *erythema marginatum*.

19. Correct choice: B

GRANULOMA FACIALE (p. 29)—Granuloma faciale is often biopsied, because clinically it may mimic sarcoidosis, infected nevus, or neoplasm. Histologically, it produces a full-thickness dermal infiltrate with neutrophils, lymphocytes, eosinophils, and plasma cells, limited by a *Grenz zone* (a clear band) from the uninvolved epidermis. The disease is self-limited. Coexistence of leukocytoclasia and nuclear dust around small vessels may generate confusion with vasculitides. Pautrier microabscesses and atypical lymphocytes (suggestive of mycosis fungoides) are absent. Marked eosinophilic infiltration is also seen in infected insect bites.

20. Correct choice: B

SKIN TUBERCULOSIS AND LEPROSY (p. 32)—Skin tuberculosis may be seen in AIDS patients, and leprosy in immigrants from Asian countries. The lepromatous form of leprosy is associated with plentiful mycobacteria within histiocytes and giant cells (the latter known as *lepra* or *Virchow cells*), whereas Hansen bacilli are absent in tuberculoid leprosy. Lupus vulgaris results from reactivation tuberculosis and is most commonly associated with nonnecrotizing granulomas, in which acid-fast bacilli (AFBs) are difficult to demonstrate by special stains. If pseudoepitheliomatous hyperplasia is a prominent feature, consider chromoblastomycosis or other fungal infections (e.g., blastomycosis), which may simulate tumoral lesions.

21. Correct choice: C

PALISADING GRANULOMAS (p. 33)—This form of granulomatous inflammation is thought to arise as a reaction to a focus of collagen degeneration and is characterized by a central region of necrosis and a peripheral rim of palisading histiocytes. The nodules of rheumatic fever also exhibit this histopathologic pattern. *Granuloma annulare* presents as painless pale red annular plaques, often grouped in a circinate fashion, most commonly on the dorsal surfaces of hands and feet. *Necrobiosis lipoidica* manifests as pink-brown, depressed plaque on the anterior legs of diabetic patients.

Rheumatoid nodules develop on the extensor surfaces of patients with rheumatoid arthritis.

22. Correct choice: D

LICHEN SCLEROSUS ET ATROPHICUS (p. 38)—This condition may affect males and females from infancy to late adulthood, but onset in perimenopausal age is most frequent. It affects the labia majora, labia minora, perianal region, and trunk. When confined to the vulva, it is designated as *kraurosis vulvae*, whereas the penile form is known as *balanitis xerotica obliterans*. Grossly, white papules coalesce to form plaques, which in time result in a smooth, ivory-colored surface. Pruritus is frequent. Salient features include the following: hyperkeratosis with follicular plugging, atrophy of the stratum malpighii, and hydropic degeneration of the basal layer; edema and collagen degeneration in the upper dermis; and chronic inflammatory infiltrate in the middermis.

23. Correct choice: A

ERYTHEMA NODOSUM (p. 41)—Clinical presentation and histopathologic features are those of erythema nodosum (EN). EN is a form of panniculitis with predominant *septal* involvement. The granuloma arranged around a central cleft is characteristic of early stages and known as *Miescher radial granuloma*. Bacterial infections (usually streptococcal), are the most frequent predisposing conditions. Sarcoidosis, fungal infections, tuberculosis, inflammatory bowel disease, leukemia, pregnancy, estrogen use, and so on, are also associated with EN.

CHAPTER 2

1. Correct choice: C

ORGANOID NEVUS (p. 49)—Verrucous hyperplasia consists of papillomatous hyperplasia of the epidermis and hyperkeratosis. This change is associated with a number of benign skin conditions, including *organoid nevus* (nevus sebaceus of Jadassohn), which manifests in childhood as a patch of alopecia. In the area of alopecia, we find abortive follicular structures, large sebaceous units in connection with the epidermis, and verrucous hyperplasia. Choice A is associated with molluscum contagiosum, choice B with clear cell acanthoma, choice D with seborrheic keratosis, and choice E with all forms of verruca.

2. Correct choice: C

SEBORRHEIC KERATOSIS (p. 50)—In its usual form, this common benign lesion occurs on the trunk of adults. However, the sudden appearance of numerous foci of seborrheic keratosis is often a sign of an underlying visceral malignancy. The *acanthotic* type is the most frequent histologic form of seborrheic keratosis: it is characterized by an increased number of basal-like keratinocytes, horny pseudocysts, and variable pigmentation. An important diagnostic feature is that the lesion lies *above* the level of adjacent normal epidermis.

3. Correct choice: A

ACTINIC KERATOSIS (p. 51)—This sunlight-related lesion appears as scaly erythematous papules with a characteristic sandpaper-like surface. Presence of cytologic atypia in the epidermis is associated with aberrant keratinization. There are several variants, the most common of which is the *hypertrophic* form, where the alternating pattern of keratinization becomes most pronounced: adnexal structures are covered by light keratin (orthokeratotic) while intervening actinic epidermis is covered by a column of dark keratin (parakeratotic). Choice B is the *atrophic* variant, choice C is the *lichenoid* type, and choice D is the *acantholytic* variant. Regarding choice E, pigmented actinic keratosis may mimic solar lentigo. Actinic keratosis presenting with a pattern similar to Bowen disease (full-thickness atypia) is referred to as *bowenoid variant.*

4. Correct choice: E
BOWEN DISEASE/CARCINOMA *IN SITU* (p. 53)—Carcinoma *in situ* of the epidermis is still a controversial concept. Morphologically, it may indicate various skin conditions, such as *Bowen disease, erythroplasia,* or *bowenoid papulosis.* (a) *Bowen disease* is *in situ* carcinoma predominantly affecting sun-unexposed skin. Grossly, it is characterized by slowly enlarging, irregular, erythematous plaques; cytological atypia involves the full thickness of the epidermis, but dermal invasion is rare. (b) *Erythroplasia* indicates lesions similar to Bowen disease but located on the glans penis, vulva, and oral mucosa and more often invasive. (c) *Bowenoid papulosis* describes pigmented papular lesions in the anogenital region resembling condiloma acuminatum and associated with human papillomavirus type 16 (HPV 16): they show full-thickness cellular atypia, but usually regress spontaneously. Finally, *actinic keratosis* exhibiting prominent cellular atypia is referred to as the *bowenoid* variant.

5. Correct choice: A
KERATOACANTHOMA (p. 56)—Keratoacanthoma usually grows rapidly (4 to 6 weeks) and undergoes rapid regression (4 to 6 weeks). Keratoacanthoma can be thought of as a well-differentiated form of squamous cell carcinoma. The architecture of keratoacanthoma is characteristic. In its full-blown appearance, keratoacanthoma is a dome-shaped mass with a central keratin-filled crater, overhanging edges, and pushing borders. Keratinization is absent in early stages, whereas lichenoid infiltrate is characteristic of late lesions. Cytologic atypia and mitotic activity are similar to well-differentiated squamous cell carcinomas. Peripheral eosinophilic infiltration is highly suggestive of keratoacanthoma, being infrequent in squamous cell carcinoma.

6. Correct choice: A
BASAL CELL CARCINOMA AND VARIANTS (p. 57)—Basal cell carcinoma (BCC) is a very common, usually indolent skin neoplasm most often developing in the head and neck. Metastatic spread is exceptional. There are several variants: the *basaloid* variant has the features described in the question stem and is probably analogous to the cloacogenic (basaloid) form of anal carcinoma. Of the rare cases of metastatic BCC reported in the literature, this variant is more frequently represented than all others. The *sclerosing* form is associated with a florid desmoplastic reaction (hence the designation "morphea-like") and results in considerable problems of surgical management.

7. Correct choice: A
SQUAMOUS CELL CARCINOMA AND VARIANTS (p. 58)—The *adenoid* variant acquires a pseudoglandular appearance from lack of cell cohesiveness (acantholysis). The *spindle cell* variant arises on sun-exposed areas, especially on the lips (it should be differentiated from melanoma and atypical fibroxanthoma). The *verrucous* variant is well differentiated, almost always located in the foot, and rarely associated with spread to regional nodes. In contrast to basal cell carcinoma, squamous cell carcinoma cells express *U. europaeus* binding sites.

8. Correct choice: D
MERKEL CELL CARCINOMA (p. 59)—This carcinoma is a small round cell tumor that occurs predominantly in the face and neck. It derives from epidermal Merkel cells, neuroendocrine cells involved in tactile sensation. Histologically, it closely mimics malignancies such as small cell carcinoma of the lung, lymphoma, and lymphoepithelioma. Neoplastic cells are immunoreactive for keratin, especially CK20, and neurofilaments: a perinuclear dotlike keratin reactivity is characteristic (but not pathognomonic) of this neoplasm. Electron microscopy (EM) demonstrates neurosecretory granules, which supports a neuroendocrine origin. In addition, neoplastic cells express neuron-specific enolase and CD44.

9. Correct choice: B
SWEAT GLAND CARCINOMAS (p. 60)—Sweat gland carcinomas represent a small percentage of all adnexal tumors and most commonly arise in adulthood. Most of them have lost the morphologic features of their original benign counterpart. A prominent ductal architecture or clear cell appearance may mimic metastatic breast carcinoma or, respectively, renal cell carcinoma. Of those cases retaining features of normal sweat gland differentiation, *malignant eccrine poroma* is the most frequent and most aggressive type. Prominent basaloid features may simulate basal cell carcinoma, whereas marked pigmentation may suggest melanoma. Chondroid syringoma has features identical to mixed tumors of the salivary glands. Eccrine spiradenoma is strikingly similar to thymoma. Metastatic potential varies according to morphologic features.

10. Correct choice: D
TRICHOEPITHELIOMA (p. 61)—Trichoepithelioma is a benign tumor originating from the hair follicle, often developing in childhood as single or multiple papules around the nose and mouth. It may be transmitted as an autosomal dominant trait. The most important differential diagnosis is with basal cell carcinoma. Lack of the artifactual clefts around the tumor islands, a papillary configuration, and the presence of small cysts containing laminated keratin are distinctive features differentiating trichoepithelioma from basal cell carcinoma.

11. Correct choice: B
CYLINDROMA (ECCRINE CYLINDROMA; p. 61)—The most impressive clinical appearance of cylindroma is that of multicentric coalescing tumors of the scalp, giving rise to a hatlike growth that has received the picturesque designation of *turban tumor.* However, its most common presentation is that of an isolated nodule of the head or neck (in a minority of cases in other sites). This tumor is thought to be of apocrine origin. Histologically, it shows a distinctive lobular configuration with conspicuous deposition of basement membranelike material within and around the lobules. The epithelial lobules seem to fit together like a jigsaw puzzle.

12. Correct choice: B
SPIRADENOMA (p. 61)—This adnexal skin tumor is frequently painful (like glomus tumor) and may occur anywhere in the body. It consists of two cell types, epithelial and myoepithelial cells, and contains a rich infiltrate of lymphocytes, especially within perivascular spaces. These features make this tumor similar to thymoma. The conspicuous vessels and the dense cellularity may generate confusion with metastatic tumors or vascular neoplasms.

13. Correct choice: A
PILOMATRICOMA (p. 61)—Also called *calcifying epithelioma of Malherbe,* this lesion occurs most commonly on the head and neck of young individuals. It is a well-circumscribed tumor consisting

of small basaloid cells, which undergo abrupt keratinization without an intermediate granular layer. Keratinized cells retain their outline, resulting in characteristic "ghost" or "shadow" cells. Foreign body giant cell reaction and calcifications are frequent. Foci of extramedullary hematopoiesis may be seen as well.

14. Correct choice: D

SYRINGOMA (p. 63)—Syringoma is a benign tumor of eccrine gland origin, whose most common clinical presentation is that of multiple tan papular lesions on the face, particularly on the lower eyelids of women. Histologically, it is composed of clusters of small ducts lined by two layers of epithelial cells. The ducts have commalike projections, giving a tadpole appearance.

15. Correct choice: A

CHONDROID SYRINGOMA (p. 63)—This tumor has light microscopic, immunohistochemical, and ultrastructural features strikingly similar to mixed tumors of salivary glands. It develops most frequently on the face and neck. *Syringoma* is composed of small ductlike structures with a two-cell lining showing characteristic comma-shaped extensions.

16. Correct choice: B

DERMATOFIBROMA (FIBROUS HISTIOCYTOMA) AND DERMATOFIBROSARCOMA PROTUBERANS (pp. 64 and 66)—Dermatofibroma develops as a single firm nodule with a red-brown or black color (depending on the amount of hemosiderin) in the extremities. Located within the dermis, it is poorly circumscribed and composed of spindly cells. A clear (Grenz) zone separates the overlying epidermis from the neoplasm. Foamy and multinucleated histiocytes, sometimes of the Touton type (peripheral nuclei), are scattered within the spindly component. Densely cellular dermatofibromas acquire a storiform appearance suggestive of DFSP. *CD34 is positive in DFSP and negative in dermatofibroma.* Factor XIIIa (a marker of dermal *dendrocytes*) is frequently positive in dermatofibroma and focally positive in DFSP as well. Actin is inconstantly positive in DFSP, and HMB-45 is negative in both tumors.

17. Correct choice: B

DERMATOFIBROSARCOMA PROTUBERANS (p. 66)—DFSP is a slowly growing dermal tumor of intermediate malignancy that develops on the trunk or upper extremities of elderly patients as polypoid, often multinodular, lesions. Neoplastic cells are spindly and arranged in a storiform pattern. The neoplasm occupies the dermis and infiltrates the surrounding subcutis, imparting a honeycomblike appearance to fat lobules. A moderate or high mitotic rate is present, but there is little hemosiderin and there are few foamy histiocytes. The storiform (cartwheel) pattern is highly characteristic, yet not pathognomonic, of DFSP. Positive immunoreactivity for CD34 is helpful in differentiating DFSP from similar dermal tumors.

18. Correct choice: A

SUPERFICIAL MALIGNANT FIBROUS HISTIOCYTOMA (ATYPICAL FIBROXANTHOMA; p. 67)—This tumor is relatively common, arising preferentially on sun-exposed areas of elderly people. The histological features are those described in the question stem. Its histology appears in stark contrast to its usually indolent growth and clinically benign behavior. It may show a locally aggressive behavior and occasionally metastasize. Its histogenesis and classification have not yet been settled, but some authors view this tumor as a superficial well-differentiated variant of malignant fibrous histiocytoma.

19. Correct choice: C

CUTANEOUS LEIOMYOMA (p. 69)—This tumor may arise in the nipple or scrotum, from arrectores pilorum muscles (usually multiple), or from vascular structures. Grossly, the lesion is a pink ill-defined nodule, which is often very painful and tender on pressure. Microscopically, the tumor is composed of well-differentiated smooth muscle cells arranged in interweaving fascicles. *Neurothekeoma* is a tumor of presumed peripheral nerve sheath origin with a characteristic myxoid background. Other benign skin lesions that are often painful: *erythema nodosum, glomus tumor, angiolipoma, eccrine spiradenoma,* and *verruca plantaris.*

20. Correct choice: E

LOBULAR CAPILLARY HEMANGIOMA (PYOGENIC GRANULOMA; p. 69)—This vascular lesion is of a reactive nature, often developing after a minor trauma in the face, hands, and especially lips of children or young adults. *Epulis of pregnancy* is a pyogenic granuloma developing on the lips of pregnant women. The lobular architecture, with a central branching vessel giving rise to multiple smaller vessels, is characteristic. This feature is shared by a number of other *benign* vascular lesions, including infantile hemangioendothelioma, venous stasis, verruga peruana, and bacillary angiomatosis. Pyogenic granuloma spontaneously regresses or stabilizes, and only occasionally recurs after excision.

21. Correct choice: B

BACILLARY ANGIOMATOSIS (p. 70)—Histopathologic features and the presence of silver-positive small bacilli are consistent with *bacillary angiomatosis*. Bacillary angiomatosis results from an opportunistic infection due to *B. henselae* (Rochalimaea henselae), transmitted to humans by the cat flea. The cat is the permanent host of this microorganism. It manifests in immunocompromised patients (including AIDS) with nodular lesions in the skin and visceral organs (including bone and brain). *B. quintana* is the etiologic agent of *trench fever,* whereas *B. bacilliformis* causes *verruga peruana.*

22. Correct choice: A

ANGIOLYMPHOID HYPERPLASIA WITH EOSINOPHILIA (p. 71)—Also called *histiocytoid/epithelioid hemangioma,* this benign vascular neoplasm of the skin is characterized by proliferating blood vessels with prominent epithelioid-like endothelial cells. The stroma contains an abundant lymphocytic and eosinophilic infiltrate. It belongs to the same category as epithelioid hemangioendothelioma (of intermediate malignancy) and angiosarcoma (malignant). Epithelioid hemangioendothelioma preferentially affects deep tissues, whereas epithelioid hemangioma involves the skin.

23. Correct choice: B

KAPOSI SARCOMA (p. 72)—There are five main variants of Kaposi sarcoma (KS): (i) *classical (European),* occurring mostly in older males of Mediterranean descent; (ii) *epidemic (AIDS associated),* affecting 25% of AIDS patients, especially homosexual males; (iii) *postimmunosuppression (transplant associated),* occurring in immunosuppressed individuals following transplantation; (iv) *lymphangiopathic,* presenting as a primary lymph node involvement; (and) *African,* affecting Bantu children in endemic form. Morphological features are similar: spindly cells with interspersed slitlike vascular spaces and interstitial round eosinophilic bodies. The tumor is immunoreactive for endothelial markers and CD34. The classical form preferentially affects the skin; the AIDS-associated variant involves visceral organs and runs a more aggressive course. Herpesvirus type 8 has been shown to play a crucial pathogenetic role in the AIDS-associated variant.

24. Correct choice: B

MYCOSIS FUNGOIDES (p. 80)—Mycosis fungoides (MF) is a T-cell neoplasm derived from the CD4 subset of T lymphocytes.

■ *Premycotic* stage: scaly, erythematous, and pruritic patches; histology shows nondiagnostic dermatitis-like infiltration.

■ *Mycotic* stage: raised plaques; histology shows dermal infiltrate of atypical lymphocytes extending to the epidermis.

■ Small intraepidermal collections of lymphocytes (called *Pautrier microabscesses*) are most characteristic of MF, but single-cell infiltration along the dermal–epidermal junction in a "string-of-pearl" distribution is the most frequent change. Atypical lymphocytes have irregular cerebriform nuclear contours. Single-cell epidermotropism is also seen. Choice A indicates *cutaneous lymphoid hyperplasia*, choice C indicates *Munro microabscesses* of psoriasis, and choice E indicates *lymphomatoid papulosis*.

CHAPTER 3

1. Correct choice: E

BENIGN MELANOCYTIC LESIONS (p. 89)—Of the five features, symmetry of growth is the most characteristic of benign melanocytic proliferations: The dermal component of the melanocytic expansion is roughly equal, in lateral diameter, to the epidermal component. This can be appreciated on low-power examination. In contrast, nuclear atypia is usually absent in benign lesions, with Spitz nevus being a notable exception. Neurotization (also called schwannian differentiation) is a common manifestation of senescence in such lesions. Pagetoid spread is seen in melanomas, but also in Spitz nevi. A "shoulder" of melanocytic hyperplasia located at the margins of a melanocytic lesion is more often associated with malignancy.

2. Correct choice: D

CONGENITAL MELANOCYTIC NEVI (pp. 93 and 99)— Congenital melanocytic nevi are relatively infrequent, found in 1% of newborns. Grossly, they generally appear larger and more irregular than acquired nevi. Histologically, nevus cells extend deep into the dermis up to the subcutis, around pilosebaceous units and arrector pili muscles. Otherwise, the morphology of congenital nevi is similar to that of acquired nevi.

3. Correct choice: E

SPITZ NEVUS (SPINDLE AND EPITHELIOID CELL NEVUS; p. 93)—The microscopic features are highly suggestive of Spitz nevus, a benign melanocytic lesion that bears similarities to melanoma because of marked cytologic atypia, mitotic activity, and occasional pagetoid spread. Melanin is usually scanty or absent. The architectural features are very important in differentiating it from melanoma: symmetric growth, triangular shape, fascicles oriented perpendicular to the epidermal surface, and downward maturation of nevus cells. A prominent vascular network may lead to a diagnosis of hemangioma. Head and neck are the most common sites.

4. Correct choice: C

BLUE NEVUS (p. 96)—This entirely intradermal nevus is composed of spindle-shaped and dendritic cells, containing usually large amounts of pigment. There is a clear zone between the nevus and the overlying epidermis, which is uninvolved. If the pigment is mistaken as hemosiderin, a blue nevus may be erroneously diagnosed as fibrous histiocytoma. In common blue nevus, melanin is indeed more abundant within melanophages (histiocytes), which may obscure the accompanying dermal melanocytic component. Choice A is characteristic of Spitz nevus, choice B of dysplastic nevus, choice D of congenital nevus, and choice E of minimal deviation melanoma.

5. Correct choice: C

VERTICAL GROWTH PHASE: CLARK'S SYSTEM (p. 103)— The Clark system is based on evaluation of the level of invasion of melanomas into the underlying dermis and subcutis.

• *Level I:* intraepidermal melanoma, that is, *in situ* melanoma.

• *Level II:* invades into the papillary dermis.

• *Level III:* fills the papillary dermis, but stops at the interface between papillary and reticular dermis.

• *Level IV:* infiltrates the reticular dermis.

• *Level V:* extends into the subcutaneous fat.

This grading system has a good correlation with the 5-year survival rate and likelihood of regional metastases.

6. Correct choice: B

BRESLOW'S SYSTEM (p. 105)—This system is based on measurement of melanoma thickness from the top of the granular layer to the deepest level of invasion of the tumor. It assumes that the overlying epidermis is intact, not ulcerated. This microstage system has a definite correlate with prognosis and likelihood of lymph node metastases. Three categories have been identified:

1. *Low risk:* thickness less than 0.76 mm
2. *Intermediate risk:* thickness greater than 0.76 but less than 1.5 mm
3. *High risk:* thickness greater than 1.5 mm

7. Correct choice: C

COMPARISON BETWEEN CLARK'S AND BRESLOW'S SYSTEMS (p. 105)—It is still recommended that both Clark's level and Breslow's thickness be included in the diagnostic report of melanomas, because, as the present example shows, such staging systems are not equivalent. This melanoma would be classified as a level III according to Clark's system and within the high-risk category according to Breslow's. The implications are significant. The 5-year survival rate predicted by Clark's would be close to 90%, whereas the 5-year survival rate based on Breslow's would be approximately 50%. The likelihood of regional node metastases would be similar in both systems.

8. Correct choice: D

SUPERFICIAL SPREADING MELANOMA (p. 104)—This is the most common clinicopathological form of melanoma in white persons. It may develop anywhere in the body and appears as a variably colored flat lesion with irregular notched borders. The most characteristic feature of this form is the pagetoid spread of atypical melanocytes within the epidermis, with nest formation and presence of melanin up to the horny layer (*pigmented parakeratosis*). Development of vertical growth is manifested by the appearance of a nodule within the lesion.

9. Correct choice: C

LENTIGO MALIGNA (p. 104)—Also called *Hutchinson freckle*, this form of melanoma typically grows on the cheeks (or otherwise sun-exposed areas) of elderly white persons. The designation of lentigo maligna derives from the characteristic lentiginous distribution of atypical melanocytes along the dermo–epidermal junction, either singly or in small nests. Lentigo maligna is an actinic-induced melanocytic lesion, which could be viewed as the melanocytic counterpart of actinic keratosis.

10. Correct choice: A
ACRAL LENTIGINOUS MELANOMA (p. 104)—This form is most frequent in Blacks and Asians. It develops most commonly in palms, soles, and subungual areas, but also along mucocutaneous junctions and the anal region. Microscopically, it is similar to lentigo maligna (Hutchinson freckle), but the overlying epidermis is hyperplastic instead of atrophic as in the latter. Acral lentiginous melanoma has a more aggressive behavior compared to the lentigo maligna and superficial spreading forms.

CHAPTER 4

1. Correct choice: E
REACTION TO INJURY: MYOPATHIC VERSUS DENERVATION CHANGES (pp. 114 and following)—One of the major questions to address when examining a muscle biopsy is whether the pathologic changes result from a myopathic process (i.e., a *primary* muscle disease) or from denervation (i.e., a *neurogenic* condition). Changes favoring a myopathic condition include the following: increased internal nucleation, necrosis and regeneration of myofibers, endomysial fibrosis, and myofiber splitting. Myofiber atrophy is seen in almost every form of muscle disease, but its pattern is a helpful diagnostic feature. In myopathies, atrophic fibers with round contours are distributed at random throughout the muscle. In contrast, neurogenic atrophy leads to grouping of atrophic fibers (group atrophy), which additionally display an angular shape.

2. Correct choice: B
REACTION TO INJURY: NEUROGENIC ATROPHY (p. 119)—In neurogenic atrophy (resulting from axonal damage or motorneuron loss), atrophic fibers are angulated and usually clustered in groups (*group atrophy*). If reinnervation takes place, the same neuron will reinnervate neighboring myofibers, imparting the same fiber phenotype (either type I or type II) to a large group of myofibers: hence *fiber type grouping*. The endomysial compartment is not expanded by fibrosis or fatty infiltration. Necrosis, regeneration, and fiber splitting are characteristic of primary muscle diseases (myopathic changes). Ragged red fibers are due to accumulation of abnormal mitochondria (e.g., *nemaline rod myopathy*, p. 121). Chronic inflammation is associated with inflammatory myopathies such as *polymyositis* (p. 117).

The following table compares biopsy findings of neurogenic and myopathic conditions.

3. Correct choice: D
MITOCHONDRIAL MYOPATHIES (pp. 122 and 131)—Ragged red fibers constitute the morphologic expression of mitochondrial diseases. Although rare, these conditions are often suspected when clinical investigations are inconclusive. Neuropathologists frequently receive muscle biopsies with comments such as "rule out mitochondrial disease." A modified Gomori staining is most helpful in identifying morphologic evidence of abnormal mitochondria, which may be entirely inapparent on H&E. Ultrastructural, and above all, biochemical and genetic investigations are necessary to achieve a specific diagnosis.

4. Correct answer: C
DUCHENNE MUSCULAR DYSTROPHY (p. 124)—This condition is caused by mutations of the X-linked gene encoding *dystrophin*. Lack of expression of this protein results in *Duchenne* muscular dystrophy (DMD), whereas partial expression of dystrophin leads to *Becker* muscular dystrophy (BMD). H&E changes in muscle biopsies from patients with DMD are characteristic, but diagnostic certainty can be achieved with immunohistochemistry (or immunoblot) for dystrophin. In DMD, there is complete absence of the normal sarcolemmal immunoreactivity, whereas in BMD immunoreactivity is patchy and discontinuous.

5. Correct choice: B
INCLUSION BODY MYOSITIS (p. 129)—Inclusion body myositis (IBM) is an inflammatory myopathy that afflicts men

Changes	Neurogenic	Myopathic	Stains
Atrophic myofibers	Angular contour	Round contour	H&E
Group atrophy	Present	Absent	H&E
Endomysium	Normal	Expanded (fibrosis, fatty infiltration, inflammation)	H&E; Gomori trichrome
Fiber type grouping	Present	Absent	ATPase histochemistry
Degeneration/ necrosis	Absent	Present	H&E; other stains
Regeneration	Absent	Present	H&E; alkaline phosphatase
Nuclei	Subsarcolemmal	Internalized	H&E
Target fibers	Present (25% cases)	Absent	NADH histochemistry
Inflammation	Absent or scanty	May be present, depending on etiology	H&E; acid phosphatase
Inclusions	Absent	May be present, (e.g., inclusion body myositis)	H&E; Gomori trichrome

more often than women in the age range 50 to 70. Both clinically (distal weakness) and pathologically (angular fiber atrophy, group atrophy, etc.), IBM may mimic neurogenic atrophy. Inflammatory infiltration is usually scanty, and ragged red fibers may be seen. *Rimmed vacuoles* represent the most characteristic H&E changes, consisting of intrasarcoplasmic vacuoles surrounded by and containing dustlike granular material. Intranuclear inclusions are less apparent on H&E. Ultrastructural studies demonstrate intranuclear filamentous inclusions. In contrast to polymyositis, IBM is poorly responsive to steroid treatment.

CHAPTER 5

1. Correct choice: C
EVALUATION OF SOFT TISSUE LESIONS (p. 137)—To avoid diagnostic mistakes in soft tissue lesions, the following step-by-step evaluation is suggested.

1. One should assume that the lesion is of a reactive nature, because reactive lesions may display features mimicking neoplasms (*pseudosarcomas*). Mitoses or pleomorphism cannot be used to discriminate between pseudosarcomatous lesions and soft tissue neoplasms.
2. The lesion should be considered benign until proven otherwise: necrosis is the most reliable sign of malignancy.
3. If malignant, a lesion may not be a sarcoma after all: consider a pseudosarcomatous carcinoma or melanoma, and rule out these differentials by appropriate immunostains.
4. The issue of histogenesis should be addressed after the previous questions.
5. The mitotic rate is important in separating benign from malignant forms of certain tumors.

2. Correct choice: B
DIFFERENTIAL DIAGNOSIS BETWEEN SARCOMAS AND PSEUDOSARCOMAS (p. 138)—A number of features may help ruling in sarcomas and ruling out pseudosarcomas, but high vascularity and necrosis are generally features of malignant soft tissue tumors. Note: The vascular network may not be readily apparent. Highly pleomorphic, bizarre nuclei may be present in a number of benign soft tissue lesions (e.g., leiomyoma, schwannoma, etc.). Lobular architecture in a vascular mass generally favors a benign lesion (e.g., pyogenic granuloma). "Floret" cells are seen in benign soft tissue lesions (e.g., pleomorphic lipoma). Rapid growth of a small mass is usually a manifestation of benign lesions (e.g., nodular fasciitis).

3. Correct choice: C
SPINDLE CELL MELANOMA (DESMOPLASTIC) MELANOMA (p. 139)—Melanoma is one of the great mimics. It may mimic sarcomatous tumors, too, especially in its spindle cell/desmoplastic variant. Desmoplastic melanomas have a propensity to spread along peripheral nerves, thus reinforcing the impression of a primitive peripheral nerve tumor. Desmoplastic melanoma is characterized by diffuse S100 immunoreactivity, whereas S100 expression is patchy or focal in MPNST. A rich reticulin network should favor MPNST (because of basement membrane around neoplastic cells), but desmoplastic melanoma may as well have abundant reticulin. HMB-45 is often negative in desmoplastic melanomas.

4. Correct choice: C
CD34 MARKER (p. 145)—CD34 is a transmembrane protein expressed by hematopoietic and endothelial cells. CD34 immunohistochemistry is used as a diagnostic tool in pathologic evaluation of STTs. It is expressed by a wide variety of neoplasms, including *solitary fibrous tumors, gastrointestinal stromal tumors,* and *dermatofibrosarcoma protuberans.* Pseudosarcomatous carcinoma, melanoma, atypical fibroxanthoma, and synovial sarcoma (all of which may mimic sarcomas) are CD34-negative.

5. Correct choice: E
NODULAR FASCIITIS (p. 153)—Nodular fasciitis (NF) is a reactive process akin to myositis ossificans. Its rapid growth helps distinguish this highly cellular lesion from sarcomatous tumors. The wavy collagen bundles lined by spindly cells are similar to those of a keloid scar. Nuclear pleomorphism and mitotic activity may be marked, but cellular components are heterogeneous, including fibroblasts, myofibroblasts, inflammatory cells, and vascular endothelial cells. Quite characteristic is the architecture, in which several zones are identifiable: a peripheral capillary-rich rim, an intermediate myxoid area, and a central hypocellular core. Cells are positive for smooth muscle actin. Proliferative fasciitis is seen in people over 50 years of age and is morphologically similar to NF.

6. Correct choice: E
SPINDLE CELL LIPOMA (p. 155)—This is a lipoma with a substantial spindle cell component. It occurs most often in the neck and shoulder regions of elderly men. Differential diagnosis includes neurofibroma and fibrous histiocytoma. Spindle cell lipoma is S100- and CD34-immunoreactive.

7. Correct choice: C
LIPOBLASTOMA (p. 156)—Lipoblastoma is a rare pediatric tumor that may be confused with myxoid liposarcoma. It is histologically similar to fetal adipose tissue and consists of lipoblasts in a myxoid stroma with plexiform vessels. Its lobular architecture and characteristic capillary network are not seen in liposarcoma, a tumor exceedingly rare in children.

8. Correct choice: B
RHABDOMYOMA (p. 157)—Rhabdomyomas can be divided into *fetal* and *adult* forms. The fetal form is found in the head and neck region (retroauricular) of children less than 3 years of age and in the genital region of middle-aged women. Fetal rhabdomyoma consists of immature skeletal myocytes in a myxoid matrix. The main differential diagnosis is with well-differentiated rhabdomyosarcoma. The adult form is seen in the oral cavity of adults and consists of vacuolated cells intermixed with so-called *spider cells.*

9. Correct choice: B
PAPILLARY ENDOTHELIAL HYPERPLASIA (p. 157)—This peculiar lesion develops in ectatic veins (varicose veins or hemorrhoids) or in vascular tumors. It consists of endothelium-lined papillary structures protruding into the vascular lumen. *Malignant endovascular papillary angioendothelioma* is an extremely rare type of angioendothelioma (sometimes mistaken for malignant vascular tumors), with histology similar to papillary endothelial hyperplasia. Features favoring papillary endothelial hyperplasia include intravascular location, bland nuclear morphology, and well-demarcated borders.

10. Correct choice: A
ELASTOFIBROMA (p. 161)—This lesion is often bilateral and found close to the apex of the scapula, deep to the muscle layer. A

history of hard labor and familiality are often present. The presence of cylindrical structures composed of immature elastic fibers is the defining histologic feature. It is probably a reactive process accompanied by defective formation of elastic fibers.

11. Correct choice: A

FIBROUS PROLIFERATIONS OF CHILDHOOD (p. 161)—These lesions develop in pediatric age and include calcifying aponeurotic fibroma, fibrous hamartoma of infancy, infantile digital fibromatosis, fibromatosis colli, and so on. Histological *and* clinical features are the most important clues to the correct diagnosis. Calcifying aponeurotic fibroma occurs in the dorsal hand or wrist of children/adolescents and is considered of chondroid origin. It can be thought of as the cartilaginous equivalent of fibromatosis. Morphologically, fibromatosis, rheumatoid nodule, and schwannoma are the main differentials.

12. Correct choice: C

FIBROMATOSIS (p. 163)—Fibromatosis is a group of disorders characterized by proliferation of myofibroblasts, with a tendency for local recurrence but no metastatic behavior. Ultrastructural features of myofibroblasts include nuclei with distinctive indentations (strangulations) and a cytoplasmic contractile system similar to that of smooth muscle cells. Adherens and tight junctions are present. Filamentous proteins can be demonstrated by immunohistochemistry, including vimentin, α-smooth muscle actin, desmin, and smooth muscle myosin heavy chain. The clonal origin of these lesions supports a neoplastic origin.

13. Correct choice: A

FIBROSARCOMA (p. 165)—Fibrosarcomas are rare malignant tumors that vary from well-differentiated to poorly differentiated forms. They may arise from superficial or deep sites. They consist of fibroblast-like cells with oval nuclei. The most characteristic architectural feature is a *herringbone* pattern, in which fascicles of neoplastic cells intersect at acute angles. Reticulin staining demonstrates reticulin fibers investing each cell (similar to hemangiopericytoma). Ultrastructural studies reveal fibroblastic/myofibroblastic features. A diagnosis of fibrosarcoma should be questioned if multinucleated giant cells are found.

14. Correct choice: A

DERMATOFIBROSARCOMA PROTUBERANS (p. 167)—A cartwheel or storiform arrangement is highly characteristic of DFSP. This pattern may be seen focally in a number of tumors (e.g., malignant fibrous histiocytoma, peripheral nerve sheath tumors, fibromatosis, nodular fasciitis, etc.). In DFSP, however, this pattern is present in each and every field. Local recurrence is frequent, but this tumor does not metastasize. Remember the typical immunohistochemical profile of DFSP: positive for CD34 and negative for factor XIIIa (vice versa in fibrous histiocytoma).

15. Correct choice: D

MALIGNANT FIBROUS HISTIOCYTOMA (p. 169)—Malignant fibrous histiocytoma (MFH) is considered the most frequent malignant soft tissue tumor. The mixture of highly anaplastic spindle cells in a storiform arrangement with multinucleated bizarre giant cells is the most characteristic feature. However, many of the cases once considered typical MFH were poorly differentiated forms of liposarcomas, leiomyosarcomas, rhabdomyosarcomas, and synovial sarcomas. Thus, a diagnosis of MFH should be reserved for soft tissue tumors where light microscopical, immunohistochemical, or ultrastructural studies fail to reveal evidence of specific tissue differentiation. MFH usually occurs in elderly peo-

ple, and the thigh is the most frequent site. This cancer is locally aggressive and metastasizes in up to 50% of cases.

16. Correct choice: A

VARIANTS OF MFH (pp. 171–173)—There are six variants of MFH. Angiomatoid MFH contains blood-filled cystic spaces frequently associated with large collections of lymphocytes. These are more often found at the periphery of the tumor and may form lymphoid follicles simulating lymph nodes. The angiomatoid variant is the most benign form of MFH and tends to occur in young patients. Choice B is similar to giant cell tumor of bone. Choice C has a rich *neutrophilic*, not lymphocytic, infiltrate. Choice D is characterized by a widespread myxoid background: this condition also has a good prognosis. Choice E is the classic and most common type.

17. Correct choice: A

VARIANTS OF LIPOMA (p. 174)—Angiolipoma is characterized by abundant vascularity, often more prominent at the periphery, and hyaline thrombi. The tumor often manifests with pain. Fibrolipoma contains bundles of mature connective tissue. Myxolipoma shows a myxoid background. Chondroid lipomas contain areas of chondroid matrix. Angiomyolipoma consists of a variable mixture of mature adipose tissue with smooth muscle vascular channels: Cells are immunoreactive for HMB-45.

18. Correct choice: B

HISTOLOGIC TYPES OF LIPOSARCOMA (p. 175)—The myxoid variant is the most common. The hypocellularity, chicken-wire capillary network, and myxoid matrix are characteristic of myxoid liposarcoma, which is easily recognized on frozen section. Lipoblasts are usually scanty, however. Note that the term "dedifferentiated liposarcoma" does not refer to a specific histologic variant, but rather to the emergence of an undifferentiated component in an otherwise well-differentiated liposarcoma. Myxoid and well-differentiated liposarcomas have a better prognosis than the pleomorphic and round cell types.

19. Correct choice: A

SOFT TISSUE LEIOMYOSARCOMA (p. 179)—The histologic criteria used to differentiate leiomyosarcoma from leiomyomas of soft tissues are different from those applied to uterine tumors. Mitotic count is the most important parameter, but size, necrosis, and depth of location should also be considered. These criteria may differ considerably in relation to site (deep versus superficial). An association of leiomyosarcomas with Epstein-Barr virus is observed in AIDS patients, but not in those affecting immunocompetent hosts. Superficial (skin-based) leiomyosarcomas have a striking male predominance, while deep tumors (retroperitoneum, inferior vena cava) are more frequent in females. Superficial leiomyosarcomas have an excellent prognosis.

20. Correct choice: E

RHABDOMYOSARCOMA (180)—This small round cell tumor develops in children between 3 and 12 years of age and is most frequently located in the head/neck region and urogenital tract. Tumors located close to a mucosa (nasal cavity, vagina, conjunctiva, etc.) are characterized by a cellular condensation beneath the epithelium (*cambium layer of Nicholson*) and around blood vessels. Deeper, submucosal tumors, such as *botryoid rhabdomyosarcoma*, are loosely textured and contain the characteristic "strap" cells. The *embryonal* variant consists of sheets of small, poorly differentiated cells with eccentric nuclei and eosinophilic cytoplasm. The *alveolar* variant is characterized by thin fibrous septa forming a round cavity lined by discohesive tumor cells.

21. Correct choice: A

PROGNOSIS OF RHABDOMYOSARCOMA (pp. 180 and 181)—Rhabdomyosarcoma behaves as a highly aggressive malignancy. In regard to treatment response and survival, rhabdomyosarcomas can be classified into "favorable" versus "unfavorable" groups. Most cases of embryonal tumors (including the rare pleomorphic variant) and botryoid tumors are "favorable" with a 2-year survival rate approaching 90%. The alveolar form has the worst prognosis.

22. Correct choice: D

LYMPHANGIOMYOMA (p. 190)—This tumor consists of a mixture of lymphatic channels and smooth muscle bundles. It is encountered in association with tuberous sclerosis (TS), in which angiomyolipomas (positive for HMB-45) are also found. Lymphangiomyomatosis is a diffuse form that most commonly involves the lungs. Rhabdomyoma of the heart is also frequently associated with tuberous sclerosis, but does not express HMB-45. The common theme of TS-related lesions is their hamartomatous nature.

23. Correct choice: E

HEMANGIOPERICYTOMA AND SYNOVIAL SARCOMA (pp. 190 and 191)—Although increasingly controversial, hemangiopericytoma is still recognized as a distinct entity. The staghorn pattern is a nonspecific vascular arrangement found in a variety of soft tissue neoplasms, including synovial sarcoma, fibrosarcoma, solitary fibrous tumor, peripheral nerve sheath tumors, chondrosarcoma, and so on. Generous sampling can help in ruling out synovial sarcoma, because in this tumor, immunoreactivity for epithelial markers is often focal. A *diagnosis of exclusion* is advised in identifying hemangiopericytoma: a spindle cell tumor exhibiting a staghorn pattern *throughout*, positive for CD34, and negative for smooth muscle, nerve sheath (S100), and epithelial markers.

24. Correct choice: C

SYNOVIAL SARCOMA (p. 191)—Synovial sarcoma (SS) preferentially develops *around* (but not *within*) knee and ankle joints of young adults. Characterized by a distinctive biphasic pattern, it consists of epithelial cells arranged in glandular formation scattered within a sarcomatous spindle cell component. Ninety percent of cases possess a translocation between chromosomes X and 18, involving two genes of unknown function, SSX1 or 2 (on chromosome X) and SYT (on chromosome 18). A *monophasic* variant (consisting exclusively of the mesenchymal component) may mimic fibrosarcoma, malignant peripheral nerve sheath tumor, and mesenchymal chondrosarcoma. A favorable prognosis is associated with a glandular component greater than 50%, diploid tumors, and tumors with the SSX2 gene translocation.

25. Correct choice: A

SCHWANNOMA (p. 194)—The classic light microscopic features, with alternating Antoni A/B areas and the parallel cellular palisades of *Verocay bodies*, combined with S100 immunoreactivity are usually sufficient for diagnosis. Schwann cells are surrounded by a continuous basal lamina. In the intercellular space, long-spaced collagen fibers may form bodies characterized by a peculiar cross-banded pattern, known as *Luse bodies*, at the ultrastructural level. Variants are *granular cell schwannoma* (synonymous with granular cell tumor) and *cellular schwannoma* (highly cellular, mitotically active, but benign).

26. Correct choice: C

GRANULAR CELL TUMOR (pp. 194 and 201)—The tongue is the most frequent location of this benign neoplasm, which is indeed a schwannoma because of its presumed origin from Schwann cells. It has been reported in a variety of locations, most often the tongue. Ultrastructural studies have shown that the granules are modified lysosomes containing hydrolytic enzymes such as acid phosphatase. Benign and *malignant* forms of granular cell tumor are often morphologically indistinguishable, so that only metastatic spread can be used as evidence of malignancy.

27. Correct choice: C

NEUROFIBROMA (p. 195)—Although Schwann cells constitute the predominant cell component, neurofibromas consist of all the histologic elements of a peripheral nerve, including fibroblasts and axons. Schwann cells and axons can be identified by S100 and neurofilament immunoreactivity, respectively. Schwannomas are entirely composed of neoplastic Schwann cells and do not contain axons.

28. Correct choice: B

MALIGNANT PERIPHERAL NERVE SHEATH TUMOR (MPNST; p. 196)—This highly malignant neoplasm originates from Schwann cells, frequently from malignant degeneration of neurofibromas in the context of neurofibromatosis type 1. Although the microscopic features tend to be those of an undifferentiated sarcoma, the previously mentioned microscopic characteristics are strongly suggestive of MPNST. Pseudopalisading necrosis is similar to that seen in glioblastoma multiforme. In addition, patchy often focal S100 immunoreactivity is usually seen. Desmoplastic (spindle cell) melanoma is one of the most important differential diagnoses, but often histologic and immunohistochemical features alone are not sufficient to distinguish between MPNST and desmoplastic melanoma.

29. Correct choice: B

ALVEOLAR SOFT PART SARCOMA (p. 200)—This sarcoma most commonly arises in the deep thigh or leg of young females. Microscopically, the nesting pattern and the tendency of central cells to be noncohesive impart the alveolar configuration. The cytoplasmic needlelike structures and crystalloid inclusions are characteristic. Several immunohistochemical and ultrastructural features appear consistent with a myogenic origin of this tumor.

30. Correct choice: B

RHABDOID TUMORS (p. 201)—This tumor occurs in the kidney, soft tissues, and peripheral nerves. The cells have a striking eosinophilic cytoplasm that on EM appears filled with masses of intermediate filaments, especially in paranuclear locations. Rhabdoid tumor is probably not a specific neoplasm, but a morphologic variant of different types of tumors. The emergence of a rhabdoid phenotype appears to be associated with an aggressive course.

31. Correct choice: B

CLEAR CELL SARCOMA (p. 203)—Also called *melanoma of soft parts*, this neoplasm develops from tendons or aponeuroses, most commonly in the feet of young adults. The cells have a conspicuous nucleolus and contain both iron and melanin. A nesting or fascicular pattern is common. Immunoreactivity for S100 and HMB-45 is consistently present, in analogy with skin melanomas.

32. Correct choice: A

DESMOPLASTIC SMALL CELL TUMOR (p. 204)—DSCT affects young adult males. The cytological features are those of a small cell tumor, with scanty cytoplasm, uniform nuclei, and inconspicuous nucleoli. Tumor cells are arranged in a nesting pattern with prominent desmoplasia (hence the designation). The peculiarity of this tumor lies in the characteristic immunohisto-chemical profile, which includes reactivity for desmin (in a dotlike perinuclear pattern), epithelial markers, and neuronal markers. Because fetal mesothelium expresses both desmin and epithelial markers, DSCS is believed to be a malignant neoplasm of mesothelial origin (renamed *mesothelioblastoma*). The prognosis is grim.

CHAPTER 6

1. Correct choice: B
DEGENERATIVE JOINT DISEASE (OSTEOARTHRITIS; p. 224)—The articular cartilage is the component primarily affected by degenerative joint disease. Matrix alterations close to the synovial surface are the earliest phenomena observed in the arthritic joint. This change can be highlighted by the use of special stains for sulfated proteoglycans (e.g., safranin O). Degeneration and thinning of cartilage is then followed by eburnation of exposed bone and development of osteophytes and loose bodies. In contrast to inflammatory forms (rheumatoid arthritis, psoriatic arthritis, and ankylosing spondylitis), lymphomonocytic infiltration of the synovium is mild and represents a secondary phenomenon.

2. Correct choice: D
RHEUMATOID NODULE (pp. 228 and 229)—This form of granuloma is found in 25% of cases of rheumatoid arthritis, but also in rheumatic disease and systemic lupus erythematosus. The palisading arrangement of histiocytes and central necrosis with fibrin deposition are characteristic features.

3. Correct choice: A
GOUT AND URATE CRYSTALS (p. 232)—Deposition of urate crystals in and around involved joints may lead to massive destruction of cartilage and bone. Tophi are localized nodules of urate deposition, consisting of multiple foci of urate crystal surrounded by a florid giant cell reaction. Without alcohol fixation, the crystals may not be easy to appreciate. These water-soluble crystals are easily washed out by routine staining methods. Alcohol fixation, instead, allows optimal preservation of monosodium urate crystals, which appear as *needle shaped* and doubly refractile.

4. Correct choice: B
CALCIUM PYROPHOSPHATE CRYSTAL DEPOSITION DISEASE (CPPD; p. 232)—Also called *pseudogout* or *chondro-calcinosis*, this condition generally manifests with symptoms and signs similar to degenerative osteoarthritis, usually beginning in the fourth decade of life. Calcium pyrophosphate crystals are needle shaped and have a color pattern under a red compensator opposite to that of urate crystals. Deposition of calcium pyrophosphate in the articular cartilage results in degenerative joint disease. The term "pseudogout" is commonly reserved for cases manifesting acutely with joint swelling and pain similar to gout.

5. Correct choice: E
HOFFA DISEASE (p. 237)—Also called *synovial lipomatosis*, this condition is characterized by extensive fatty growth within the subsynovial tissue. It affects the knee and is related to expansion of the infrapatellar fat pad. Choice A is characteristic of gout and pseudogout, choice B of degenerative osteoarthritis, choice C of rheumatoid arthritis, and choice D of avascular necrosis.

6. Correct choice: D
PIGMENTED VILLONODULAR SYNOVITIS (PVNS; p. 238)—Also called *giant cell tumor of the tendon sheath*, PVNS

affects the flexor joints of the wrist and the knee. The major cellular component (polygonal cells) has immunohistochemical and ultrastructural features of synoviocytes. A characteristic papillary architecture is observed in the adjacent synovium, which is interpreted as a hyperplastic response. Hemosiderin- and fat-laden macrophages are seen at the periphery of the lesion, probably resulting from reactive changes. This lesion must be distinguished from *hemosiderotic synovitis*, which develops in patients with chronic bleeding diathesis (hemophilia). *Primary synovial chondromatosis* is characterized by cartilage nodules within the synovial membrane, involving only one joint, usually hips or knees.

CHAPTER 7

1. Correct choice: B
OSTEOGENESIS IMPERFECTA (p. 249)—This bone disorder is due to mutations of collagen type 1. It is characterized by recurrent fractures that begin *in utero* in the most severe fatal forms. Short stature and disproportionately shortened limbs characterize the cases manifesting in childhood. Innumerable fractures affecting the growth plate lead to cartilage nodules that produce a "bag of popcorn" appearance on x-rays. Choice A is indicative of *osteomalacia/rickets*, hypophosphatasia, and aluminum toxicity; choice C of *osteopetrosis*, an inherited disorder also resulting in shortening of long bones and propensity to fractures; choice D of *achondroplasia*, an inherited disorder manifesting with dwarfism secondary to premature sealing of growth plates and due to genetic abnormalities in signal transduction; and choice E of osteoporosis.

2. Correct choice C
OSTEITIS FIBROSA CYSTICA (p. 253)—Also called *Recklinghausen disease*, this is the most severe manifestation of skeletal changes due to hyperparathyroidism. Bone resorption affects the whole skeletal system, but lesions are more frequent or evident in the mandible. It is characterized by cystic areas of osteolysis associated with reactive bone formation and accumulation of hemosiderin and osteoclast. *Brown tumor* refers to deposits of hemosiderin associated with reactive fibroblastic, osteoclastic, and vascular proliferation, and a large number of giant cells. Osteitis fibrosa cystica of the mandible is virtually identical to a lesion unrelated to hyperparathyroidism, that is, *central giant cell reparative granuloma:* Diagnosis thus rests on clinical history. In contrast to brown tumors, giant cells are evenly distributed within *giant cell tumors*.

3. Correct choice: E
PAGET DISEASE (OSTEITIS DEFORMANS; p. 254)—This bone condition affects up to 10% of the general population in some European countries and the United States. Paget first suspected a viral origin. Recent studies have shown the presence of paramyxovirus-like capsids in osteoclasts, paramyxovirus antigens in osteoclasts, and viral transcripts in various cell types. The disease may be monostotic or polyostotic. The most frequently involved sites include skull, vertebral column, and axial skeleton. Ribs and small bones are rarely affected. Histologically, we find a haphazard mosaic-like pattern of *cement lines*, representing the borders between adjacent areas of newly formed lamellar bone. Giant cell osteoclasts are typical of Paget disease. In *fibrous dysplasia*, cement lines are present, typically accompanied by eccentric bone atrophy.

4. Correct choice: C

MYOSITIS OSSIFICANS CIRCUMSCRIPTA (p. 260)—A zonal architecture is characteristic of this lesion, with a central highly cellular sarcoma-mimicking region, surrounded by osteoid deposition and a peripheral shell of well-formed bone. The lesion is akin to nodular fasciitis, and 50% of cases are preceded by a history of recent trauma. The most frequent locations are flexor muscles of the upper arm, quadriceps femurs, adductor muscles of the thigh, gluteal muscles, and soft tissues of the hands. Without clinical radiologic information, myositis ossificans may be difficult to differentiate from sarcomas, but the fact that osteosarcoma is less mature at the periphery (in contrast to myositis ossificans) is a helpful feature.

5. Correct choice: C

ACUTE (PYOGENIC) OSTEOMYELITIS (p. 262)—This infection follows hematogenous spread or, less commonly, spread by contiguity from adjacent foci. Patients with sickle cell disease are prone to developing two types of bone complications, that is, infarcts and pyogenic osteomyelitis. The latter is most frequently caused by *Salmonella* species, an infrequent etiologic agent in patients without sickle cell disease, except intravenous drug abusers. The great majority of osteomyelitis in the general population is caused by staphylococci. Chronic osteomyelitis is often mistaken for a malignant process on clinical and radiologic grounds.

CHAPTER 8

1. Correct choice: C

BONE TUMOR STAGING (p. 267)—Staging of bone neoplasms is based on the system originally proposed by Enneking and includes three parameters: grade, anatomical location, and distant metastasis. Low-grade tumors are considered stage I and high-grade tumors stage II. Presence of metastasis is equivalent to stage III, regardless of grade. Each stage is subclassified as A (involvement of one compartment) or B (more than one compartment involved).

2. Correct choice: D

MULTIPLE MYELOMA (p. 268)—MM represents approximately 1% of all malignant neoplasms and 10% of all hematologic malignancies. This plasma cell neoplasm retains cytologic similarities to the cell of origin and leads to production of a monoclonal type of immunoglobulin (Ig) or fragments of Ig. It usually presents as multiple osteolytic lesions, most commonly involving the vertebrae, skull, ribs, and pelvis.

3. Correct choice: D

MULTIPLE MYELOMA (p. 268)—Each bone lesion of multiple myeloma characteristically appears on x-rays as sharply circumscribed punched-out areas of osteolysis. This is by no means pathognomonic of multiple myeloma, but it suggests the diagnosis in the presence of typical laboratory findings, for example, monoclonal spike in the γ region of the serum protein electrophoresis. Choice A is often associated with (though not specific of) osteosarcoma, choice B is highly characteristic of chondrosarcoma, choice C is frequently associated with Ewing sarcoma, and choice E is typical of osteoid osteoma.

4. Correct choice: B

EWING SARCOMA (p. 272)—This case sums up the main clinical, morphologic, and immunohistochemical features of this soft tissue/bone neoplasm: monomorphic round cells, immunoreactivity for CD99, predilection for young people, and preferred localization in the shaft of long bones. The onionskin pattern, detectable on x-rays, results from progressive periosteal bone apposition. The tumor has a soft, fleshy texture. CD99 expression, although characteristic of this tumor, is also detected in other neoplasms, such as lymphoblastic lymphoma and other sarcomas. Ewing sarcomas have specific cytogenetic abnormalities, the most frequent of which is t(11;22), detectable on fresh frozen tissue.

5. Correct choice: B

OSTEOCHONDROMA (p. 274)—This is the most frequent benign bone tumor. Osteochondroma probably originates from the abnormal (nonneoplastic) growth of superficial chondroid foci. It develops in the metaphysis of long bones, especially the distal femur, proximal tibia, and proximal humerus. Radiologically, it appears as a sessile or pedunculated mass growing away from the joint. The histopathologic appearance is characteristic: a nidus of mature bone surrounded by a well-differentiated cap of mature cartilage. In fact, it is the peripheral rim of cartilage that matures into the central core of the bone. The medullary cavity is in direct continuity with the stalk. Usually asymptomatic, it may produce deformities or impinge on adjacent tendons, nerves, or vessels. Choice A is characteristic of *chondroblastoma*, choice C of *fibrous dysplasia*, choice D of *osteoid osteoma*, and choice E of *chondroma*.

6. Correct choice: C

CHONDROMA (pp. 275–277)—This benign lesion is composed of mature cartilage organized in a lobular pattern. Sporadic chondromas occur predominantly in the short tubular bones of hands and feet. The most important differential diagnosis is with low-grade chondrosarcoma. Radiologic appearance is essential in distinguishing a chondroma from its malignant counterpart. Innumerable chondromas are found in Maffucci syndrome and Ollier disease, usually unilaterally. In Maffucci syndrome, chondromas are associated with multiple soft tissue hemangiomas. In both conditions, chondromas have an increased propensity to degenerate into chondrosarcomas.

7. Correct choice: A

CHONDROBLASTOMA (p. 277)—This benign tumor develops before the age of 20, usually in the distal femur, proximal tibia, or proximal humerus. The previous histological description applies to the majority of chondroblastomas, but these tumors show great morphological variability. Occasionally, the prevalence of giant cells or high cellular density leads to a mistaken diagnosis of giant cell tumor or, respectively, chondrosarcoma. The chicken-wire pattern of calcification, glycogen-rich cytoplasm, thick cell membrane, and reticulin pattern are all helpful clues. The x-ray appearance is highly characteristic: a well-circumscribed epiphyseal mass extending to the metaphysis. The tumor manifests with pain and needs ample surgical debridement and bone grafting.

8. Correct choice: B

CHONDROMYXOID FIBROMA (p. 278)—This rare benign tumor of cartilaginous origin usually develops in the metaphysis of long bones, most commonly in the feet, and preferentially between 10 and 25 years of age. Its cellular pleomorphism may suggest a diagnosis of chondrosarcoma. Important low-power features favoring a diagnosis of chondromyxoid fibroma include well-circumscribed margins, a lobular architecture, and a biphasic pattern due to islands of chondromyxoid appearance surrounded by fibroblastic septa. Local recurrence is seen in 25% of cases.

9. Correct choice: B

CHONDROSARCOMA (p. 279)—This sarcoma has, by definition, areas of chondroid differentiation. The age range is 30 to 60 years. It most frequently develops in the pelvis, shoulder girdle, and ribs, manifesting radiologically with osteolytic areas admixed with radioopaque (flocculent) areas of blotchy calcification. The Codman triangle, instead, is more often associated with osteosarcoma. The degree of differentiation varies from well-differentiated (difficult to distinguish from chondromas) to poorly differentiated tumors. In contrast to osteosarcoma, grading is of crucial importance for prognosis. Survival rate is approximately of 80%, 50%, and 20% for low-, intermediate-, and high-grade lesions.

10. Correct choice: E

VARIANTS OF CHONDROSARCOMA (p. 282)—The *dedifferentiated* variant is thought to arise from anaplastic degeneration of an otherwise well-differentiated tumor. The dedifferentiated region is at the periphery of the lesion. Choice A is characteristic of *chordoma* or the myxoid variant, resembling chordoma; choice B of the *clear cell* variant, composed of cords and nests of clear cells with sharply defined borders; and choice C of the *mesenchymal* variant, most common in younger patients and characterized by the coexistence of two sharply demarcated patterns, a well-differentiated chondrosarcoma, and a small cell anaplastic component showing a hemangiopericytoma-like pattern.

11. Correct choice: D

OSTEOID OSTEOMA (p. 284)—The clinical history is suggestive of osteoid osteoma, with nocturnal pain relieved by aspirin. The radiolucent nidus surrounded by marked osteosclerotic reaction is also characteristic and occasionally prompts a mistaken clinical diagnosis of Garré osteomyelitis. The histology is diagnostic, characterized by osteoid and woven bone trabeculae lined by plump osteoblasts and enmeshed in a densely vascular stroma. Choice B, *Osteoblastoma,* is morphologically identical to osteoid osteoma, but it usually develops in the spinal skeleton.

12. Correct choice: B

OSTEOMA (p. 286)—This rare benign tumor is composed of well-developed lamellar bone. It is probably a hamartomatous rather than a neoplastic lesion. *Gardner syndrome* is characterized by intestinal polyposis, multiple osteomas, epidermal cysts, and fibromatosis. The condition is autosomal dominant (like FAP), and intestinal polyps are identical to those associated with FAP. Aside from those occurring with Gardner syndrome, osteomas are usually solitary and involve facial bones, for example, the maxilla and mandible.

13. Correct choice: C

CONVENTIONAL OSTEOSARCOMA (p. 287)—Production of variably calcified osteoid is the defining feature of osteosarcomas. Care should be taken to distinguish between bone entrapped by the neoplastic growth and bone/osteoid produced by tumor cells. Fibroblastic or chondroblastic components are often present and may occasionally be predominant. Immunoreactivity for vimentin is consistently present, but nonspecific. Osteosarcoma is also positive for osteonectin and bone morphogenetic protein; the chondroblastic foci are immunoreactive for S100. Giant cells are present in one-third of cases and may be extremely numerous (*giant cell variant*). Most osteosarcomas are nowadays resected after chemotherapy and thus contain necrotic areas. The extent of necrosis after chemotherapy has prognostic significance.

14. Correct choice: C

RISK FACTORS FOR OSTEOSARCOMA (p. 287)—Osteosarcoma has two peaks of incidence, one in childhood/adolescence and the second in middle/elderly age. The majority of the latter cases develop in association with *Paget disease*. Other recognized risk factors include radiation exposure, chemotherapy, foreign bodies, and various bone conditions (i.e., fibrous dysplasia and chondromatosis). Also, hereditary retinoblastoma leads to increased risk of osteosarcomas. *De novo* cases of osteosarcoma outnumber those arising as a complication of radiation therapy or in association with Paget disease and fibrous dysplasia.

15. Correct choice: B

VARIANTS OF OSTEOSARCOMA (p. 291)—The *parosteal* (or *juxtacortical*) variant is peculiar in its mode of growth. The tumor originates from the metaphysis, grows outward as a lobulated mass, and eventually may surround the whole bone. This type of tumor grows very slowly and is associated with a good prognosis. Histologically, it is a well-differentiated sarcoma that may mimic myositis ossificans and osteochondroma. Remember that osteochondroma grows in continuity with the bone. Choice A, *gnathic* osteosarcoma of the jaw, is considered a clinical variant because of its better prognosis. Choice C, *Paget associated*, usually multicentric, is as aggressive as conventional osteosarcoma. Choice D, *periosteal*, grows *within* the cortex, shows minimal involvement of the medullary canal, and has a predominant chondroblastic component.

16. Correct choice: D

GIANT CELL TUMOR (p. 293)—This locally aggressive tumor occurs in patients between 20 and 40 years of age, usually in the proximal tibia, distal radius, distal femur, and sacrum (any other site should suggest some other giant cell–rich tumor). It appears as a lytic expansile mass that extends into the subchondral bone plate. Two points should be stressed: (i) the multinucleated giant cells of a giant cell tumor are *uniformly* scattered throughout the lesion; (ii) mononuclear cells (of histiocytic origin?) are the true neoplastic element, whereas giant cells arise from fusion of mononuclear cells. Multinucleated giant cells in other bone lesions and neoplasms are *unevenly* distributed. In contrast to most bone tumors, the giant cell tumor is more common in females.

17. Correct choice: A

ANEURYSMAL BONE CYST (p. 302)—An aneurysmal bone cyst develops most often in vertebrae and flat bones, but also in the shaft of long bones. Radiologically, it appears as an eccentric, expansile, radiolucent, cystic mass. The lesion is composed of spaces separated by septa that lack endothelial lining and consist of a mixed fibroblastic/myofibroblastic/histiocytic population. When located in the mandible, the main differential diagnosis is with *giant cell reparative granuloma*. The choices include the conditions most important in the differential diagnosis of a cystic hemorrhagic bone lesion.

18. Correct choice: E

SIMPLE CYST (p. 304)—The proximal humerus and proximal femur are the most common sites of this cystic lesion affecting predominantly children and adolescents. This is a unilocular pseudocyst filled with clear or hemorrhagic fluid and lined by a vascular fibrous tissue. Hemosiderin-laden macrophages, cholesterol clefts, and scattered multinucleated giant cells are additional features. It may manifest with pathologic fractures. It is unusual to receive a surgical specimen of simple cysts for pathologic evaluation, as the treatment of choice consists of intracystic injection of methylprednisolone.

19. Correct choice: A

GANGLION CYSTS (p. 304)—This common lesion develops as a result of myxoid degeneration within the joint capsule or tendon sheath. The dorsal aspect of the carpal area is the most frequent location, followed by the volar aspect of the wrist. The lesions consist of a fibrous wall without synovial lining containing mucous fluid.

20. Correct choice: C

FIBROUS DYSPLASIA (p. 305)—Sporadic forms of fibrous dysplasia affecting the jaw tend to occur in young adults and manifest as painless swelling of the jaw. Irregularly shaped (C-shaped or Chinese letter–shaped) trabeculae of woven bone *not* rimmed by osteoblasts and immersed in a fibrous stroma are the histological hallmarks. In *ossifying fibromas*, trabeculae are contoured by osteoblasts; by psammoma bodies in *cementifying fibromas. Juvenile ossifying fibroma* occurs in young females, shows highly cellular stroma, and has an aggressive behavior. Lesions classified in the *fibroma* category tend to be well circumscribed, in contrast to fibrous dysplasia.

21. Correct choice: A

FIBROUS DYSPLASIA, OSTEOFIBROUS DYSPLASIA, AND ALBRIGHT SYNDROME (p. 305)—The previously described bone lesions are consistent with fibrous dysplasia. Fibrous dysplasia can be monostotic (70%) or polyostotic (30%). Of the latter, a minority is due to *Albright syndrome* (also called *McCune-Albright syndrome*), caused by somatic mutations of *c-fox* gene and manifesting with multiple endocrinopathies, precocious puberty, and unilateral skin hyperpigmentation and fibrous dysplasia. In osteofibrous dysplasia, the bone trabeculae are rimmed by osteoblasts.

22. Correct choice: D

METAPHYSEAL FIBROUS DEFECT (p. 306)—Clinical presentation, age, and microscopic features are consistent with a metaphyseal fibrous defect. This is a condition of uncertain etiology (neoplastic, reparative?) and is most often seen in male adolescents in the proximal tibia or distal femur. A *storiform* pattern is the most important clue to diagnosis. Other features, such as hemosiderin deposits and collections of multinucleated giant cells, are nonspecific.

23. Correct choice: C

LANGERHANS CELL HISTIOCYTOSIS (EOSINOPHILIC GRANULOMA; p. 308)—This lesion (also called *eosinophilic granuloma*) appears on x-rays as a well-circumscribed osteolytic lesion mimicking a metastatic carcinoma. Histologically, the differential diagnosis is with *osteomyelitis* and bone involvement by *sinus histiocytosis with massive lymphadenopathy* (Rosai-Dorfman disease). In the latter, predominance of plasma cells and histiocytes is the salient diagnostic feature. Immunoreactivity of Langerhans cells for CD1a and S100, and presence of Birbeck granules on EM, are diagnostic. Solitary involvement of the lungs is seen in up to 50% of cases.

CHAPTER 9

1. Correct choice: D

BREAST IN PREGNANCY (p. 331)—Pregnancy changes of the breast are due to the combined effects of estrogens, progesterone, prolactin, and growth hormone. They consist of marked enlargement/dilatation of lobules, due to increased number of acini, and cytoplasmic vacuolization of luminal cells reflecting increased secretory activity. The cells vary from columnar to cuboidal. Inexperience may result in erroneous diagnosis of malignancy, especially in consideration of occasional areas of necrosis due to infarction.

2. Correct choice: B

BENIGN BREAST DISEASE (BBD; p. 332)—BBD refers to a wide spectrum of morphological changes, some of which are well-defined pathological entities (e.g., fibroadenoma and duct papilloma), whereas others probably represent extreme variations in normal breast morphology rather than pathologic states. *Fibrocystic change* is analogous to BBD, because it encompasses various morphological alterations that differ in pathogenesis and clinical significance. Choice A is characteristic of *epithelial hyperplasia*, choice C of *cysts*, choice D of papilloma, and choice D of *epithelial metaplasia*.

3. Correct choice: D

FIBROCYSTIC CHANGES AND EPITHELIAL HYPERPLASIA (pp. 332 and 338)—Epithelial hyperplasia is the parameter that, depending on degree and type, is correlated with risk of breast cancer development. Epithelial hyperplasia refers to an increased number of ductal epithelial cell layers. Florid epithelial hyperplasia leads to an increased risk of developing carcinoma, especially if there is associated cellular atypia *(atypical ductal hyperplasia)*. *Apocrine metaplasia* is the most common metaplastic change seen in normal breast.

4. Correct choice: E

SCLEROSING ADENOSIS/RADIAL SCAR (p. 334)—Adenosis is an increased number of glandular elements. Pregnancy-related adenosis is physiological. Pathological forms of adenosis cover a spectrum including *sclerosing adenosis* and *radial scar*. This condition may generate confusion with lobular carcinoma (on low power) and with tubular carcinoma (on high power), because of its disorganized, poorly circumscribed, seemingly infiltrative pattern. A low-power view is often more informative than closer examination. The architecture is that of a central focus of fibrosis surrounded by an increased number of acini. The acini appear compressed in the central region and dilated in the peripheral region. The lobular architecture is preserved. The designation of *radial scar* is used when the central region of fibrosis and hyalinization is prominent, and that of *sclerosing papilloma* if papillary formations are conspicuous. In sclerosing adenosis, glandular elements retain a double-cell epithelial layer, but myoepithelial cells may be difficult to appreciate without special immunostains.

5. Correct choice: B

MICROGLANDULAR ADENOSIS (p. 337)—This infrequent form of adenosis lacks the two-layer lining (epithelial–myoepithelial) typical of benign lesions. It consists of tubules containing PAS-positive material. The lack of myoepithelial lining is evident when compared to normal adjacent lobular units. Staining for myoepithelial markers confirms this feature. Myoepithelial cells, in contrast, are present in intraductal papilloma, radial scar, sclerosing adenosis, and tubular adenoma, in which lesions the myoepithelial layer may not be readily apparent on H&E.

6. Correct choice: A

BLUNT DUCT ADENOSIS (p. 338)—This diagnosis is rather controversial, but most authors agree that it refers to an increased number of acini without disruption of lobular architecture. Hypertrophic changes of both epithelial and myoepithelial cells are present. A frequent concomitant change is columnar cell metaplasia, in which luminal cells are tall and have apical snouts. Stromal hyperplasia is seen in the other form of adenosis, that is, sclerosing adenosis.

7. Correct choice: B

EPITHELIAL HYPERPLASIA AND DUCTAL CARCINOMA IN SITU (pp. 338 and 341)—Epithelial hyperplasia refers to an increased number of epithelial cells within preexisting glandular units. *Usual ductal hyperplasia* (UDH) is the term recommended by the World Health Organization (WHO). It runs a spectrum of increasingly severe changes, from mild (increase in thickness up to four cell layers), to moderate (occasional bridging), to severe (complete obliteration of lumen). Severe forms of hyperplasia may be difficult to distinguish from DCIS. It is generally agreed that there is a biological continuum that makes it difficult to operate such a distinction in each individual case. Atypical ductal hyperplasia represents an intermediate stage between severe UDH and DCIS. A number of morphologic criteria may help in differentiating between atypical ductal hyperplasia and DCIS.

10. Correct choice: E

SOLITARY INTRADUCTAL PAPILLOMA (p. 349)—This lesion usually manifests with bloody discharge. It arises from large lactiferous ducts and is composed of branching papillary fronds that fill the lumen. Monoclonality of the lesion has been demonstrated. A myoepithelial layer is present, evident on H&E or immunostaining for myoepithelial markers. The branching papillae contain a fibrovascular core and are lined by cells with oval, regular nuclei and rare mitotic figures. Fibrovascular core and two-cell type lining (epithelial–myoepithelial) are the two most important criteria for distinguishing a benign papillary lesion from papillary carcinoma. Apocrine metaplasia is common in papillomas. Infarction is not rare, accounting for nipple discharge.

11. Correct choice: A

LOBULAR CARCINOMA *IN SITU* (LCIS; p. 352)—LCIS is characterized by expansion of lobules by a monomorphic cell population showing no mitotic activity or necrosis. Cells are often positive for mucin staining, immunoreactive for keratin and EMA, and occasionally for S100. Extension to the ducts may be seen. LCIS

	Epithelial Hyperplasia	DCIS
Architectural features	Slitlike peripheral spaces	Round, rigid spaces throughout the lesion
	Nuclei oriented along the axis of bridges	Nuclei oriented randomly or across bridges
	Streaming pattern present	Streaming pattern absent
Cytological features	Polymorphic cell population: "myoepithelial" cells present	Uniform cell population: "myoepithelial" cells absent
	Indistinct cell margins (syncytium-like)	Cell margins more evident
	Nuclear overlapping and irregular spacing	Even, monotonous nuclear spacing
Additional features	Malignant features absent	Malignant features present
	Apocrine metaplasia may be present	No apocrine metaplasia
	Necrosis rare	Necrosis sometimes conspicuous
Adjacent changes	Periductal fibrosis absent	Periductal fibrosis common
	Gradual transition with other benign lesion	Abrupt transition with benign lesion

8. Correct choice: D

LOBULAR CANCERIZATION (p. 346)—The description indicates lobular cancerization, which results from spread of a ductal carcinoma into the lobular component. Whether this theory is correct or not, the finding of lobular cancerization should prompt a search for an otherwise typical ductal carcinoma in other parts of the specimen. Malignant cells usually expand and distort the lobular unit, often accompanied by a certain degree of fibrosis. A diagnostic error of invasion is particularly likely to occur if lobular cancerization involves an area of sclerosing adenosis, which exaggerates distortion of the acinar architecture.

9. Correct choice: E

DCIS, LOW GRADE AND HIGH GRADE (p. 348)—High-grade, poorly differentiated DCIS shows the features listed here in answers A through D. DCIS cells are seldom positive for estrogen/progesterone receptors. In contrast, low-grade DCIS usually does not express c-*erb*-B2 oncoprotein or p53 oncoprotein; in addition, it has a low proliferation rate and fewer stromal vessels.

is frequently bilateral (70% of cases), and the risk of subsequent breast cancer (ductal or lobular) is increased by eight to ten times compared to the general population. Clinical follow-up is thus necessary. Mastectomy may be advisable in selected instances (e.g., positive family history for breast cancer).

12. Correct choice: A

LOBULAR CANCERIZATION VERSUS LCIS (p. 354)—This differential diagnosis is based mainly on cytological features. Cells of DCIS spreading through the acinar system retain their pleomorphic appearance and large size, and they are cohesive; those of LCIS are smaller and uniform, and they tend to lose their cohesiveness. Lobular architecture is preserved in both, whereas necrosis is more frequent in cancerization. Fibroplasia and inflammatory reactions are more intense around ducts involved by cancerization by DCIS.

13. Correct choice: A

BENIGN BREAST DISEASE AND RISK OF BREAST CANCER (p. 353)—Severe (florid) ductal epithelial hyperplasia is associated with only slightly increased risk of cancer (up to two times). If cellular atypia is present (*atypical epithelial hyperplasia*), breast cancer risk increases substantially, up to four to five times. This risk relates to both breasts. In contrast, DCIS treated by biopsy alone is associated with subsequent development of breast cancer in a very high percentage of patients, from 25% to 75%. The risk in DCIS is related to the *ipsilateral* breast. In DCIS, the probability of regional node metastasis at the time of presentation is approximately 1%. The risk of breast cancer in LCIS treated by biopsy is within the range of 20% to 35% and relates to *both* breasts.

14. Correct choice: A

GRADING OF INFILTRATING DUCTAL CARCINOMA (pp. 357 and 358)—The system developed by Bloom and Richardson, modified by Elston and Ellis, is based on three parameters: nuclear morphology, mitotic count, and tubule formation. The details given in the question stem correpond to a grade 1 (well-differentiated) carcinoma. Grading of breast carcinoma may be accomplished by two approaches: a combined method considering architecture (i.e., tubule formation), nuclear grading, and mitotic rate; or nuclear grading alone. Although the former method (Bloom and Richardson) is applicable to ductal carcinomas only, the latter can be used for all breast cancer types. Expression of estrogen and progesterone receptors is valuable in predicting response to hormonal therapy. Vascular invasion has prognostic significance as well.

15. Correct choice: A

PROGNOSTIC AND PREDICTIVE FACTORS IN BREAST CANCER (p. 358)—*Prognostic* factors are used to assess the prognosis at the time of diagnosis; *predictive* factors instead correlate with response to a specific treatment. All of the choices are prognostic factors, of which metastatic lymph node status is the most significant. The absence of axillary lymph node metastases is associated with 80% survival at 10 years. With up to three nodes involved, the survival rate is approximately 40%, and 15% with more than ten nodes involved. Expression of estrogen/progesterone receptors is a predictive factor, useful in assessing the likelihood of a favorable response to tamoxifen therapy. Measurement of HER2/*neu* gene expression has been recently accepted in clinical management to select patients for treatment with a monoclonal antibody that targets the HER2/*neu* protein.

16. Correct choice: B

INFILTRATING LOBULAR CARCINOMA (p. 358)—This type represents approximately 10% of invasive breast cancer. The arrangement in single lines of cell and targetoid formations is highly characteristic. Infiltrating lobular carcinoma has the following clinicopathological features: often bilateral and multicentric; a marked propensity to infiltrate surrounding tissue in a diffuse manner; a high frequency of metastatic spread to cerebrospinal fluid, ovary, pleura, peritoneum, and bone marrow; mutations and lack of expression of *E-cadherin* gene. Low cellular density, lack of necrosis, and infrequent mitoses may lead to false-negative diagnoses, particularly during intraoperative consultation. Several variants are described: solid, alveolar, tubulolobular, and pleomorphic. Interestingly, the classic type of infiltrating lobular carcinoma usually does not overexpress HER2/*neu* gene, whereas the pleomorphic type does.

17. Correct choice: E

TUBULAR CARCINOMA (p. 360)—Tubular carcinoma is a rare subtype of breast adenocarcinoma, which is composed of well-differentiated regularly formed tubules with a characteristic angular outline. Occasionally, the well-differentiated appearance of the neoplastic tubules is erroneously interpreted as a benign change. Axillary metastases are infrequent at the time of diagnosis (less than 10% of cases). The prognosis is good. This tumor type is often confused with sclerosing adenosis and microglandular adenosis.

18. Correct choice: B

MUCINOUS CARCINOMA (p. 361)—Mucinous carcinoma is characterized by abundant extracellular mucin production, so that neoplastic cells seem to float in a sea of mucin. This variant (less than 5% of all breast cancer) occurs predominantly in elderly women and is associated with a lower rate of nodal metastasis and longer survival. Grossly, mucinous carcinomas are well circumscribed. Tumor cells frequently express hormone receptors.

19. Correct choice: E

PROGNOSIS OF MUCINOUS CARCINOMA (p. 361)—It is generally agreed that a specific type of breast cancer may be diagnosed if at least 90% of the tumor shows that given pattern. However, mucinous tumors are an exception, because a favorable prognosis applies only to those cases in which the *entire* tumor is composed of mucinous carcinoma.

20. Correct choice: B

MEDULLARY CARCINOMA (p. 362)—This variant is infrequent (2% to 3% of all breast cancer), tends to affect younger women, and is disproportionately represented in women carrying BRCA-1 mutations. Histologically, it is characterized by marked pleomorphism and mitotic activity. However, it is well circumscribed and surrounded by a florid lymphoplasmacytic reaction. The tumor has a soft texture, which accounts for its designation. It is associated with a better prognosis than conventional ductal carcinoma. Retention or overexpression of adhesion molecules may account for its pushing pattern of growth, cohesiveness of tumor cells, and limited metastatic potential.

21. Correct choice: C

MICROPAPILLARY CARCINOMA (p. 363)—This rare form of breast cancer is characterized histologically by tubuloalveolar or micropapillary formations lacking fibrovascular cores and surrounded by a clear space. Lymphatic/vascular invasion is observed in 33% to 67% of cases. Most cases of micropapillary carcinoma are found in association with infiltrating ductal carcinoma (NOS) or mucinous carcinoma. Presence of a micropapillary pattern is a negative prognostic indicator.

22. Correct choice: A

ADENOID CYSTIC CARCINOMA (p. 364)—Some breast tumors exhibit morphological features virtually identical to analogous tumors of salivary or sweat glands. Adenoid cystic carcinoma exhibits glandular lumina along with pseudocysts containing basement membrane–like (glassy and eosinophilic) material. The large pseudocystic spaces contain Alcian blue–positive, PAS-negative material (hyaluronic acid), whereas the true glandular lumina contain PAS-positive, Alcian blue–negative material (neutral mucin). The pseudocystic spaces are immunoreactive with antibodies to basement membrane components. In contrast to the salivary gland tumor, breast adenoid cystic carcinoma has a good prognosis.

23. Correct choice: D

SECRETORY (JUVENILE) CARCINOMA (p. 364)—The secretory type is the most common malignant breast tumor in childhood, but otherwise a rare form of cancer. It is characterized by irregular epithelial islands containing numerous glandular lumina with PAS-positive secretions. Nuclear pleomorphism is mild and mitotic figures are inconspicuous.

24. Correct choice: A

APOCRINE CARCINOMA (p. 365)—This rare variant is characterized by large cells with prominent cytoplasmic eosinophilia, conspicuous nucleoli, apical snouts, and numerous mitochondria on EM. Because focal apocrine differentiation is often present in other types of breast carcinoma, a diagnosis of apocrine carcinoma is justified when the apocrine changes involve at least 90% of the mass. An interesting feature is frequent expression of GCDFP-15, a marker of apocrine differentiation. This marker is probably prolactin-inducible protein (PIP).

25. Correct choice: E

INFLAMMATORY BREAST CANCER (p. 367)—This form is associated with a rapidly growing cancer that infiltrates dermal lymphatics. This leads to swelling and erythema of the breast simulating an inflammatory condition (hence the clinical designation). It should be noted that *inflammatory* carcinoma is not a histopathologic subtype. It is a clinical manifestation that may be associated with different types of invasive breast carcinoma. It implies, however, a poor prognosis.

26. Correct choice: E

PAGET DISEASE OF THE NIPPLE (p. 367)—Paget disease of the breast refers to spread of an underlying breast carcinoma to the epidermis of the nipple. Up to two-thirds of cases are associated with an underlying carcinoma, which may be in situ or invasive. Prognosis depends on the extent of the underlying carcinoma. Paget cells have abundant slightly eosinophilic vacuolated cytoplasm and prominent nucleoli. They are immunoreactive for EMA, low-molecular-weight keratin, and typically for HER2/*neu*, but not for S100 or HMB-45. Melanoma and Bowen disease should be considered in the differential diagnosis. Clinically, the condition manifests with crusted erythema of the nipple and areola. Paget cells should not be confused with *Toker clear cells*, normally found in the nipple epidermis.

27. Correct choice: C

CARCINOMA OF MALE BREAST (p. 367)—Male breast cancer accounts for less than 1% of all cases of breast cancer. It usually develops in elderly men, and gynecomastia is *not* a risk factor. The majority of cases express hormonal receptors. Prognosis is superimposable to that of women. Patients with Klinefelter syndrome have an increased risk for breast carcinoma.

28. Correct choice: A

FIBROADENOMA (p. 370)—This benign lesion (only less than 1 out of 1,000 cases show malignant transformation) typically occurs in young women and manifests as a well-demarcated mobile nodule within the breast parenchyma. As the designation implies, histologically the lesion is composed of both a stromal and an epithelial component. The stromal component appears to be the true neoplastic element. *Complex fibroadenoma* refers to fibroadenomas containing cystic change, sclerosing adenosis, papillary apocrine metaplasia, or epithelial calcifications: These are said to have increased risk of malignant behavior.

29. Correct choice: D

JUVENILE FIBROADENOMA (p. 371)—This variant of fibroadenoma is characterized by three features: the young patient's age, large size, and hypercellularity of the stromal and/or epithelial component. A characteristic tufted or gynecomastoid pattern is seen in the tubular component, in which tufts of epithelial cells protrude into the lumen. Juvenile fibroadenoma is more frequent in blacks. It often recurs after excision. It is important to distinguish it from *phyllodes tumor*, which affects older women and is characterized by high cellularity and increased mitoses in the stroma.

30. Correct choice: D

PHYLLODES TUMOR (p. 373)—The phyllodes tumor shares similarities with fibroadenoma: It originates from intralobular stroma and is accompanied by a nonneoplastic glandular component. Nodules of proliferating stroma are lined by epithelium in a leaflike configuration. This tumor affects older women (45 years is the median age of incidence) and has a propensity to recur and occasionally metastasize. Its metastatic potential is in relation to the degree of cellular anaplasia. Thus, cellular density of stroma, cytological atypia, and mitotic activity are prognostically relevant factors. High-grade lesions are similar to poorly differentiated sarcomas. Extensive sampling is recommended to assess malignant features, because histological heterogeneity is in phyllodes tumors the rule rather than the exception.

31. Correct choice: D

PERILOBULAR HEMANGIOMA (p. 375)—This is the most common form of breast vascular lesions and is so named because of its characteristic perilobular arrangement. Thin-walled capillary channels surround, but do not invade, lobular units and are devoid of atypia or mitoses. The most important task is to differentiate perilobular hemangiomas from angiosarcomas, which are composed of anastomosing channels that invade the lobules and show atypia and mitoses.

32. Correct choice: A

LYMPHANGIOSARCOMA (p. 376)—Most cases arise in the setting of long-standing lymphedema, such as after surgical excision of lymph nodes for cancer (breast cancer: *Stewart-Treves syndrome*) or chronic infections (filariasis). A smaller percentage arises following radiation, and a few around foreign bodies. Thorotrast and PVC exposure have been associated with angiosarcomas of the liver. Angiosarcomas usually occur in the skin of the head and neck of elderly men.

33. Correct choice: C

NIPPLE ADENOMA (p. 377)—Also called *florid papillomatosis of the nipple*, this lesion presents with nipple discharge and occasionally erosions (clinically, it may be confused with Paget disease). It is composed of florid glandulopapillary formations filling the large ducts. The main differential diagnosis is with syringomatous adenoma (characteristic comma-shaped glands) and with tubular carcinoma. Dual-cell population (epithelial and myoepithelial), oval nuclei, and peripheral clefts are features favoring a benign process. Foci of necrosis should not be interpreted as evidence of malignancy, as in intraductal papillomas.

34. Correct choice: A

ADENOMYOEPITHELIOMA (p. 380)—This rare tumor arises, in part, from myoepithelial cells, which appear as cuboidal cells expressing myoepithelial markers (S100 protein, actin, etc.). It may recur, but rarely metastasizes. The malignant counterpart is designated as myoepithelial carcinoma, which is characterized by obvious cytological atypia. Myoepithelial cells may be seen in other types of breast neoplasms.

35. Correct choice: E

ACUTE PURULENT MASTITIS (p. 381)—Purulent inflammation with neutrophil collection within the lumen of a large duct, with subsequent abscess formation, is generally due to *S. aureus* and develops almost exclusively in the lactating breast.

36. Correct choice: B
FAT NECROSIS (382)—This benign lesion often develops after trauma, accidental or surgical. An area of necrotic fat is surrounded by a rim of lipid-laden macrophages. Eventually, organization ensues, with granulation tissue and formation of a fibrous capsule. Foreign body giant cells, calcium deposits, and hemosiderin are frequent.

37. Correct choice: D
MAMMARY DUCT ECTASIA (p. 382)—This condition (also known as *periductal mastitis*) presents in multiparous women in their forties or fifties as a poorly circumscribed subareolar nodule, often accompanied by nipple retraction. Because of these features, it is often biopsied to rule out malignancy. Histologically, it consists of dilated ducts filled with inspissated secretion and surrounded by florid chronic inflammation. Plasma cells are numerous, justifying the old designation of plasma cell mastitis. A granulomatous reaction and fibrosis may develop, resulting in nipple retraction.

38. Correct choice: E
DIABETIC MASTOPATHY (p. 383)—This obscure inflammatory breast condition is morphologically equivalent to *lymphocytic lobulitis*. It occurs predominantly in women with type I diabetes and is characterized by perilobular chronic inflammation leading to lobular atrophy and diffuse fibrosis. Multifocal painful nodules represent the most usual clinical presentation. Choice A describes *duct ectasia*, in which a periductal chronic inflammation is associated with marked dilatation of ducts; choice B, *chronic granulomatous mastitis*, of uncertain pathogenesis and associated with a granulomatous reaction centering on lobules; and choice D, *fat necrosis*.

39. Correct choice: E
PSEUDOANGIOMATOUS HYPERPLASIA (p. 385)—This benign lesion is of a reactive nature and probably due to hormonal influences. The slitlike spaces result from artifactual retraction. The characteristic immunophenotype includes positivity for CD34 and vimentin and lack of factor VIII–related antigen. This lesion may be confused with angiosarcoma.

40. Correct choice: C
COLLAGENOUS SPHERULOSIS (p. 386)—This change may be associated with other breast lesions such as sclerosing adenosis. It consists of a focus of epithelial/myoepithelial hyperplasia surrounding characteristic round spherules that contain basement membrane–like material, and thus stain positively for collagen type IV. This benign change should not be confused with adenoid cystic carcinoma or other epithelial cancer.

CHAPTER 10

1. Correct choice: E
REACTIVE GLIOSIS AND ROSENTHAL FIBERS (p. 408)—Rosenthal fibers result from accumulation of α-B-crystallin and glial fibrillary acidic protein (GFAP) in hypertrophic processes of reactive astrocytes. They are seen in any form of reactive gliosis, as well as in association with certain tumors (particularly in *pilocytic astrocytomas*) and around brain neoplasms (e.g., *craniopharyngioma* and *hemangioblastoma*). Some nonneoplastic conditions, such as hemangiomas and old infarcts, may elicit florid reactive gliosis

containing Rosenthal fibers. Alexander disease is a rare form of hereditary leukodystrophy due to GFAP gene mutations: It is associated with innumerable Rosenthal fibers in the white matter, perivascular, and subpial regions. Note: Reactive gliosis may accompany any central nervous system (CNS) lesion.

2. Correct choice: C
HSV ENCEPHALITIS (p. 417)—Viral encephalitides produce similar chronic inflammatory changes, regardless of the underlying etiologic agent. Perivascular lymphocytic cuffing, aggregates of microglial, histiocytic, and lymphocytic cells (*microglial nodules*), neuronal degeneration, and reactive gliosis are the usual features. HSV encephalitis is the most common *sporadic* (nonepidemic) form of viral encephalitis. A correct pathologic diagnosis is essential because effective therapy is available. The most important morphologic clue as to the underlying etiology is the *Cowdry type A* inclusions, which are nuclear eosinophilic inclusions surrounded by a clear halo seen in neurons and glia. Polymerase chain reaction (PCR) may be used for rapid HSV identification.

3. Correct choice: E
PROGRESSIVE MULTIFOCAL ENCEPHALOPATHY (p. 418)—PML is due to a papovavirus known as JC virus (from the initials of the first patient in whom the virus was identified). The virus affects oligodendroglia, causing widespread and multifocal white matter destruction mimicking multiple sclerosis. Histologically, multifocal myelin degeneration, bizarre astrocytes, and oligodendroglia with intranuclear inclusions are appreciated. Sometimes, a biopsy of PML lesions may be erroneously interpreted as malignant glioma because of bizarre astrocytes. Knowledge of the clinical history (immune depression) and MRI findings (multifocal white matter lesions) assist in the diagnosis.

4. Correct choice: B
HIV ENCEPHALITIS (p. 419)—HIV encephalitis (clinically referred to as *AIDS-associated cognitive/motor complex* or *AIDS dementia complex*) results from the direct spread of HIV to the CNS through macrophages. The typical histopathologic features are those mentioned in this case. Multinucleated giant cells in the context of multifocal chronic inflammation and microglial nodules are virtually pathognomonic of HIV encephalitis.

5. Correct choice: A
HIV AND TUMORS (p. 420)—There is no increased risk of developing any type of glial tumors in patients with HIV infection. The most common AIDS-related neoplasms are non-Hodgkin lymphomas and Kaposi sarcoma. The incidence of cervical squamous cell carcinoma is definitely increased in HIV-positive women, and there is recent evidence that leiomyosarcoma is associated with Epstein-Barr virus in HIV-positive patients. A cerebral ring-enhancing lesion in an AIDS patient is either lymphoma or toxoplasma abscess until proven otherwise.

6. Correct choice: D
CAVERNOUS ANGIOMA (p. 426)—The two most common vascular lesions that come to the surgical pathologist include cavernous angioma and arteriovenous malformation (AVM). Cavernous angioma consists of thin-walled dilated vessels with little or no intervening brain parenchyma, so that their walls are frequently back to back. Hemosiderin deposition resulting from discrete bleeding is often seen around the lesion. Seizures are the most common clinical presentation of cavernous angiomas, which are frequently asymptomatic. AVM consists of a conglomerate of abnormal vascular structures that include arteries, veins, and

dysplastic vessels with discontinuous elastic lamina. Acute hemorrhage is the most common presentation of AVMs.

7. Correct choice: A

CEREBRAL AMYLOID ANGIOPATHY (CAA; p. 427)—Bleeding due to CAA is commonly seen in elderly patients, with or without associated Alzheimer-type dementia. Because CAA affects cortical and leptomeningeal vessels, hemorrhage is cortical based and displays a "lobar" distribution. It is due to the accumulation of *amyloid A4* (beta-amyloid) within the vascular walls. Congo red staining and/or immunohistochemistry for amyloid A4 confirms the diagnosis. The most frequent causes of intracerebral bleeding include the following:

- Hypertension (basal ganglia, cerebellum, and pons)
- Bleeding diathesis (petechiae in white matter)
- Vascular malformations (particularly arteriovenous malformations)
- Infections (multiple bleedings, white matter, and/or gray–white matter junction)
- Trauma (usually associated with parenchymal contusion)
- Amyloid angiopathy

Rupture of berry aneurysms may lead to intraparenchymal bleeding as well.

8. Correct choice: C

RELATIVE INCIDENCE OF BRAIN TUMORS (p. 429)—Approximately 50% of brain tumors are *metastatic*. The following table contains a simplified classification of primary brain tumors with their relative incidence rates (note that *gliomas* account for 50% of primary brain tumors; of these, glioblastoma multiforme (GBM) is the most common).

9. Correct choice: A

PILOCYTIC ASTROCYTOMA (PA; p. 437)—This tumor occurs predominantly in children and young adults. The cerebellar hemisphere and the hypothalamic/suprasellar region are the most common locations. The biphasic pattern of alternating densely fibrillary and loosely structured areas is highly characteristic. Like all astrocytomas, this tumor is immunoreactive for GFAP. Rosenthal fibers are typically found in this tumor. Nuclear pleomorphism may be marked, and some mitotic activity may be found, but the tumor is usually well-circumscribed and slow growing. Thus, a grade 1 is attributed to PA in the WHO system. Tumors in a diencephalic location, however, may be less amenable to total resection and have a worse prognosis.

10. Correct choice: B

GRADE 2 (DIFFUSE) ASTROCYTOMA (p. 438)—In evaluating a brain biopsy for neoplasms, the following step-by-step method is advisable:

- Is it normal brain tissue? The cellular density of normal brain is rather low: Gray matter usually shows a mixture of large and small neurons plus glial cells. White matter is mainly composed of oligodendroglia (small uniform cells with a perinuclear halo).
- If the cellular density is increased, is it a tumor or a reactive process? Reactive processes are characterized by mildly increased cellularity with uniformly distributed hypertrophic astrocytes and, depending on the condition, inflammatory cells. Neoplastic lesions are characterized by increased cellularity, nuclear pleomorphism, and other features of anaplasia.
- If this is a neoplasm, is it primary or metastatic? Primary brain neoplasms (gliomas) retain the morphology of normal cellular

Tissue of origin	Neoplasms	Frequency
Glial cells: Gliomas	Astrocytes: astrocytomas	80%
	Oligodendrocytes: oligodendroglioma	5%–50%
		10%
	Ependymal cells: ependymoma	8%
	Choroid plexus epithelium: choroid plexus papilloma	1%–2%
Meninges (arachnoid)	Meningioma	15%
Primitive neuroectodermal precursors	Primitive neuroectodermal tumors (PNET), including:	6%–8%
	Medulloblastoma (posterior fossa)	
	Pineoblastoma (pineal gland)	
	Retinoblastoma (retina)	
	Central neuroblastoma (cerebral hemispheres)	
Anterior pituitary	Pituitary adenoma	6%–8%
Schwann cells (cranial or spinal nerves)	Schwannoma	6%
Neuronal (ganglionic) precursors	Ganglioglioma (mixed neuronal and glial neoplasm)	0.5%–1%
	Gangliocytoma (pure neuronal neoplasm)	
	Central neurocytoma	
Misplaced embryonal rests	Odontogenic epithelium: craniopharyngioma	3%
	Germ cells: dysgerminoma, teratoma, etc.	1%–2%
	Endoderm (intestinal epithelium): colloid cyst	0.5%–1%
	Skin: epidermoid and dermoid cysts	0.5%–1%
Uncertain origin	Hemangioblastoma	1%–2%
Lymphocytes	Lymphoma	1%
Notochord (remnants)	Chordoma	<0.5%

components, astrocytes (*astrocytomas*), oligodendroglia (*oligodendrogliomas*), or ependyma (*ependymomas*). *Gliomas* (the most common intracerebral neoplasms) show a characteristic fibrillary background.

- If this is a primary brain tumor, is it astrocytic or oligodendroglial? (Ependymomas are found in specific locations and age groups.) Astrocytic tumors have irregular nuclear features and a dense fibrillary background, whereas oligodendrogliomas are characterized by the fried-egg appearance of cells and a delicate fibrillary background.
- If this is a glioma, is it low grade or high grade? Low-grade gliomas have increased cellular density and cytological pleomorphism, but no mitotic activity, microvascular proliferation, or necrosis.

11. Correct choice: D

SUBEPENDYMAL GIANT CELL ASTROCYTOMA (SEGA) AND TUBEROUS SCLEROSIS (p. 440)—SEGA is a peculiar tumor that grows from the walls of the lateral ventricles. It is pathognomonic of *tuberous sclerosis* (TS), which is due to mutations of TSC1 or TSC2 genes. TS manifests with multiple hamartomatous lesions in the skin, CNS, and visceral organs. Cortical tubers are malformative (hamartomatous) nodules, probably resulting from faulty cortical development. Other lesions include shagreen patches and ash-leaf patches of the skin, cardiac myomas, renal angiomyolipomas, and so on.

12. Correct choice: D

OLIGODENDROGLIOMA (p. 441)—Tumors of oligodendroglial origin resemble normal oligodendroglia in their cytological phenotype: Round uniform nuclei and perinuclear halos make these cells appear like fried eggs. Generally, oligodendrogliomas are slowly growing tumors located in subcortical white matter of the cerebral hemispheres. Calcifications are frequent. Although slowly growing, oligodendrogliomas ultimately have a negative prognosis. Their infiltrative behavior prevents complete surgical resection. Like astrocytomas, these tumors eventually progress to more malignant forms. However, oligodendrogliomas are responsive to chemotherapy and have a better prognosis than astrocytomas of the same grade.

13. Correct choice: D

GLIOBLASTOMA MULTIFORME/GRADE 4 ASTROCYTOMA (p. 443)—The two major grading systems of astrocytomas are those of *Daumas-Duport* (also referred to as *St. Anne-Mayo*) and the *WHO*. They are similar.

- *Grade 2 astrocytoma* is well differentiated and characterized by increased cellular density and cellular atypia (nuclear pleomorphism), but *no* mitotic activity.
- *Grade 3 astrocytoma* shows mitotic activity, but *no* necrosis or microvascular hyperplasia.
- *Grade 4 astrocytomas* (also called *glioblastoma multiforme*) has cytological anaplasia, mitotic activity, *plus* necrosis and/or microvascular proliferation.

Microvascular hyperplasia consists of hyperplasia of the endothelial/perithelial cells in capillary vessels, often leading to glomeruloid formations.

14. Correct choice: B

EPENDYMOMA (p. 448)—Ependymomas derive from ependymal cells and thus develop in proximity to cerebral ventricules.

Neoplastic cells tend to arrange themselves around small vessels as *perivascular pseudorosettes* or around a small lumen as *ependymal rosettes*. Ependymoma is a grade 2 tumor according to the WHO classification. Although slowly growing and well demarcated, the tumor has a propensity to recur as a progressively more malignant, less differentiated glioma.

15. Correct choice: B

MYXOPAPILLARY EPENDYMOMA (p. 450)—This variant of ependymoma is grade 1. It is characterized by spindly ependymal cells arranged in a fascicular and papillary pattern within a myxoid intercellular matrix. It usually occurs in the distal segment of the spinal cord, that is, the *conus medullaris*. A definitive cure is achieved by total excision.

16. Correct choice: C

MEDULLOBLASTOMA (p. 458)—This neoplasm is composed of uniform small cells with high nucleocytoplasmic ratio and molding nuclei. A helpful morphological feature is the presence of *Homer-Wright rosettes* (neuroblastic type), consisting of a fibrillary core surrounded by tumor cells. Medulloblastoma is the most common of PNETs, affecting infancy and childhood and including medulloblastoma, pineoblastoma, retinoblastoma, central neuroblastoma, and ependymoblastoma. These tumors are thought to derive from a putative primordial cell precursor. Some authors prefer to use the term PNET for all these neoplasms. PNETs are WHO grade 4 tumors, that is, highly aggressive. PNETs may show neuronal differentiation (synaptophysin expression), astrocytic (GFAP), both, or neither.

17. Correct choice: E

MENINGIOMA (p. 460)—Meningioma is the most common benign primary intracranial tumor. It is attached to the dura and pushes the underlying brain, without infiltrating the parenchyma. Most sporadic meningiomas show monosomy of chromosome 22. Loss of the NF-1 gene on chromosome 22 is associated with meningiomas occurring in the neurofibromatosis type. Meningiomas exhibit a wide range of morphological patterns, the most frequent being meningotheliomatous, transitional, and fibrous (the latter shown in this case). Diagnostic features include a syncytial appearance of tumor cells, whorl formation, intranuclear pseudoinclusions, and psammoma bodies. The most common variants are grade I tumors. The *papillary, chordoid*, and *clear cell* variants are grade 2 and behave more aggressively than the most common forms. Choice A is frequent in olfactory neuroblastoma, choice B is most frequent in medulloblastomas, choice C is present in 90% of oligodendrogliomas, and choice D is frequent in anaplastic astrocytoma progressing to GBM.

18. Correct choice: C

CHORDOMA (p. 469)—This tumor arises from notochordal remnants distributed along the midline, from the base of the skull (clivus) to the sacrum. The clivus and sacrum are the first and second most common sites. Cellular composition is characteristic: vacuolated cells arranged in chords and nests within a mucinous background. Positivity for epithelial markers (EMA and keratin) is typically associated with immunoreactivity for S100. The lesion is bone destructive and usually recurs after surgical resection. Occasionally, it may give rise to lung, lymph node, or skin metastases. The most important differential diagnosis is with chondrosarcoma. Chondroid differentiation can be usually appreciated on H&E. Chondrosarcomas are immunoreactive for S100, but not for EMA or keratin.

19. Correct choice: B
GERM CELL TUMORS of CNS (p. 473)—The great majority of germ cell tumors develop in the sellar/suprasellar region: most of them are *germinomas* and *teratomas*. Mature teratoma is the most common type of sacrococcygeal germ cell tumor. Up to 90% of them occur in females. If present at birth, they are most often benign; if the tumor becomes clinically apparent after 2 months of age, it is usually malignant. The most common malignant form in the sacrococcygeal region is the yolk sac tumor. There is no particular association with spina bifida.

20. Correct choice: E
HEMANGIOBLASTOMA (pp. 479–481)—This benign neoplasm of uncertain histogenesis develops most frequently in the posterior fossa, but may occur in supratentorial and spinal regions. It is composed of foamy, vacuolated cells (the true neoplastic elements) amid a rich vascular network. Patients with von Hippel-Lindau may develop cerebellar and retinal hemangioblastomas as well as renal cell carcinoma. Choice A is associated with dysplastic cerebellar gangliocytoma (a malformative rather than neoplastic lesion); choice B with neurofibromas; choice C with various brain tumors, especially schwannomas of the eighth nerve; and choice D with cortical tubers and SEGA.

21. Correct choice: D
BRAIN METASTASES (p. 482)—The three metastatic brain tumors that most frequently manifest with intracranial bleeding include renal cell carcinoma, melanoma, and choriocarcinoma. Intracerebral hemorrhage may also be the initial manifestation of primary brain neoplasms, particularly glioblastoma and oligodendroglioma. Metastatic tumors are often multiple, sharply circumscribed, and localized at the junction between gray and white matter. Primary tumors that most often metastasize to the brain are those of *lung, breast, melanoma, kidney*, and *colon*. Although rare, choriocarcinoma displays a striking tendency to spread to the brain.

22. Correct choice: A
COLLOID CYST (p. 488)—A colloid cyst contains mucinous or protein-rich fluid and is typically located in the midline of the third ventricle. It probably develops from endodermal remnants, accounting for its respiratory-type epithelium. This lesion usually manifests with recurrent signs and symptoms of increased intracranial pressure in middle-aged patients (headache and nausea). Increased intracranial pressure is secondary to obstruction of the *foramen of Monro*.

23. Correct choice: B
CYSTS WITH MURAL NODULE (pp. 436, 437, 452, 479)—Such gross appearance, appreciable on CT/MRI scans is characteristic of at least three tumors, all of which are benign (WHO grade 1). These include *pilocytic astrocytoma, hemangioblastoma,* and *ganglioglioma*. The mural nodule is contrast enhancing. Craniopharyngioma also contains multiple cysts. Epidermoid tumor is usually composed on a unilocular cyst with uniform thin walls and keratin-filled lumen. All PNETs (medulloblastoma, pineoblastoma, etc.) have a solid pattern. Oligodendroglioma and low-grade astrocytomas are intraparenchymal tumors with a diffuse, mostly solid growth. GBM characteristically shows a variegated gross appearance with areas of hemorrhage and necrosis. Metastases may be partially cystic.

24. Correct choice: A
ALZHEIMER DISEASE (p. 490)—The intraneuronal inclusions described are neurofibrillary tangles (NFTs), which consist of paired helical filaments derived from altered *tau* protein. These changes are not pathognomonic of Alzheimer disease (AD) as they are present, in small numbers, in the brains of intellectually normal individuals. However, finding numerous NFTs in the neocortex is virtually diagnostic of AD. It should be noted that a diagnosis of AD relies on special stains that demonstrate NFTs and senile plaques (SPs). SP consists of a core *amyloid A4* deposit surrounded by dystrophic neuronal processes and reactive glia. Both NFT and SP can be demonstrated by using Bielschowsky or analogous silver impregnation techniques. Alternatively, immunohistochemistry for tau or amyloid A4 may be used to visualize NFT and, respectively, SPs.

25. Correct choice: C
PARKINSON DISEASE (p. 492)—Parkinson disease can be confirmed at autopsy by demonstrating loss of dopaminergic (pigmented) neurons in the substantia nigra as well as typical neuronal inclusions referred to as *Lewy bodies*. These are round eosinophilic intracytoplasmic bodies on H&E. Lewy bodies contain α-synuclein, detectable by immunohistochemistry. Choices A and B are found in pyramidal neurons of the hippocampus in normal aging and Alzheimer disease, choice D in intranuclear eosinophilic bodies of unknown significance in substantia nigra neurons, and choice E in *rabies*, particularly in Purkinje neurons and hippocampal pyramidal neurons.

CHAPTER 11

1. Correct choice: E
GENERAL NEUROENDOCRINE MARKERS (pp. 508 and 509)—The general markers are found in most neuroendocrine neoplasms, even though they may lack both sensitivity and specificity. Neuron-specific enolase is characteristic of nerve cells and is found in neuroendocrine and nonneuroendocrine cells. Chromogranins are associated with dense-core granules, but are difficult to demonstrate in cells that contain only a few dense-core granules, such as small cell carcinoma of the lung. Bombesin is found in gastrointestinal (GI) and pulmonary neoplasms. Leu-7 is found in many neuroendocrine neoplasms, but is also seen in lymphoid cells. ACTH, though a specific hormone, has widespread expression among neuroendocrine neoplasms, but represents a specific peptide hormone.

CHAPTER 12

1. Correct choice: C
PITUITARY ADENOMA (p. 529)—A pituitary adenoma may have sheetlike, papillary, and trabecular patterns. Typical of pituitary adenomas is the loss of the reticulin network of the normal adenohypophysis, as evident in the picture, which demonstrates a peripheral rim of compressed pituitary gland. Pituitary adenomas account for approximately 10% of intracranial neoplasms. *Microadenomas* measure less than 1 cm, and *macroadenomas* measure more than 1 cm. *Functioning* adenomas are usually microadenomas and become clinically apparent with an endocrine syndrome related to the specific hormone produced. In contrast, macroadenomas are usually hormonally inactive and manifest by compression of nearby structures, for example, chiasm with visual deficits. Prolactinomas are the most frequent of functioning adenomas.

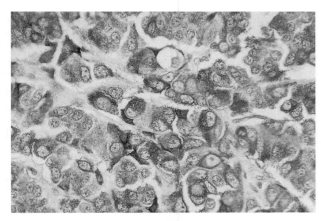

ANSWER 12.1

Hyperprolactinemia manifests with amenorrhea galactorrhea in women.

2. Correct choice: D
PROLACTINOMA AND BROMOCRIPTINE (pp. 533–535)—Almost 50% of all functioning pituitary adenomas secrete prolactin (growth hormone, GH, and ACTH follow in order of frequency). Prolactinomas can be treated with dopamine agonists such as bromocriptine, which inhibits prolactin secretion. Bromocriptine results in gradual shrinkage of the tumor with diffuse interstitial fibrosis, without evidence of tumor necrosis or generation. Because bromocriptine is not tumoricidal, the treatment is not curative. Apoplexy refers to hemorrhage within a pituitary adenoma or hypertrophic pituitary (e.g., in pregnancy), which results in rapid expansion of the pituitary gland.

3. Correct choice: D
CRANIOPHARYNGIOMA (p. 542)—This histologically benign tumor is thought to arise from misplaced odontogenic epithelium and is morphologically similar to adamantinoma (ameloblastoma). It develops in the suprasellar region and often contains cystic spaces and abundant calcium deposits. Children are most often affected. Histologically, it contains tongues of well-differentiated epithelium with peripheral palisading and central *stellate reticulum*, multifocal deposits of *wet keratin* (i.e., with ghost keratinized cells), and calcifications. A *papillary* variant is described, which tends to affect middle-aged persons. Craniopharyngiomas do not metastasize, but recur frequently after surgery.

4. Correct choice: A
EMPTY SELLA SYNDROME (p. 549)—The *primary* form is due to an arachnoidal diverticulum that herniates through a defect of the sellar diaphragm and exerts a compression on the pituitary gland. Approximately 50% of adults have an incompetent sellar diaphragm, and 5% have an empty sella. Choices B through E are the most common causes of the *secondary* form. Clinical manifestations include visual deficits due to chiasmal prolapse and impaired endocrine function secondary to traction on the pituitary stalk.

CHAPTER 13

1. Correct choice: E
HETEROTOPIC THYROID (p. 557)—Heterotopic thyroid tissue can be found anywhere in the region of the thyroglossal duct and below the thyroid in the substernal region, the so-called *Wölfler's triangle*, with the base at the mandible and the apex at the aortic arch. Thyroid tissue may be found in lymph nodes, esophagus, larynx, trachea, heart, and great vessels, but the most frequent location is the posterior tongue close to the foramen cecum. Here, heterotopic thyroid is present in up to 10% of individuals. Conversely, parathyroid, salivary gland, thymus, adipose, and muscle tissue may be found in the thyroid.

2. Correct choice: E
SUBACUTE (GRANULOMATOUS) THYROIDITIS (p. 559)—Also called *de Quervain thyroiditis*, this condition affects mostly female patients aged 30 to 50 usually following an episode of upper respiratory infection. It presents with neck pain exacerbated by swallowing, thyroid enlargement, transient hyperthyroidism, and systemic symptoms. The clinical picture resolves spontaneously. Nonnecrotizing granulomas constitute the histopathologic hallmark of de Quervain thyroiditis. Histiocytes and multinucleated giant cells often contain colloid material. Coxsackievirus, mumps, measles, and adenovirus are suspected to trigger this condition.

3. Correct choice B
HASHIMOTO THYROIDITIS (p. 560)—Extensive lymphocytic inflammation with germinal centers and Hürthle cells are characteristic of Hashimoto thyroiditis. Hürthle cells are follicular cells with abundant eosinophilic granular cytoplasm and clear nuclei similar to those of papillary carcinoma. It manifests initially with thyroid enlargement and symptoms of hyperthyroidism, and later (the burnout phase) with hypothyroidism. Hashimoto thyroiditis is the most frequent cause of hypothyroidism. The mechanism is autoimmune, principally mediated by a type 2 hypersensitivity reaction. Autoantibodies to a variety of fixed thyroid antigens are produced, triggering inflammation and destruction of thyroid tissue. You may recall that a type 2 reaction is characterized by antibodies directed against *fixed* antigens, whereas a type 3 reaction is mediated by *soluble* antigen/antibody complexes.

4. Correct choice: A
GRAVES DISEASE (p. 561)—Hyperplasia/hypertrophy of follicular cells is the most important histological feature in Graves disease, associated with lymphocytic infiltration. Such hyperplastic changes regress after antithyroid treatment and are often absent in thyroidectomy specimens. Thus, thyroidectomy specimens often show lymphocytic infiltration, occasional Hürthle cells, and lymphoid follicles with germinal centers. Graves disease may be seen as a manifestation of autoimmune thyroid disease. It shares features with Hashimoto thyroiditis, such as a genetic defect in suppressor T cells that leads to a proliferation of B cells producing antithyroid autoantibodies. These antibodies (*TRAbs*: thyroid receptor antibodies) are directed against thyrotropin receptors, thus stimulating growth and function.

5. Correct choice: E
RIEDEL THYROIDITIS AND RELATED SCLEROSING CONDITIONS (p. 562)—Riedel thyroiditis is characterized by diffuse, yet asymmetric fibrosis of the thyroid. Fibrotic areas have a stony hard consistency. Fibrosis extends beyond the thyroid parenchyma, resulting in fixation of the organ to adjacent tissues. Histologically, inflammatory infiltration is relatively mild, with predominance of lymphocytes and eosinophils. This process is sometimes associated with similar fibrosclerosing conditions, including retroperitoneal and mediastinal fibrosis and sclerosing cholangitis.

It has no relationship with other forms of thyroiditis nor to amyloid deposition.

6. Correct choice: D

PAPILLARY CARCINOMA (pp. 564 and 565)—This is the most common thyroid malignancy. The most characteristic histopathological features include a papillary architecture, nuclear clearing with pseudoinclusions (so-called *Orphan Annie-eyed nuclei*), nuclear crowding, and psammoma bodies. There is virtually no other thyroid lesion that contains psammoma bodies. Thus, a finding of psammoma bodies in tissue sections or cytological preparations suggests the presence of a papillary carcinoma. Psammoma bodies probably arise from progressive calcification and mineral deposition in necrotic cells. Hürthle cell tumors may contain intrafollicular accumulation of inspissated colloid that may resemble psammoma bodies.

7. Correct choice: E

VARIANTS OF THYROID PAPILLARY CARCINOMA (p. 570)—Among such variants, the rare *tall cell variant* is associated with a more aggressive behavior than other subtypes. The cells lining the papillary projections have a height at least double their width. The *diffuse sclerosing* type involves the thyroid parenchyma in a diffuse fashion and is characterized by fibrosis and abundant psammoma bodies. This variant has a worse prognosis than the classic type. The *encapsulated* variant is entirely surrounded by a capsule and has a good prognosis. The *follicular* variant consists of follicles, but neoplastic cells have the above mentioned nuclear features: The prognosis is the same as conventional papillary carcinoma. A *papillary microcarcinoma* is less than 1 cm in greatest diameter. A *Warthinlike* variant has been recently described, showing a morphology similar to Warthin cell tumors of the salivary gland.

8. Correct choice: D

DIFFERENTIAL DIAGNOSIS BETWEEN NODULAR GOITER AND FOLLICULAR ADENOMA (pp. 573 and 574)—This is a classic diagnostic problem in thyroid pathology. Features favoring *adenoma* include the following: an isolated nodule, compression of surrounding parenchyma, a complete capsule, and follicles smaller than those of a normal gland. Features favoring a *dominant nodule* in nodular goiter include the following: multiple nodules, lack of compression of surrounding parenchyma, absence of a complete capsule, and follicles of variable size and often larger than a normal gland. Adenoma is monoclonal, whereas a dominant nodule is polyclonal.

9. Correct choice: E

FOLLICULAR ADENOMA (p. 574)—This common lesion is of monoclonal origin and appears as a solitary encapsulated mass. Mitotic figures are usually rare. *Follicular* adenoma is the most common morphological form. Trabecular, colloid, atypical (i.e., spindle cell), and papillary forms are rare morphological variants. Dysregulation of thyroid-stimulating hormone (TSH) receptor function is crucial in the pathogenesis of these tumors. Somatic mutations in one of the TSH receptor units results in increased cAMP levels and clonal expansion. DNA ploidy has no prognostic relevance. Careful microscopical evaluation should rule out capsular invasion, the single most important predictor of malignant behavior.

10. Correct choice: D

FOLLICULAR CARCINOMA (p. 576)—Follicular carcinoma of the thyroid refers to all thyroid carcinomas displaying a follicular pattern, excluding the follicular variant of papillary carcinoma, Hürthle cell carcinoma, and other rarer tumors. Assessment of capsular and blood vessel invasion is the most crucial step with regard to prognosis. Based on this parameter, follicular cancers are subclassified into *minimally invasive* (good prognosis) and *widely invasive* (poor prognosis). Blood-borne metastasis is the preferred route of spread, with lungs and bones the most frequent targets. *Ras* mutations are more frequent in follicular than in papillary neoplasms, but are not correlated with prognosis. Lymphatic metastases are characteristic of papillary carcinoma.

11. Correct choice: B

HÜRTHLE CELL TUMORS (p. 578)—This morphologically distinct category of thyroid neoplasms is characterized by prominent oncocytic changes. Cells display eosinophilic granular cytoplasm, which is packed with mitochondria. These tumors are usually encapsulated and have a characteristic tan-brown cut surface. Most of them have a follicular architecture, but others exhibit papillary or solid patterns. Whether a thyroid tumor should be called adenoma or carcinoma depends on the presence of capsular/vascular invasion. The majority of Hürthle cell neoplasms are adenomas. It should be noted that the WHO classification does not recognize Hürthle cell neoplasms as a separate category. Clear cell changes may occur in thyroid neoplasms (including Hürthle cell tumors) and are due to accumulation of lipids, glycogen, or thyroglobulin (*signet-ring neoplasm*).

12. Correct choice: E

MEDULLARY CARCINOMA (p. 580)—Medullary carcinoma of the thyroid arises from calcitonin-secreting C cells. The form of amyloid found in this tumor derives from *calcitonin*, and tumor cells are usually immunoreactive for calcitonin. However, all of the named markers are often positive as well. On the other hand, thyroglobulin is consistently negative. Ultrastructurally, the presence of dense-core granules confirms the neuroendocrine nature of this tumor. H&E features may be extremely diverse. The classic pattern is that of a tumor consisting of cells with amphophilic cytoplasm, arranged in nests separated by fibrous septa. However, many other histologic patterns have been described, including an *oncocytic* subtype that mimics Hürthle cell tumor.

13. Correct choice: C

INSULAR CARCINOMA (p. 584)—This newly recognized variant of thyroid cancer is a carcinoma of intermediate differentiation between follicular/papillary carcinomas and anaplastic carcinomas of the thyroid. An interesting aspect of this neoplasm is its unique geographic distribution, being more frequent in some parts of Europe and South America. The designation suggests its histology, characterized by solid nests of small cells, with occasional follicle formation. Although poorly differentiated, this neoplasm displays immunoreactivity for thyroglobulin (common to both follicular *and* papillary carcinomas). The prognosis is poor, but it is still unclear whether it is better than anaplastic carcinoma.

14. Correct choice: A

ANAPLASTIC CARCINOMA (p. 584)—Also referred to as *undifferentiated carcinoma*, this highly malignant tumor may have several patterns, including *squamouslike*, *spindle cell* and *giant cell* types. The morphology described here is consistent with the spindle cell type. This is occasionally confused with mesenchymal neoplasms, including those mentioned previously. Immunohistochemical or ultrastructural evidence of epithelial differentiation may help clinch the diagnosis. Thyroglobulin immunoreactivity is absent in poorly differentiated cases.

15. Correct choice: A
PARATHYROID HISTOLOGY (p. 595)—It may be useful to review the normal histology of parathyroids. Adipose tissue is virtually absent in the newborn, appears during adolescence, and increases in amount until about 40 years, after which it remains constant. There is significant variability in the proportion of adipose tissue between individuals, and smaller glands actually contain a lower proportion of fat. The principal cell types include *chief, oxyphil,* and *water-clear* cells. Transitional cell types are also described. Chief cells have dark round nuclei, scanty cytoplasm, and abundant secretory granules. Oxyphil cells have abundant granular cytoplasm with numerous mitochondria. Water-clear cells have glycogen-rich clear cytoplasm. All of the cell types are derived from chief cells and reflect different physiological activities.

16. Correct choice: B
PARATHYROID ADENOMA (p. 597)—Parathyroid adenomas affect mostly women in the fourth decade and manifest with hypercalcemia and recurrent urinary stones. Although chief cells are usually predominant, other types are present in varying mixtures. The presence of clusters of cells with bizarre nuclei is relatively common and does not indicate malignancy. Likewise, lymphocytic infiltration and occasional mitotic figures are common findings in otherwise benign parathyroid tumors. A diffuse pattern of growth is the most frequent, but follicular, nesting, or pseudopapillary patterns may be encountered. A trabecular architecture, instead, is suggestive of carcinoma. Capsular and intravascular infiltration are clear signs of malignancy.

17. Correct choice: B
PRIMARY PARATHYROID CELL HYPERPLASIA (p. 599)—Differentiating adenoma from chief cell hyperplasia is crucial to clinical management. There is no specific morphological feature (size of lesion, cell types, etc.) that allows a definite diagnosis, except for the finding of a rim of compressed but normal parathyroid tissue around an adenoma and/or identification of a normal parathyroid gland during surgery. Indeed, the pathological approach to this problem varies from center to center. It is recommended that histological examination should be performed on the largest parathyroid gland resected *in toto* plus a biopsy of at least one normal appearing gland.

18. Correct choice: E
WATER-CLEAR CELL HYPERPLASIA (p. 599)—This form of hyperplasia is rare. It may produce massive glandular enlargement, especially of the superior parathyroids. It is predominantly composed of water-clear cell types. These cells have clear cytoplasm and distinct cell borders. It manifests with hyperparathyroidism. This condition is not associated with any known familial syndrome such as multiple andocrine neoplasia (MEN). A lipoadenoma is an adenoma with abundant adipose tissue.

19. Correct choice: D
PARATHYROID CARCINOMA (599)—Parathyroid carcinomas are rare and account for 1% to 2% of primary hyperparathyroidism. They are usually large tumors (average weight: 12 g) that tend to adhere to adjacent structures. Nuclear pleomorphism and mitotic activity are histological criteria distinguishing carcinoma from adenoma, whereas capsular invasion is not. Large adenomas,

in fact, may develop focal hemorrhage, which results in areas of fibrosis that entrap tumor cells.

CHAPTER 14

1. Correct choice: B
CORTICAL HYPERPLASIA (p. 630)—PPNAD is a rare form of adrenocortical hyperplasia most likely related to circulating autoantibodies that bind ACTH receptors, thus stimulating adrenal growth and function. ACTH-producing adenomas or hypothalamic overstimulation of pituitary ACTH cells by CRH account for *Cushing disease*. Bronchial carcinoids and small cell carcinomas cause most cases of cortical hyperplasia due to ectopic production of ACTH or corticotropin-like factors.

2. Correct choice: B
ADRENOCORTICAL ADENOMA (p. 631)—This benign lesion is usually of small size, rarely exceeding 5 cm. It is composed of well-differentiated cells closely resembling the zona fasciculata. Adrenal adenomas are usually asymptomatic. They may give rise to Cushing, Conn, or adrenogenital syndromes in cases of overproduction of glucocorticoids, mineralocorticoids, or sex hormones, respectively. The differential diagnosis between adenoma and carcinoma favors adenoma when the size is small, mitotic activity absent or minimal, and vascular and capsular invasion not detectable. Combined cytokeratin and vimentin expression is characteristic of adenoma, whereas cytokeratin expression is often focal or absent in carcinoma. EMA is expressed by renal cell carcinoma, but not by adrenal tumors.

3. Correct choice: E
SPIRONOLACTONE BODIES AND CONN SYNDROME (p. 632)—*Spironolactone bodies* are often detected in aldosterone-secreting adrenal adenomas excised from patients previously treated with spironolactone. Ultrastructurally, they are composed of a concentric arrangement of membranes. By immunohistochemistry, aldosterone has been found in spironolactone bodies. The clinical diagnosis of primary hyperaldosteronism (Conn syndrome) is based on clinical and laboratory findings (i.e., hypertension combined with hypokalemia, hyperkaluria, and increased plasma renin activity). Adenomas are responsible for over two-thirds of cases of hyperaldosteronism.

4. Correct choice: B
ADRENOCORTICAL CARCINOMA (p. 634)—By the time of diagnosis, this tumor has usually acquired a large size and has often spread to regional lymph nodes, liver, lungs, and other organs. The cut surface is characteristically variegated, with multifocal hemorrhage and necrosis. Mitotic figures are frequent, including atypical mitoses (in contrast to cortical adenoma), but glandular formations are absent (in contrast to most renal cell carcinoma). There are two peaks of incidence: one in the fourth decade and a smaller one in childhood.

5. Correct choice: A
PROGNOSTIC FACTORS OF NEUROBLASTOMA (p. 648)—Numerous independent as well as interrelated prognostic factors have an influence on the prognosis of neuroblastoma. The most important of these allow the classification of patients into three distinct groups of good, intermediate, and poor prognosis (see the table that follows).

1st Group (>90% Cure Rate)	2nd Group (25%–50% Cure Rate)	3rd Group (5% Cure Rate)
Young children; early stage	Older children; advanced stage	Older children; advanced stage
Hyperdiploid tumors	Diploid or tetraploid tumors	Diploid tumors
Lack of MYCN amplification	Lack of MYCN amplification	Presence of MYCN amplification
High levels of TRK-A	Low levels of TRK-A	Low levels of TRK-A
Lack of chromosome 1 deletions	Presence of chromosome 1 deletions	Presence of chromosome 1 deletions

6. Correct choice: E

GANGLIONEUROBLASTOMA AND GANGLIONEU-ROMA (pp. 649 and 650)—These tumors represent better-differentiated stages than neuroblastoma, tend to occur in increasingly older age groups, and develop most commonly from the sympathetic chain of retroperitoneal and mediastinal space. Ganglioneuroblastoma consists of variable mixtures of immature, neuroblastic-like elements and well-differentiated ganglion cells. The neoplasm is further classified into *imperfect* (where ganglion cells cover the full range of differentiation) or *perfect* (where there is a sharp gap between well-differentiated ganglion cells and immature elements). Ganglioneuroma is composed of mature ganglion cells surrounded by Schwann cells and affects adults.

7. Correct choice: A

PHEOCHROMOCYTOMA (p. 655)—Unfortunately, there is no reliable morphological or clinical method for distinguishing between benign and malignant pheochromocytomas except metastatic spread. Capsular and vascular invasion is seen in both benign and malignant cases. However, greater tumor size, extensive necrosis, and lack of cytoplasmic hyaline globules tend to be more frequent in malignant than in benign pheochromocytomas.

8. Correct choice: C

FAMILIAL PHEOCHROMOCYTOMA (p. 655)—Familial pheochromocytomas are often bilateral and multicentric and occur at an earlier age than sporadic forms. Up to 50% of patients with MEN type 2 (*a* or *b*) develop pheochromocytomas. This tumor is also seen in up to 20% of patients with VHL and up to 5% of patients with von Recklinghausen disease. Genetic screening of sporadic pheochromocytomas shows that one-fifth of cases occur in carriers of familial syndromes.

CHAPTER 15

1. Correct choice: B

MALIGNANCY IN PARAGANGLIOMAS (pp. 671 and 687)—This is a carotid body paraganglioma (CBP). Paragangliomas may arise from paraganglia of the head and neck (related to the parasympathetic system) or from those in the abdominal/pelvic cavities (related to the sympathetic system). Paragangliomas of the head and neck are morphologically similar, regardless their location. Their characteristic lobular arrangement ("zellballen") is demonstrated

by the picture. Histomorphological parameters are unreliable for assessing the malignant potential of these neoplasms, and a diagnosis of malignant paraganglioma may be made on the basis of metastatic spread.

2. Correct choice: D

EXTRAADRENAL PARAGANGLIOMAS (p. 679)—These tumors arise from extraadrenal chromaffin tissue histologically and functionally analogous to the adrenal medulla. The distribution of extraadrenal paraganglia follows that of the sympathetic nervous system. The highest concentration of extraadrenal paraganglia is found in the retroperitoneal paraaortic regions from the origin of the inferior mesenteric arteries to aortic bifurcation. They are known as *organs of Zuckerkandl.* Most commonly, extraadrenal parangliomas develop from paraganglia in this region. A trabecular arrangement is the most common histological pattern. Abdominal extraadrenal parangliomas have a malignant behavior in 25% to 50% of cases. The malignancy rate in pheochromocytoma (adrenal medullary paraganglioma) is in the range of 2% to 14%.

CHAPTER 16

1. Correct choice: B

SEROUS ATROPHY (p. 703)—*Serous atrophy* is a frequent finding in AIDS patients as well as in patients suffering from extreme malnutrition, cachexia, starvation. The gelatinous eosinophilic appearance of the extracellular substance combined with atrophy of the adipose tissue are diagnostic features.

2. Correct choice: A

GRANULOMAS (p. 703)—The named conditions include causes of bone marrow granulomas. In the majority of cases (probably up to 80%), the underlying etiology remains unclear despite all appropriate investigations, that is, special stains and cultures. A very common form of bone marrow granuloma is *lipid granuloma*, analogous to that observed in other organs of the reticuloendothelial system (spleen, liver, and lymph nodes). Histiocytes in lipid granulomas contain intracytoplasmic lipid droplets.

3. Correct choice: A

AML VERSUS ALL (p. 707)—All of the previous morphological features are helpful in distinguishing AML from ALL, but only *unequivocal Auer rods* (present in two-thirds of AML cases) can definitively establish a diagnosis of AML. Auer rods appear as cytoplasmic, eosinophilic, needle-like inclusions within myeloid cells. AML affects middle-aged persons and is subdivided into seven types, depending on blast maturation, morphology, and cytogenetic abnormalities.

4. Correct choice: D

MYELODYSPLASTIC SYNDROMES (MDS; p. 719)—These are heterogeneous bone marrow conditions that share the following features:

- Usually manifest with cytopenia in patients over 50
- Result from maturation defects of one or more myeloid lines leading to ineffective hematopoiesis
- Have a tendency to degenerate into acute myeloid leukemia

The bone marrow is usually hypercellular. A useful diagnostic feature is the finding of myeloid precursors away from their normal paratrabecular location. The WHO classification divides MDS into two groups, *primary* and *therapy related.*

5. Correct choice: E
CHRONIC IDIOPATHIC MYELOFIBROSIS WITH MYELOID METAPLASIA (p. 726)—This is characterized by progressive fibrosis and obliteration of functioning marrow. (i) Initially, the marrow is hypercellular with an increase in granulocytic precursors and megakaryocytes; fibrosis may not be readily apparent, unless reticulin staining is used, and the blood cell count is normal or increased. (ii) At later stages, the increase in bone marrow fibrosis is patchy and accompanied by a progressive reduction in functioning marrow; the blood cell count begins to drop, with associated splenomegaly and extramedullary hematopoiesis. (iii) Advanced stages are characterized by extensive bone marrow fibrosis, teardrop erythrocytes in peripheral blood, massive splenomegaly, and compensatory extramedullary hematopoiesis.

6. Correct choice: D
MASTOCYTOSIS (p. 727)—The systemic form of mast cell disease involves the bone marrow in the majority of cases (90%), most frequently in a patchy manner. A bone marrow biopsy is usually performed to confirm a clinical diagnosis. Mast cells are spindly cells similar to histiocytes or fibroblasts and can be identified on toluidine blue staining. Immunocytochemistry for mast cell tryptase, however, is the most sensitive and specific method for identification of mast cells.

7. Correct choice: B
BONE MARROW INVOLVEMENT IN NHL (p. 729)—NHLs involve the bone marrow in up to 50% of cases. Bone marrow biopsies are usually performed for staging purposes. Marrow involvement by NHL can be categorized in five patterns: focal paratrabecular, focal random, interstitial, diffuse, and intravascular/intrasinusoidal. The focal paratrabecular pattern is the most common. Some types of NHLs display a specific predilection for one or the other pattern. Examples:

- *Focal paratrabecular:* Follicular lymphoma, predominantly small cell lymphoma, mixed small and large cell lymphoma
- *Focal random:* Small lymphocytic lymphoma
- *Interstitial and diffuse:* Burkitt and lymphoblastic lymphoma
- *Intravascular:* Large cell lymphoma

8. Correct choice: C
HODGKIN LYMPHOMA (p. 743)—HL involves the bone marrow in 10% of cases at the time of clinical presentation. The pattern of involvement is usually diffuse. Aspiration smears are ineffective in detecting HL in the bone marrow, in contrast to trephine iliac biopsies, especially when done bilaterally. A "dry tap" is usually caused by extensive bone marrow fibrosis. Reed-Sternberg (RS) cells can be more easily detected in areas with the typical cellular background of HL or areas of fibrosis. Immunostains for CD15 and CD30 are positive on RS cells and may help identify them in difficult cases. LCA (CD45) is negative on RS cells.

9. Correct choice: E
LYMPHOCYTIC AGGREGATES AND OTHER BENIGN LYMPHOID LESIONS (p. 745)—Lymphocytic aggregates represent the most common reactive lymphoid lesion in the bone marrow. Found in up to 47% of all marrow biopsies, lymphocytic aggregates increase in frequency with age, but have no pathological significance. Their round configuration and well-demarcated outline help distinguishing them from lymphomas. Other reactive lymphoid infiltrates include:

- *Reactive polymorphous lymphohistiocytic lesions* (lymphocytes, transformed lymphocytes, plasma cells, and histiocytes): AIDS, rheumatoid arthritis, and so on
- *Germinal centers:* immune or inflammatory disorders
- *Systemic polyclonal immunoblastic proliferations:* diffuse increase in lymphocytes, immunoblasts, and plasma cells associated with peripheral smear abnormalities; unknown pathogenesis

10. Correct choice: C
MULTIPLE MYELOMA (MM; pp. 749–751)—The diagnosis of MM relies on serum and urine protein electrophoresis and quantitation, immunoelectrophoresis, radiographic studies, and bone marrow examination. The diagnostic criteria for MM in the bone marrow have not been standardized, but identification of atypical plasma cells and infiltrative sheets of plasma cells are highly suggestive. The rule of 10% of plasma cells in marrow smears as a minimum for a diagnosis of MM is not always valid, because the involvement of bone marrow may be patchy. Light chain restriction by immunohistochemistry is often useful in confirming the monoclonal nature of plasma cells. Ratios greater than 16:1 are usually associated with MM, whereas ratios less than 16:1 are found in reactive plasmacytosis and MGUS. No bone lesions are present in MGUS, a condition seen in up to 3% of persons over 70.

11. Correct choice: C
VARIANTS OF MYELOMA (p. 752)—The *osteosclerotic* variant is associated with sclerotic bone lesions, sometimes with *p*olyneuropathy, *o*rganomegaly, *e*ndocrinopathy, *m*onoclonal gammopathy, and *s*kin lesions (POEMS syndrome); the prognosis is good. *Smoldering* and *indolent myeloma* have the same features as classic MM but no progression, even without treatment. *MGUS* affects up to 3% of persons older than 70 with no bone lesions, no light chains in the urine, and progression to MM in 25% of cases within 10 years. The *nonsecretory* variant is rare; there is no monoclonal protein in the blood or urine, but monoclonal light chains are detectable in marrow plasma cells by immunohistochemistry.

12. Correct choice: B
GAUCHER DISEASE (p. 755)—This is an autosomal recessive disorder manifesting with hepatosplenomegaly, painful bone lesions, pancytopenia due to bone marrow failure, and accumulation of glucocerebroside-laden histiocytes (*Gaucher cells*), which have a characteristic crumpled paper-like cytoplasm. It is common among Jewish people of East European descent and results from *glucocerebrosidase* deficiency. Choice C is due to *sphingomyelinase* deficiency, resulting in the accumulation of sphingomyelin in the nervous system and visceral organs (liver and spleen) and death before 3 years. Choice D is due to 1,4-glucosidase deficiency, resulting in the accumulation of glycogen in all organs, especially the heart. Choice E is due to *hexosaminidase* deficiency, resulting in accumulation of G_{M2} ganglioside in neurons and the retina, with mental retardation and neurologic deterioration beginning in the first year of life.

13. Correct choice: B
BONE MARROW NECROSIS (pp. 703 and 758)—Bone marrow necrosis may be observed in a variety of disorders, including infections, lupus erythematosus, sickle cell disease, leukemias, and lymphomas. However, metastasis is the most common cause of marrow necrosis. When viable tissue is obtained, the presence of a metastatic tumor is usually easily identifiable as islands of neoplastic tissue sharply demarcated from normal marrow cells. The

most common tumors metastasizing to bone in adults and children (760) include:

- Adults: breast, prostate, lungs, GI tract, kidney, and thyroid
- Children: neuroblastoma, Ewing sarcoma, rhabdomyosarcoma, and retinoblastoma

In adults, marrow metastases frequently induce a sclerotic reaction and may be mistaken for *myelofibrosis*. Small round cell tumors in children and adults may mimic *lymphomas/leukemias*.

CHAPTER 17

1. Correct choice: D
ARCHITECTURAL PATTERNS IN HOGDKIN AND NON-HOGDKIN LYMPHOMAS (p. 782)—Lymphomas with a characteristic appearance on low magnification include nodular-sclerosing HL (NSHL), the nodular variant of lymphocyte-predominant HL (LPHL), and follicular center cell (FCC) lymphoma. The following should be noted:

- FCC lymphoma may be confused with the nodular variant of LPHL because of the sclerosing pattern and the similarity between activated FCC and Reed-Sternberg cells.
- T-cell lymphoma may be mistaken for HL and vice versa, because the monoclonality of T cells cannot be established by surface antigen immunohistochemistry, and HL may contain numerous T lymphocytes.

2. Correct choice: A
FOLLICULAR HYPERPLASIA IN RHEUMATOID ARTHRITIS (p. 784)—Reactive lymphadenopathy occurs in collagen vascular diseases such as rheumatoid arthritis, Still disease, Sjögren syndrome, and systemic lupus erythematosus (SLE). It is characterized by follicular hyperplasia and abundant interfollicular plasma cells. In SLE, follicular hyperplasia is often associated with paracortical necrosis without neutrophilic infiltration. Choice C is indicative of *AIDS* lymphadenopathy, choice D of *Castleman disease*, and choice E of *cat-scratch disease*. The table on p. 171 summarizes proposed reactive lymphadenopathies.

3. Correct choice: C
HISTIOCYTIC NECROTIZING LYMPHADENITIS (p. 785)—Also called *Kikuchi-Fujimoto disease*, this condition affects not only young Asian women as previously believed, but also men and women in non-Asian countries. The most common presentation is the one outlined in the question stem. Plasmacytoid monocytes are CD4 + cells with an open nucleus and small nucleoli, three to four times larger than mature lymphocytes. Large areas of necrosis surrounded by lymphocytes, histiocytes, and plasmacytoid monocytes are characteristic. Neutrophils are absent in necrotic areas, in contrast to cat-scratch disease.

4. Correct choice: A
CAT-SCRATCH DISEASE (p. 786)—*B. henselae*, a small bacillus identifiable by Warthin-Starry staining, is the etiologic agent of cat-scratch disease. This condition is characterized by follicular hyperplasia associated with a specific pattern of necrosis and granulomatous inflammation. Necrotic areas are located in the subcapsular region, surrounded by palisading histiocytes and infiltrated by neutrophils. Capsulitis is consistently present. This pattern is not pathognomonic of cat-scratch disease, as it is found in

other infectious conditions, for example, tularemia, lymphogranuloma venereum, and Yersinia infection. Choice B is characteristic of *Rosai-Dorfman disease,* choice C of *rheumatoid arthritis* and *Sjögren syndrome,* choice D of *infectious mononucleosis,* and choice E of *sarcoidosis.*

5. Correct choice: D
ANGIOFOLLICULAR HYPERPLASIA (CASTLEMAN DISEASE; pp. 788–790)—This condition is characterized by small germinal centers organized around hyalinized vessels. An "onionskin" arrangement of lymphocytes around small vessels is an eye-catching feature. Plasma cells are polyclonal; the pathogenetic role of HHV-8 is still debated. Castleman disease may be subclassified into *hyaline-vascular* and *plasma cell* variants (see the table that follows).

Hyaline-Vascular Variant	Plasma Cell Variant
Angiofollicular hyperplasia predominant	Interfollicular sheets of plasma cells
Presents as a large mediastinal mass, often in asymptomatic young individuals	Associated with systemic disease: fever, hypergammaglobulinemia, multiorgan failure
Good prognosis: surgical resection is usually curative	Poor prognosis: often progresses to Kaposi sarcoma or lymphoma

6. Correct choice: E
INFECTIOUS MONONUCLEOSIS (p. 790)—Infectious mononucleosis is due to Epstein-Barr virus infecting B lymphocytes. Cytotoxic (CD8 +) T lymphocytes represent the majority of atypical lymphocytes in peripheral smears. This condition may lead to *partial* effacement of lymph node follicular architecture, with a pattern mimicking either nodular-sclerosing Hodgkin disease or high-grade non-Hodgkin lymphomas. Large numbers of *immunoblasts*, with abundant cytoplasm and prominent nucleoli, are the hallmark of infectious mononucleosis. Transformed immunoblasts may mimic Reed-Sternberg cells or the neoplastic lymphocytes of immunoblastic lymphoma.

7. Correct choice: B
POSTTRANSPLANTATION LYMPHOPROLIFERATIVE DISORDER (PTLD; p. 791)—PTLD is a B-cell proliferation that may be polyclonal or monoclonal (i.e., lymphoma). Epstein-Barr virus (EBV) is associated with this complication, and the EBV genome can be identified in most cases. Immunosuppressive therapy is probably the underlying predisposing factor. Cytomegalovius (CMV) infection causes hepatitis characterized by microabscesses and characteristic inclusions. Recurrence of hepatitis B, C, or D virus is a frequent posttransplantation event.

8. Correct choice: A
ROSAI-DORFMAN DISEASE (p. 792)—The most typical presentation is that of a young Black male with massive cervical lymphadenopathy. Extranodal involvement is seen in 25% of cases. The lymph node sinuses are expanded by numerous histiocytes, some showing *emperipolesis*, that is, phagocytosis of blood elements (mostly lymphocytes). Histiocytes are S100 protein positive. The etiopathogenesis of this condition is obscure. Differential diagnosis: Langerhans cell histiocytosis and melanoma. Choice

Follicular Hyperplasia without Necrosis

Rheumatoid arthritis, Sjögren syndrome, Still disease	Prominent interfollicular plasmacytosis
Angiofollicular hyperplasia (Castleman disease)	Small follicular centers with central hyalinized small vessels and surrounding follicular center cells in an onionskin pattern
Kimura disease	Interfollicular eosinophilia and proliferation of interfollicular small vessels
HIV infection	Large germinal centers with typical serpiginous appearance and thin or absent mantle zone
Syphilis	Striking capsulitis and plasma cell infiltration

Follicular Hyperplasia with Necrosis

Systemic lupus erythematosus	Paracortical necrosis without polymorphonuclear leukocytes or granulomas; hematoxylin bodies
Kikuchi disease (histiocytic necrotizing lymphadenitis)	Extensive areas of necrosis surrounded by histiocytes; numerous plasmacytoid (CD4 +) histiocytes; no neutrophils
Cat-scratch disease, other infections (tularemia, Yersinia, lymphogranuloma venereum)	Subcapsular stellate necrotizing granulomas containing polymorphs—a microabscess within a granuloma
Toxoplasmosis	Mixed inflammatory infiltrate with frequent giant cells; toxoplasma organisms easily identified in AIDS-related cases

Interfollicular Hyperplasia

Whipple disease	Sheets of PAS-positive histiocytes
Infectious mononucleosis	Germinal centers with ragged margins, interfollicular expansion by transformed immunoblasts mimicking lymphoma
Posttransplant lymphoproliferative disorder	Somewhat similar to infectious mononucleosis, with monomorphic or polymorphic B-lymphocyte hyperplasia
Hemophagocytic syndrome	Striking erythrophagocytosis, usually in association with viral infections, non-Hodgkin lymphomas, drugs, or autoimmune disorders
Dermatopathic lymphadenopathy	Associated with skin diseases; paracortical areas expanded by melanin containing histiocytes and hyperplasia of dendritic and Langerhans cells
Sinus histiocytosis with massive lymphadenopathy (Rosai-Dorfman disease)	Marked expansion of sinuses by histiocytes and striking emperipolesis

Reactive Lymphadenopathy with Architectural Effacement

Immunoblastic lymphadenopathy (IBL) and angioimmunoblastic lymphadenopathy with dysproteinemia (AILD)	Immunoblasts and plasma cells expanding sinuses. Now classified within *angioimmunoblastic T-cell lymphoma* (AIL), p. 824
Phenytoin reaction	Changes vary in relation to stage; eosinophilia usually marked
Sarcoidosis	Numerous nonnecrotizing granulomas
Inflammatory spindle cell tumor	Mixed inflammatory infiltrate within a florid fibroblastic proliferation; most cells have histiocytic immune markers
Bacillary angiomatosis	Seen in immunosuppressed; proliferation of small blood vessels with interstitial neutrophils; etiologic agent (*B. henselae*) identifiable by Warthin-Starry

B is characteristic of immunoblastic lymphadenopathy; choice C of angioimmunoblastic lymphadenopathy; choice D of infectious mononucleosis, various viral infections, and vaccination reaction; and choice E of dermatopathic lymphadenopathy.

9. Correct choice: B

LYMPHOCYTE-PREDOMINANT HL (LPHL; p. 798)—This unique type of HL accounts for less than 5% of all HL cases. The prognosis is good. If Reed-Sternberg cells were found easily, a diagnosis of LPHL would be unlikely. "*Popcorn cells*" are plentiful and represent the defining cellular feature of LPHL. They express B-lymphocytic markers, CD45 but not CD15. Popcorn cells are referred to as *L and H cells* from the designation given to the most common subtype of LPHL, that is *lymphocytic* and *histiocytic*. The *diffuse* subtype is rare and characterized by increased numbers of T lymphocytes. The vaguely nodular growth pattern of most cases of LPHL may lead to a mistaken diagnosis of follicular center lymphoma.

10. Correct choice: C

NODULAR-SCLEROSING HOGDKIN LYMPHOMA (NSHL; p. 800)—CD15 +, CD30 +, and CD45 − immunostaining is characteristic of both *classic* Reed-Sternberg (RS) cells and the *lacunar variant* of RS cells. The lacunar variant is found in NSHL, which is the most common subtype of HD (60% of cases) and manifests in young adults with cervical or supraclavicular adenopathy. Lacunar cells are characterized by a conspicuous pericellular halo, which is due to formalin fixation and is thus absent in B5-fixed tissue. NSHL may contain large numbers of the *mononuclear* variant of RS cells. This finding is characterized by a large vesicular nucleus with a prominent nucleolus and the same immunoreactivity as classic RS cells. In contrast, the L and H variant of RS cells in LPHL is CD45 + and CD15 − .

11. Correct choice: D

MIXED-CELLULARITY HODGKIN LYMPHOMA (MCHL; p. 801)—MCHL accounts for up to 30% of all cases of HL and tends to affect patients older than those with NSHL. As its designation implies, MCHL is characterized by a mixed cellular infiltrate in which T lymphocytes are often predominant. RS cells are easily found and express CD15 and CD30, but not CD45. Thin bands of fibrosis may be seen, but these are different from the broad birefringent bands of fibrosis in NSHL. Prognosis is generally good, but worse than NSHL.

12. Correct choice: E

LYMPHOCYTE-DEPLETED HODGKIN LYMPHOMA (LDHL; p. 803)—LDHL accounts for less than 5% of all HL cases. It affects older patients (median age: 50s), who present with diffuse disease and systemic complaints. LDHL is characterized by a scanty reactive component, but RS cells display the usual CD45 − /CD15 + phenotype. There are two variants:

- *Diffuse-fibrosis type:* a disorganized pattern of fibrosis, PAS-positive intercellular matrix, rare RS cells; often diagnosed in biopsies of liver or bone marrow
- *Reticular type:* paucity of dense fibrous tissue, numerous bizarre RS cells occasionally growing in sheets, morphological similarities with other large cell neoplasms, including lymphomas or carcinomas

13. Correct choice: A

CHRONIC LYMPHOCYTIC LEUKEMIA/SMALL LYMPHO-CYTIC LYMPHOMA (p. 805)—CLL/SLL affects predominantly

elderly patients and has a slow clinical course. The neoplastic population is composed of monomorphic small lymphocytes of pre-follicular B-cell origin. Its phenotype is as follows:

- Cell markers: CD5 +, CD19 +, CD43 +, and CD10 −
- Weak and inconstant expression of surface immunoglobulin
- Immunoglobulin gene rearrangement
- Cytogenetics: variable, 13q14 deletions/translocations, 11q deletions, and trisomy 12

Choices B and E are indicative of follicular center cell lymphoma, choice C of mantle cell lymphoma, and choice D of Burkitt lymphoma.

14. Correct choice: E

LYMPHOPLASMACYTIC LYMPHOMA (p. 808)—Also called *immunocytoma*, LPL is a B-cell neoplasm sharing similarities with small lymphocytic lymphoma. Neoplastic cells of LPL retain the ability to differentiate into plasmacytoid cells and plasma cells. Often, this lymphoma is associated with leukemia. Because neoplastic plasma cells often produce monoclonal IgM (less often IgG), LPL may give rise to Waldenström macroglobulinemia and hyperviscosity syndrome. The morphological picture is characterized by a mixture of small lymphocytes, lymphoplasmacytoid lymphocytes, and plasma cells. Scattered intranuclear pseudoinclusions known as *Dutcher bodies* are frequent.

15. Correct choice: B

MANTLE CELL LYMPHOMA (MCL; p. 809)—MCL is thought to originate from prefollicular B cells. It gives rise to a characteristic mantle zone expansion resulting in a nodular pattern. This lymphoma manifests predominantly in older male patients with lymphadenopathy and marrow involvement. Translocation t(11;14) involves the genes of Ig heavy chain and cyclin D1/CCND1 (*bcl*-1), resulting in overexpression of *cyclin D1*. Cyclin D1 can be demonstrated in paraffin tissue by immunostaining. Choice A is characteristic of Burkitt lymphoma, choice C of follicular center lymphoma, and choice D of small lymphocytic lymphoma.

16. Correct choice: C

FOLLICULAR LYMPHOMA (FL; p. 810)—This is the most common NHL in the United States, presenting as generalized lymphadenopathy and marrow involvement in middle-aged patients. The genotypic hallmark of FL is a translocation involving the gene of IgH on chromosome 14 and the gene of bcl-2 on chromosome 18, leading to overexpression of the apoptosis-inhibiting bcl-2 protein. Lymphocytes of FL resemble normal germinal center B cells. In fact, neoplastic cells express CD10, but not CD5. Overexpression of bcl-2 can be detected by immunohistochemistry and is helpful in differentiating FL from normal follicles. The antiapoptotic activity of bcl-2 probably accounts for the slow growth of FL, which is, however, incurable.

17. Correct choice: A

NODAL MARGINAL ZONE LYMPHOMA (p. 814)—The nodal form of marginal zone lymphoma (MZL) may be easily mistaken for reactive lymphadenopathy because of prominent hyperplastic follicular centers. Neoplastic cells, referred to as monocytoid B cells, resemble those of the marginal/parafollicular zones: two to three times larger than small lymphocytes and with pale cytoplasm. They are negative for CD5, CD10, and CD23, but express surface Ig. NMZL has an indolent course. The MALT form of MZL is indistinguishable from the nodal form. Choice B is characteristic of follicular lymphoma, and choice D of mantle zone lymphoma.

18. Correct choice: D

DIFFUSE LARGE B-CELL LYMPHOMA (p. 815)—DLBCL accounts for approximately 20% of all NHLs. Patients present with a rapidly enlarging nodal or extranodal mass. The median age is 60, but DLBCL may affect children. Neoplastic cells are transformed lymphocytes of B-cell origin that express pan-B-cell markers such as CD19 and CD20. Expression of CD10 is infrequent and found in those cases of follicular center origin. CD5 and CD10 are usually negative. Neoplastic lymphocytes are large and have a vesicular nucleus and prominent nucleoli. The nuclei may be multilobated and simulate Reed-Sternberg cells.

19. Correct choice: C

SUBTYPES OF DIFFUSE LARGE B-CELL LYMPHOMA (p. 818)—DLBCL is a rather generic entity encompassing heterogeneous conditions. Several subtypes are recognized. The *primary effusion* form (also called *body cavity large B-cell lymphoma*) manifests in pleural or ascitic effusions rather than presenting as solid masses. HHV-8 (associated with Kaposi sarcoma) has been demonstrated in most of these cases. It is usually, but not always, seen in HIV-positive patients. Choice A is related to hepatitis B virus (HBV), choice B has a predominantly angioinvasive growth and involves the skin and nervous system, choice D is related to thymic lymphoma of probable B-thymic cell origin, and choice E means that at least 90% of the lymphocytes are T cells.

20. Correct choice: C

BURKITT LYMPHOMA (BL; p. 819)—This high-grade NHL has a MIB-1 labeling index characteristically close to 100%. There are three epidemiological variants: *sporadic*, *African* type, and *HIV associated*. The sporadic and HIV-associated forms involve extranodal sites, most commonly the GI tract, presenting as an ileocecal or peritoneal mass. The African form has a predilection for the mandible. EBV is associated in virtually all cases of the African form, 25% of HIV-associated cases, and occasional sporadic cases. The characteristic translocation in BL involves Ig loci (usually IgH on chromosome 14) and the c-*myc* gene: t(8;14). Choice A relates to mantle zone lymphoma (the bcl-1 protein is also called cyclin-D), choice B to follicular center lymphoma, choice D to lymphoplasmacytoid lymphoma, and choice E to acute T-cell lymphoblastic leukemia/lymphoma (other T-cell receptor loci are also involved).

21. Correct choice: E

PRECURSOR T-CELL LYMPHOBLASTIC LYMPHOMA/LEUKEMIA (p. 822)—This aggressive T-cell lymphoma presents typically in children or young adults as a mediastinal mass with involvement of supradiaphragmatic lymph nodes. If untreated, the condition spreads and gives rise to a leukemic phase indistinguishable from T-cell acute lymphoblastic leukemia. Neoplastic cells are positive for T-cell markers, including CD3 and CD7; 25% of cases express *common ALL antigen* (CD10). TdT (*terminal deoxytransferase*) is expressed in all cases. TdT is a special DNA polymerase expressed by precursor T and B cells.

22. Correct choice: E

PERIPHERAL T-CELL LYMPHOMA (PTCL), UNSPECIFIED (p. 823)—This T-cell lymphoma arises from mature T lymphocytes and typically manifests with generalized lymphadenopathy in adult patients with "B symptoms" (fever, weight loss, pruritus, eosinophilia, etc.). Besides pan-T-cell markers, PTCL often expresses CD4 and CD8, but is remarkably negative for TdT and CD1 (which are positive on precursor T-cell acute lymphoblastic leukemia/lymphoma). T-cell–rich (TCR) gene rearrangement is detected in a high proportion of cases. Frequent relapses and a 25% 5-year survival rate are expected. Cases associated with immunophenotypic expression of cytotoxic or natural killer cell markers behave more aggressively.

23. Correct choice: B

ANGIOIMMUNOBLASTIC T-CELL LYMPHOMA (p. 824)—AIL affects adults with "B-symptoms," as well as generalized lymphadenopathy and frequent polyclonal hypergammaglobulinemia. The salient feature of AIL, besides its T-cell composition, is the presence of a rich small-vessel meshwork with PAS-positive vessel walls. Follicular dendritic cells are abundant around such small vessels and can be identified by CD21 immunohistochemistry. T-cell monoclonality has been demonstrated in both AIL and IBL. Immunoblastic lymphadenopathy (IBL), angioimmunoblastic lymphadenopathy with dysproteinemia (AILD), and AIL probably represent aspects of the same disease spectrum. IBL and AILD develop in the context of immune dysfunction.

24. Correct choice: D

ANAPLASTIC LARGE CELL LYMPHOMA (ALCL; p. 825)—Neoplastic cells of ALCL express CD30 and T-cell antigens. Expression of *cytotoxic granule-associated protein* suggests an origin from cytotoxic lymphocytes, but it does not affect prognosis. One tenth of ALCLs express B-cell antigens. ALCL may occur in three different clinical-pathologic forms: *primary systemic*, *primary cutaneous*, and *secondary cutaneous*. It is of the utmost importance to determine whether *t(2;5)* is present in the systemic form, because this translocation has the greatest prognostic significance besides the primary site of involvement. This translocation leads to a novel fusion protein named *NPM-ALK*, resulting from the fusion of genes coding for *nucleophosmin* (NPM) and *anaplastic lymphoma kinase* (ALK). Expression of this protein can be detected immunohistochemically. EMA is often positive in ALCL. The following table presents ALCL classification and prognostic factors.

Site of Involvement + Genetics		Prognosis + Clinical
Systemic	*With* NPM-ALK fusion gene	Good prognosis: usually affects young adults
	Without NPM-ALK fusion gene	Poor prognosis: usually affects older adults
Cutaneous	*Primary*	Good prognosis
	Secondary	Poor prognosis: arising from transformation of preexisting lymphoma

25. Correct choice: E

ADULT T-CELL LEUKEMIA/LYMPHOMA (p. 826)—This T-cell neoplasm is caused by HTLV-I and is endemic in south Japan, the Caribbean islands, New Guinea, central Africa, and parts of South America. HTLV-I transmission is similar to HIV. A lifetime risk of developing leukemia is approximately 5% in seropositive persons. It may present as an *acute* form (most frequent) or as a *lymphomatous* form. Neoplastic lymphocytes express CD4 and the activation marker CD25. HTLV-I provirus can be demonstrated in neoplastic cells. This condition is characterized by circulating T cells with multilobated nuclei.

26. Correct answer: A
MYCOSIS FUNGOIDES/SÉZARY SYNDROME (p. 827)—MF/SS is a neoplasm of peripheral CD4-positive (helper) T lymphocytes. MF/SS initially involves the skin and then progresses to systemic spread. Lymph node involvement is frequent, occurring overall in 70% of cases, especially in the axillary and inguinal regions. *Sézary syndrome* refers to generalized skin involvement in the form of exfoliative erythroderma, which is associated with leukemia. Neoplastic cells have a characteristic convoluted cerebriform nucleus. Lymph node involvement may be graded according to the National Cancer Institute (NCI) scheme or the Dutch classification. Increasing degrees of nodal involvement as assessed by either of these grading schemes is correlated with increasingly poorer survival.

CHAPTER 18

1. Correct choice: B
ITP (p. 851)—Splenic disorders may be divided into those primarily affecting the white pulp or those predominantly affecting the red pulp. Reactive follicular hyperplasia is a nonspecific finding associated with various disorders, including ITP. ITP is further characterized by sheets of ceroid (lipid)-laden histiocytes in the red pulp, as evidence of active platelet phagocytosis. If this change is *not* observed, splenectomy is most likely to have a *poor* therapeutic outcome. Choice A is characteristic of thrombotic thrombocytopenic purpura; in choice C, the red pulp congestion is nonspecific, seen, for example, in hemolytic anemias; choice D is related to hemophagocytic syndromes; and choice E is classic in infectious mononucleosis.

2. Correct choice: D
LYMPHOMA INVOLVEMENT OF THE SPLEEN (pp. 852–855)—Lymphoma restricted to the spleen at clinical presentation is rare, accounting for approximately 3% of all splenectomies. Most of the cases are low-grade B-cell lymphomas, the most frequent of which is splenic marginal zone lymphoma (SMZL). SMZL is a B-cell neoplasm characterized by expanded marginal zones. These seem to surround and invade residual germinal centers, where only an attenuated rim of mantle zone lymphocytes remains visible (see picture). SMZL develops usually in elderly men. Atypical villous lymphocytes are present in peripheral blood, whereas a monoclonal peak is often present in serum and/or urine.

3. Correct choice: D
MYELOID METAPLASIA (p. 866)—Progressive fibrosis and obliteration of functioning bone marrow leads to compensatory extramedullary hematopoiesis, which involves the spleen and, less frequently, the liver. Identification of all three hematopoietic lines is a prerequisite for the diagnosis of myeloid metaplasia in the spleen. Myeloid precursors and megakaryocytes are also found in chronic myeloid leukemia.

4. Correct choice: B
HAIRY CELL LEUKEMIA (HCL; p. 867)—Patients with HCL are typically in their fifties or sixties and present with massive splenomegaly and pancytopenia. The spleen is uniformly and diffusely involved. The red pulp is infiltrated by mononuclear cells with reniform or oval nuclei and rare mitotic figures. Red "lakes" lined by neoplastic cells are characteristic. Mantle cell and marginal zone lymphomas present with a nodular pattern involving predom-

inantly the white pulp. Erythrophagocytosis is observed in chronic monocytic leukemia. The villous projections seen ultrastructurally are virtually pathognomonic of HCL and account for its designation. HCL is a cancer arising from B lymphocytes.

5. Correct choice: E
VASCULAR TUMORS OF THE SPLEEN (p. 869)—Vascular neoplasms are the most common tumors of the spleen. Littoral cell angioma is a recently described benign neoplasm consisting of sinuslike anastomosing channels lined by cells that express both endothelial cell markers (factor VIII–related antigen) and histiocytic markers (CD68). These cells are CD31-positive but CD34-negative. Papillary projections are characteristic. Occasionally, capillary or cavernous hemangiomas affect the red pulp in a diffuse manner. Choice B is associated with well-demarcated nodules of the red pulp. Splenic angiosarcomas are very rare aggressive neoplasms. Splenic lymphangioma usually occurs in the setting of systemic lymphangiomatosis.

CHAPTER 19

1. Correct choice: C
PERIPHERAL GIANT CELL GRANULOMA (pp. 881 and 882)—This lesion, probably of reactive nature, occurs most often in young women. It consists of nonencapsulated granulation tissue with numerous multinucleated giant cells. It grows in the gingiva and may erode into alveolar bone. Bilateral giant cell granulomas of the jaws are pathognomonic of *cherubism* (an autosomal dominant condition). A central giant cell granuloma of the mandible is indistinguishable from the peripheral form and overlaps in its pathological and radiological features with aneurysmal bone cyst. Choice A occurs predominantly in the tongue, choice B is also known as *intravascular papillary endothelial hyperplasia*, and choice E develops in older patients and consists of lipid-laden macrophages covered by hyperplastic epithelium.

2. Correct choice: C
ORAL SQUAMOUS CELL CARCINOMA (SCC; pp. 884 and 885)—At least half of the cases of SCC of the mouth are attributable to smoking and alcohol abuse. Ninety percent of patients are males older than 50 years who smoke and drink. Cases occurring in nonsmoking or nondrinking individuals tend to affect elderly women. Other factors, such as occupational exposure to toxins, iron deficiency (Plummer-Vinson syndrome), chronic trauma (e.g., due to ill-fitted dentures), and chronic inflammatory disorders (lichen planus and lupus erythematosus) are negligible or questionable.

3. Correct choice: E
LEUKOPLAKIA (p. 885)—*Leukoplakia* is a clinical term applied to any patch or plaque that measures at least 5 mm or greater in diameter that cannot be removed by scraping nor can it be diagnosed as a recognizable entity. The gingival gutter is the most frequently involved site. Histologically, areas of leukoplakia are due to acanthosis and/or hyperkeratosis. It may show dysplastic changes. The latter should be graded as mild, moderate, or severe. The most common pattern (*homogeneous*) is associated with a low rate of dysplastic changes (less than 10%) and transformation into neoplasia (less than 20%). Often, there is superimposed candida infection.

4. Correct choice: A
ERYTHROPLAKIA (p. 886)—Of the above lesions, erythroplakia ("red patch") would most likely harbor SCC (approximately 50%

of cases), whereas leukoplakia represents a precursor of SCC in less than 20% of cases. Note that both erythroplakia and leukoplakia are descriptive clinical terms. The red color of erythroplakia is due to dilated superficial vessels. Choice B is associated with, and probably caused by, Epstein-Barr virus. It may be a presenting sign of AIDS, but it is not directly related to HIV infection. Choice D is a benign papillomatous lesion most common on the soft or hard palate. Choice E is a trauma-related ulcer with a mixed inflammatory infiltration including numerous eosinophils.

5. Correct choice: E
HISTOLOGICAL FACTORS OF PROGNOSTIC SIGNIF-ICANCE IN ORAL SCC (p. 898)—The most important histopathological prognostic factors include the following:

- Pattern of growth and invasion: Infiltration by irregular cords or noncohesive single cells is associated with a worse prognosis than growth by solid tongues with rounded well-defined margins.
- Depth of invasion as measured with a Breslow-like method: Regional metastases are rare with a depth of invasion less than 4 mm, but frequent when greater than 8 mm.
- Vascular and perineurial invasion are negative prognostic factors.

The tumor grade is not a good predictor of lymph node metastases, nor are host response, desmoplasia, or pattern lymph node reaction.

6. Correct choice: E
VERRUCOUS CARCINOMA (pp. 902 and 903)—This variant is an extremely well-differentiated SCC of slow growth that was first identified by Ackerman in the oral cavity. It has also been found in other GI sites (nasal cavity, larynx, esophagus, anogenital areas, etc.). Approximately 5% of all SCCs are of the verrucous type. The most difficult challenge is to identify this lesion as a neoplasm because of lack of cytological markers of malignancy. It is a locally infiltrative tumor without metastatic potential. All of the patients are heavy consumers of tobacco. Choice A is a rare aggressive variant originating from the minor salivary glands with a mixed glandular-squamous pattern. Choice B is an aggressive subtype consisting of islands of basaloid cells with abrupt keratinization and peripheral palisading. Choice D is an admixture of SCC and a sarcomatous component.

7. Correct choice: I
ODONTOGENIC CYSTS (pp. 915 and 916)—Cysts of the jaw are subdivided into odontogenic and fissural. The previous list includes the most common *odontogenic cysts*. Among these, periapical cyst is the most frequent and affects adults in their 20s and 30s. Periapical cysts develop from cystic degeneration of dental gran-

ulomas. The wall cyst is lined by epithelial cells of *Malassez rests*, which are normally present within dental granulomas. The lining epithelium also contains keratinized foci, goblet cells, and peculiar hyaline bodies known as *Rushton bodies*. Periapical cysts present radiologically as well-demarcated radiolucent defects around the apex of a tooth. Maxillary incisors and mandibular molars are the most common sites. *Fissural cysts* develop at points of embryological junction between head and neck structures.

8. Correct choice: E
DENTIGEROUS CYST (p. 916)—This odontogenic cyst is one of the most common dental lesions, found in approximately 1% of adults. It develops in close association with unerupted teeth. Swelling and, less frequently, pain are clinical symptoms. The cyst is usually lined by ameloblastic-type (tooth-forming) epithelium, which is stratified and keratinizing with a conspicuous basal layer. Hemorrhage, infection, or a tangential cut may impair identification of the characteristic epithelial lining.

9. Correct choice: D
AMELOBLASTOMA (pp. 922 and 923)—This is the most common tumor arising from ameloblastic (tooth-forming) epithelium. It usually involves the jaw. In most cases, multiple cysts, whether macroscopic or microscopic, develop within the tumor. The distinguishing histological feature is the presence of epithelial islands with peripheral palisading and central loosely textured regions known as *stellate reticulum*. If cytological atypia and mitotic activity are prominent, the tumor should be diagnosed as ameloblastic carcinoma. However, the most frequently encountered problem in differential diagnosis is differentiating cystic ameloblastoma from ameloblastoid hyperplasia in dentigerous cysts.

10. Correct choice: D
ODONTOMA (p. 927)—Odontomas are characterized by the complete differentiation of ameloblasts and odontoblasts to produce enamel and dentin to form small teeth in "composite" odontomas. Complex odontomas contain enamel, dentin, and cementum.

CHAPTER 20

1. Correct choice: B
SALIVARY GLAND HETEROTOPIA (p. 933)—The most common location is within the lymph nodes of the head and neck (intranodal heterotopia). Extranodal heterotopia involves *high* sites, including ear, mandible, palatine tonsil, pituitary gland, and other

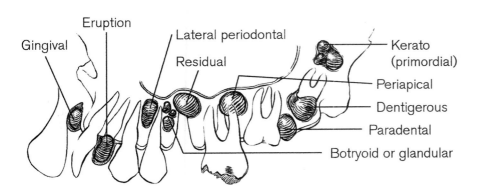

ANSWER 19.7

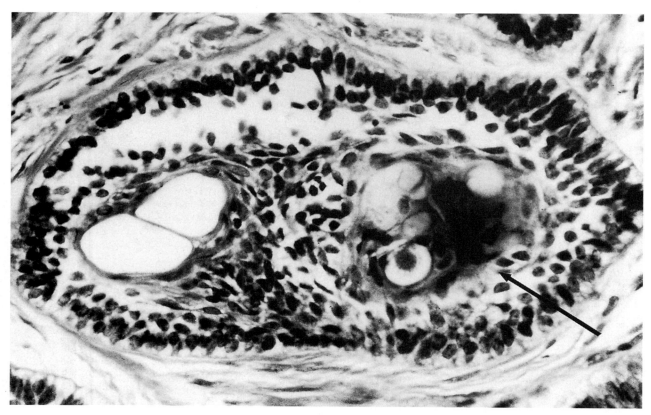

ANSWER 19.9

intracranial regions. *Low* sites of extranodal heterotopia include the right sternomastoid muscle (most frequently involved), thyroid, and cystic lesions in the neck. Awareness of intranodal salivary gland heterotopia may save the pathologist the embarrassing mistake of diagnosing metastatic tumor.

2. Correct choice: C
NECROTIZING SIALOMETAPLASIA (p. 935)—This condition is probably of ischemic origin and involves most frequently the small salivary glands of the hard palate. It presents clinically as an ulcerated lesion, which histologically may resemble squamous cell carcinoma because of prominent squamous metaplasia. Preservation of a lobular architecture is an important clue for the differential diagnosis with squamous cell carcinoma. Squamous metaplasia is observed in the center of the salivary gland, arising from preexisting ducts, whereas necrosis with accompanying inflammation involves the periphery of the glands.

3. Correct choice: E
WARTHIN TUMOR (p. 936)—Also called *cystadenoma lymphomatosum papilliferum*, this tumor develops more frequently in males (in contrast to other salivary tumors) and affects predominantly the parotid. If a parotid gland tumor is bilateral, Warthin tumor is the most likely diagnosis. Grossly, it is characterized by multiple small cysts. The histologic picture is highly characteristic (the alternative designation is virtually descriptive): cystic spaces lined by epithelium forming papillary fronds with a florid lymphocytic population forming germinal centers. Epithelial cells have a typical oncocytic appearance, being packed with mitochondria (an EM feature). Malignant transformation is rare.

4. Correct choice: C
PLEOMORPHIC ADENOMA (p. 937)—Both gross and microscopic features of this tumor are consistent with a pleomorphic adenoma, which comprises about 60% of parotid gland tumors. At least two-thirds of all parotid gland tumors are benign, and the majority of pleomorphic adenomas arise in the parotid gland. Of the previously mentioned risk factors, prior radiation is the only one correlated with increased incidence of this neoplasm. Radiation is also a known risk factor for other types of salivary gland tumors. HIV infection seems unrelated to a recent surge in the incidence of pleomorphic adenomas in the San Francisco area. EBV has been identified in the rare *lymphoepithelioma-like* variant. Smoking has been correlated with *Warthin tumor*.

5. Correct choice: C
BASAL CELL ADENOMA (p. 941)—The features summarized in the question stem correspond to an infrequent benign tumor that usually develops in the parotid gland. The *nesting* pattern is more common (two-thirds of cases) than the *tubular* pattern. Peripheral palisading is the most characteristic and diagnostically important clue, resulting in a superficial resemblance to basal cell tumors of the skin. PAS-positive material is sometimes found between epithelial cells or within the stroma. Tumor cells are immunoreactive for epithelial antigens and carcinoembryonic antigen (CEA). A tumor with these features but with cytologic atypia, mitoses, and infiltrative growth would be referred to as a *basal cell adenocarcinoma*.

6. Correct choice: E
MUCOEPIDERMOID CARCINOMA (pp. 944 and 945)—This tumor is most common in the parotid gland and relatively more frequent in children. It consists of a mixture of

three different neoplastic components, including squamous nests, mucus-producing glands, and intermediate elements referred to as "basal cells." Mucicarmine staining will highlight the mucinous component. The neoplasm can be low grade or high grade. Low-grade forms may recur but do not metastasize, whereas high-grade tumors behave aggressively. Lymphoepithelioma-like carcinoma is frequent in Eskimo and Chinese populations and is analogous morphologically and pathogenetically (i.e., EBV-related) to the nasopharyngeal counterpart.

7. Correct choice: E
ADENOID CYSTIC CARCINOMA (pp. 946 and 947)—This tumor is most common in minor salivary glands, especially of the mouth (whereas pleomorphic adenoma, Warthin tumor, and acinic cell carcinoma are typical of parotid), and may occur in lacrimal glands as well. It has a characteristic cribriform architecture, with microcysts filled with basement membrane–like material surrounded by uniform cuboidal cells as well as *true* mucus-filled glandular spaces. The combination of cystic and glandular spaces is required for diagnosis. Neoplastic cells are of myoepithelial origin and produce basement membrane–like material accumulating within microcysts. Perineurial invasion is a constant feature, resulting in tumor spread well beyond the surgical margins: this accounts for recurrences 10 to 20 years following resection, with resultant poor long-term prognosis. Pulmonary metastases are frequent, too.

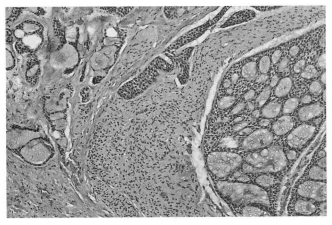

ANSWER 20.7

8. Correct choice: A
ACINIC CELL CARCINOMA (pp. 947 and 948)—This rare malignant tumor is most common in the parotid and submandibular gland. It is often well demarcated and small, sometimes multifocal (like the Warthin tumor, which is the most common bilateral/multifocal salivary gland neoplasm). The morphologic features of acinic cell carcinoma are highly variable, but the cells are usually relatively uniform and have a granular or clear cytoplasm reminiscent of serous cells. The secretory or clear vacuoles are positive for PAS. Because serous cells are rare in minor glands, the tumor is exceptional in such a location. The prognosis is related to the degree of anaplasia, but is generally poor on long-term follow-up. However, a well-encapsulated tumor of small size is likely to have a benign course.

9. Correct choice: C
HIV AND LYMPHOEPITHELIAL LESIONS (p. 954)—Lymphoepithelial cysts frequently develop in the parotid gland of

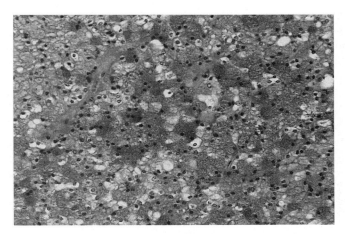

ANSWER 20.8

HIV-infected patients. They consist of multilocular cystic spaces filled with mucoid fluid and lined by glandular and/or squamous epithelium; intervening solid areas show lymphocytic infiltration with germinal centers. The pathogenesis is still debated.

10. Correct choice: E
SJÖGREN SYNDROME (p. 955)—The morphologic changes in this case, as well as the clinical manifestations, characterize *Sjögren syndrome*, which involves lacrimal and salivary glands bilaterally. Patients often have circulating anti-RNP autoantibodies (Ro and La are most frequent). The following are the newly developed *San Diego criteria* for Sjögren syndrome:

- Keratoconjunctivitis sicca
- Xerostomia
- Extensive lymphocytic infiltration of *minor* salivary glands
- Laboratory evidence of autoimmune disorder

Patients with Sjögren syndrome may have extrasalivary manifestations, with similar lesions developing in other sites. Tubulointerstitial nephritis is one of the most frequent, leading to defects in tubular function. Glomerulonephritis does not occur. Sjögren syndrome is associated with a higher risk of lymphoma, as well as primary biliary cirrhosis, sclerosing cholangitis, and interstitial lymphocytic pneumonia.

CHAPTER 21

1. Correct choice: E
RHINOSPORIDIOSIS (pp. 964 and 965)—This condition is frequent in India and occasionally seen in the United States. Rhinosporidiosis is an infectious disease whose etiologic agent appears as thick-walled sporanngia (200-μm cysts) containing thousands of spores. The nature of the infecting organism is unclear. Choice A is a rare agent of nasal infection. Choice C, also known as *phycomycosis*, is due to fungi of the genus *Mucorales*, which appear as broad, irregular nonseptate hyphae. Mucormycosis is most common in diabetic patients. Choice D is a form of foreign-body reaction to petrolatum present in preparations used for hemostatic packing. Petrolatum results in the formation of baglike spaces within the tissue containing spherules that come to resemble yeasts. Such spherules are denatured red blood cells.

2. Correct choice: B

RHINOSCLEROMA (p. 965)—Rhinoscleroma is a chronic, destructive inflammatory disease of the nose that may extend to the orbit, pharynx, larynx, and gastrointestinal tract, causing extensive ulcerations. Sheets of foamy histiocytes (*Mikulicz cells*) are characteristic of this infectious condition. *Klebsiella rhinoscleromatis* is the etiologic agent, which can be identified on tissue sections by the stains mentioned previously. Immunohistochemistry for this bacillus and serologic tests are available to establish a diagnosis. This condition should be differentiated from sinus histiocytosis with massive lymphadenopathy (*Rosai-Dorfman disease*) and leprosy. The latter condition may be histologically indistinguishable from rhinoscleroma.

3. Correct choice: D

LETHAL MIDLINE GRANULOMA (pp. 965 and 966)—This entity is in fact an umbrella including several pathogenetically unrelated conditions, characterized by extensive necrosis of midline structures of the nasopharynx, palate, paranasal sinuses, and facial skeleton. Causes include *cocaine* abuse, *Wegener granulomatosis, angiocentric lymphoma,* other forms of lymphomas, infections, and so on. The idiopathic form of LMG is a diagnosis of exclusion, and care should be taken ruling out potentially treatable conditions.

4. Correct choice: A

INFLAMMATORY NASAL POLYPS (pp. 969 and 970)—Nasal polyps can be grouped into three categories: (a) *inflammatory* (most common), (b) associated with *cystic fibrosis* (CF), and (c) *antrochoanal.* Inflammatory polyps usually manifest in patients older than 30 years and are associated with bronchospasm on aspirin consumption in 20% of cases. They are composed of edematous lamina propria infiltrated by lymphocytes, eosinophils, and plasma cells. Nasal polyps in children should arouse suspicion of CF. Antrochoanal polyps arise from cysts of the maxillary sinus protruding into the nasal cavity through the maxillary meatus. Note: CF-associated polyps contain acid mucin (Alcian blue–positive), whereas inflammatory polyps contain neutral mucin (PAS-positive).

5. Correct choice: C

SINONASAL PAPILLOMAS (p. 970)—Papillomas of the nose and paranasal sinuses can be divided into two types: squamous and schneiderian. The *squamous* type arises from the vestibule and is covered by keratinizing squamous epithelium. *Schneiderian* papillomas are more heterogeneous. They are usually lined by nonker-

atinizing squamous or transitional epithelium (less often ciliated or mucus secreting). Two main forms are recognized: fungiform and inverted. The *inverted* variant arises from the lateral wall of the nasal fossa, tends to recur following excision, and shows malignant degeneration in up to 15% of cases. The *fungiform* variant arises from the nasal septum, grows as an exophytic mass, and is not associated with malignancy. Most cases are unilateral. Association with HPV is controversial.

6. Correct choice: D

CARCINOMA OF NOSE AND PARANASAL SINUSES (pp. 973 and 974)—This rare cancer is more frequent in cigarette smokers and *nickel refiners.* Most cases arising in nickel refiners (as well as most of cases not related to occupational exposure) are squamous cell carcinomas without specific features. Instead, wood workers usually develop intestinal-type adenocarcinomas. The maxillary antrum is the most common site (58%), followed by the nasal cavity (30%) and others. The HPV genome has been detected in a minority of cases of sinonasal carcinoma, but its pathogenetic role remains unclear. Grinders and diamond polishers are exposed to cobalt and tungsten carbide (risk of asthma and lung fibrosis); battery and ammunition workers to lead (renal and peripheral nerve toxicity, anemia, and cognitive defects).

7. Correct choice: C

NASOPHARYNGEAL CARCINOMA AND EBV (pp. 974 and 975)—Nasopharyngeal carcinoma can be classified into two main histologic types: keratinizing (less frequent), and nonkeratinizing. Only the latter shows a strong association with EBV. Nonkeratinizing carcinoma of the nasopharynx is a poorly differentiated squamous cell carcinoma often containing a rich lymphocytic infiltrate, which justifies the traditional designation of *lymphoepithelioma.* The nonkeratinizing (more frequent) type may display two architectural patterns: arrangement in small nests surrounded by lymphocyte-rich fibrous septa (*Regaud* pattern A 21.7a) and diffuse sheets (*Schminke* pattern A 21.7b). The diffuse pattern may be mistaken for lymphoma. Vesicular nuclei and centrally placed prominent nucleoli support a diagnosis of carcinoma.

8. Correct choice: B

SINONASAL ADENOCARCINOMAS (p. 978)—Sinonasal malignant tumors with a glandular structure include:

■ *Salivary-type adenocarcinomas:* Adenoid cystic carcinoma is the most frequent type in this region, followed by mucoepidermoid carcinoma.

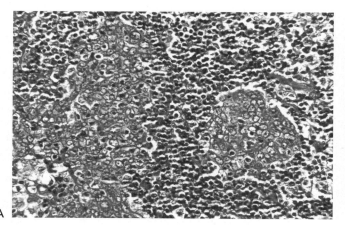

A

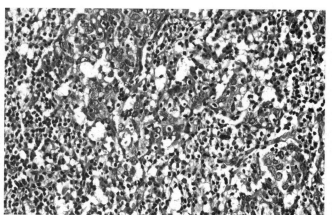

B

ANSWER 21.7

- *Low-grade adenocarcinoma* is a well-differentiated adenocarcinoma composed of tall cells without nuclear stratification.
- *Intestinal-type adenocarcinoma* is a locally aggressive neoplasm arising most commonly in the ethmoid sinus and associated with long-term exposure to fine wood dust. Morphologically, it usually resembles colonic adenocarcinoma.

9. Correct choice: D

OLFACTORY NEUROBLASTOMA (pp. 979 and 980)—The light microscopic and ultrastructural features are consistent with olfactory neuroblastoma (*esthesioneuroblastoma*), a malignant tumor that derives from the neuroepithelial cells of the olfactory mucosa. It shows morphologic characteristics of other neuroectodermal-derived tumors, such as primitive neuroectodermal tumors and adrenal neuroblastoma, including evidence of neural differentiation (i.e., *synaptophysin immunoreactivity*, Homer-Wright rosettes, neurite formation, and dense-core granules on EM). Lobular proliferation of blood vessels is sometimes seen, which may generate confusion with a vascular neoplasm. The most important differential diagnosis is with lymphoma (when a small cell population is prevalent) or poorly differentiated carcinoma (if large cells are predominant).

10. Correct choice: E

NASOPHARYNGEAL ANGIOFIBROMA (pp. 987 and 988)—This vascular lesion is encountered predominantly in males between the ages of 10 and 25. The concomitance with adolescence suggests androgen dependence, which is confirmed by the finding of testosterone receptors in the tumor. It arises always in a well-defined region of the nasal fossa from a specialized form of erectile fibrovascular tissue. Differentiation of angiofibroma from capillary hemangioma is important, considering their different evolution. Angiofibroma is composed of small vessels within irregularly arranged collagen fibers and stellate cells. Capillary hemangiomas consist of thin-walled vessels and lack abundant stroma. Spontaneous regression of angiofibromas may occur, but larger lesions need surgery and/or radiation therapy.

CHAPTER 22

1. Correct choice: B

LARYNGEAL NODULE (p. 1009)—Also called *singer's nodule*, this benign nodular lesion usually develops on the vocal cords of people who abuse their voices. In the early stages, it is composed of edematous stroma with fibroblastic hyperplasia (*gelatinous type*). Later, hyalinization of the stroma develops (leading occasionally to a misdiagnosis of localized amyloidosis) and vascular proliferation (prompting confusion with pyogenic granuloma or angioma). Almost all angiomas develop in a supraglottic location; vessels in angiomas are thick walled, whereas singer's nodule has thin-walled vessels.

2. Correct choice: D

JUVENILE LARYNGEAL PAPILLOMATOSIS (pp. 1010 and 1011)—The microscopic features and clinical history are consistent with *laryngeal papillomatosis*, a condition associated with HPV (usually 6 and 11) and manifesting with numerous laryngeal papillomas that recur repeatedly. Mild atypical changes and koilocytosis are consistently present. Those arising from the res-

piratory epithelium may not show an orderly pattern of maturation and thus may be mistaken for carcinoma in situ. The HPV genome is detectable in all cases by immunohistochemistry or *in situ* hybridization. Increased expression of epidermal growth factor receptor (not due to inherited mutations) is probably important in the pathogenesis. Exposure to alcohol, tobacco, or other irritants and voice overuse are associated with laryngitis and laryngeal keratosis.

3. Correct choice: B

ADULT LARYNGEAL PAPILLOMAS (p. 1011)—Laryngeal papillomas in adult patients are usually solitary, much less frequently associated with HPV, and do not show as high a propensity to recur as juvenile forms. However, they are more often associated with dysplastic changes and may act as precursors of squamous cell carcinomas.

4. Correct choice: C

ANATOMICAL LOCATION OF LARYNGEAL CANCER (pp. 1014 and 1018)—Anatomical location is an important prognostic determinant. Glottic tumors arise from the true vocal cord and manifest in early stages with hoarseness (A 22.4A): They have good prognosis. Tumors that cross the ventricle between the true and false vocal cord (A 22.4B) are associated with a higher rate of regional node metastasis and a worse prognosis. Supraglottic tumors arise from regions above the true cord, including false cords, epiglottis, ventricular band, and the aryepiglottic fold. Subglottic tumors arising from below the true vocal cord are rare. Those in the pyriform sinus invade the posterior edge of the thyroid cartilage and are associated with a poor prognosis. The following are approximate 5-year-survival rates according to location:

- Glottic: 90%
- Supraglottic: 65%
- Transglottic: 50%
- Subglottic: 40%

5. Correct choice: E

VERRUCOUS CARCINOMA (p. 1021)—The prognosis of laryngeal carcinoma depends mostly on location, stage, lymph node involvement, and histologic type. Verrucoid carcinoma is a rare type characterized by a polypoid gross appearance and well-differentiated microscopic features. Metastatic spread is exceptional. Basaloid squamous carcinoma is a rare extremely aggressive variant.

CHAPTER 23

1. Correct choice: A

CHONDRODERMATITIS NODULARIS HELICIS CHRONICUS (p. 1041)—This condition presents with the previously mentioned clinical and histologic features. It may recur if the nodular lesion is incompletely removed. Choice B presents with basophilic amorphous material with histiocytic and giant cell reaction. Choice C may manifest with darkly discolored wax or a dark bluish discoloration of the ear lobe in children, owing to accumulation of homogentisic acid in cartilage. Rare in the ear, choice D is characterized by sheets of macrophages with PAS-positive granules and Michaelis-Gutman bodies. Choice E, also called *granuloma fissuratum*, develops behind the ear or on the nose due to irritation from eyeglasses.

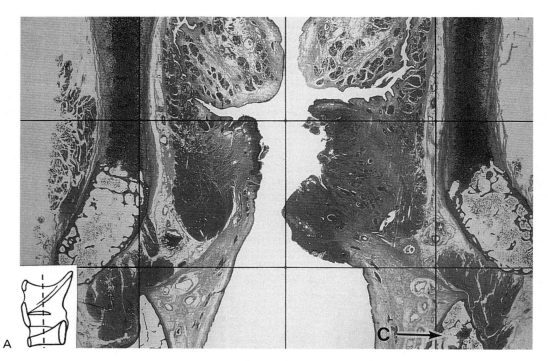

ANSWER 22.4A

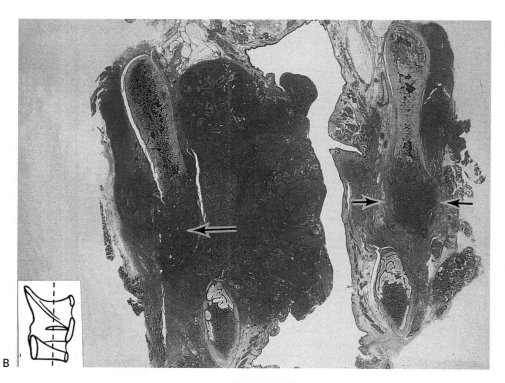

ANSWER 22.4B

2. Correct choice: B
CHOLESTEATOMA (p. 1046)—Cholesteatomas are cysts containing pearly keratin and lined by an epidermal layer devoid of adnexae. Morphologically, they are epidermoid cysts. There are congenital and acquired forms. The *congenital* form is usually closed and arises from epidermoid cell rests. The most common *acquired* form is open and develops in the context of chronic otitis media and tympanic perforation. The squamous epithelium lining the wall of the cyst is morphologically similar to epidermis, but shows an increased proliferative index, as shown by Ki-67 immunoreactivity. Cholesteatomas undergo progressive growth with erosion of the middle ear bones and ossicles. Pathogenetic mechanisms are still unclear, but probably involve epidermal invasion from the external canal into the middle ear, retraction pockets from the tympanic membrane, and trauma.

3. Correct choice: C
BASAL CELL CARCINOMA AND OTHER EPITHELIAL MALIGNANCIES (p. 1053)—Basal cell carcinoma accounts for the great majority of neoplasms in the external ear. In most cases, it arises from the pinna, and only seldom in the ear canal. Gross and histologic features of basal cell and squamous cell carcinoma of the external ear are similar to those occurring at other sites. The remaining epithelial neoplasms are most probably of ceruminous gland origin. Neoplasms of ceruminous glands are rare. Benign and malignant types are seen. The following table summarizes the features of ceruminous gland tumors.

Benign	
Adenoma (ceruminoma)	Mass blocking the ear canal
	Regular glands with two-layered epithelium (epithelial/ myoepithelial)
	Epithelial cells show apocrine features
Syringocystadenoma papilliferum	Characteristic of children-young adults
	Histologically similar to those occurring on face
Cylindroma	Morphologically similar to cylindromas in other sites
	Arrangement in a jigsaw pattern
	Differential diagnosis: adenoid cystic carcinoma

Malignant	
Adenoid cystic carcinoma	Most frequent salivary gland-type tumor
	Same features as salivary gland tumors
Mucoepidermoid carcinoma	Rare
Adenocarcinoma	Rare

4. Correct choice: C
OTOSCLEROSIS (p. 1051)—This common condition affects the otic capsule and extends to the footplate of the stapes, where the characteristic morphologic changes may be observed when a whole stapedectomy is performed. Severe forms of otosclerosis manifest with conductive hearing loss. An increased amount of new woven bone and neovascularization represent the typical microscopic findings. Because these are limited to the footplate, partial stapedectomies (limited to the crura and head) do not show any alterations. Spongiosis, with the formation of ample marrow cavities, occurs in the early stages. Other conditions mimicking otosclerosis include *Paget disease* and *osteogenesis imperfecta.*

5. Correct choice: D
JUGULOTYMPANIC PARAGANGLIOMA (JTP; p. 1060)—MRI can usually distinguish between jugular and tympanic tumors. Solitary JTPs arise in females. Sustentacular cells (highlighted by S100 immunohistochemistry) are rare in the majority of JTPs. The presence of occasional bizarre and multinucleated cells may be misleading. *Adenoma of the middle ear* consists of well-differentiated glands with a back-to-back arrangement (p. 1058). *Choristoma* is a developmental anomaly composed of salivary gland or glial tissue (p. 1048). *Meningioma* is characterized by a whorling pattern and positivity for EMA (p. 1062). *Schwannoma* of the vestibular nerve reacts strongly for S100 and is usually located in the cerebellopontine angle (p. 1061).

CHAPTER 24

1. Correct choice: A
PHTHISIS BULBI (p. 1074)—Phthisis bulbi may be defined as an end-stage condition due to a number of different eye diseases. Most of the eye bulbs submitted to pathology (with the exception of those removed because of intraocular tumors), are enucleated owing to blindness, painful conditions, or disfigurement. Phthisis bulbi is characterized by marked thickening of the sclera and disorganization of eye contents. Bone formation within a phthisical eye is common and results from metaplasia of the retinal epithelium.

2. Correct choice: A
CORNEAL DYSTROPHIES (p. 1077)—Corneal dystrophies are hereditary conditions leading to degenerative changes that affect one or more of the corneal layers, that is, the epithelium, stroma, or endothelium. Fuch's endothelial dystrophy is characterized by wartlike excrescences (guttae) of the Descemet membrane associated with loss of endothelial lining. *Granular dystrophy* is characterized by stromal deposits of an abnormal protein derived from mutation of the BIGH3 gene. *Lattice dystrophy* presents as stromal deposits of amyloid producing linear opacities. *Macular dystrophy* is indicated by accumulation of keratan sulfate–related glucosaminoglycans within the stroma and endothelium.

3. Correct choice: C
SARCOIDOSIS (p. 1083)—Sarcoidosis most commonly affects the lungs. The eyes are involved in up to 38% of patients. The conjunctiva and uvea are the most frequently involved sites, and thus a conjunctival biopsy is often used to confirm a diagnosis. Granulomatous inflammation is not associated with necrosis. Fungal and mycobacterial infections are ruled out by special stains. Tularemia and cat-scratch fever are associated with necrosis.

4. Correct choice: B
RETINOBLASTOMA (p. 1092)—This is the most common malignant tumor of the eye in childhood. Histologically, retinoblastomas are similar to other *primitive neuroectodermal tumors* (PNET) and consist of sheets of undifferentiated small cells.

Flexner-Wintersteiner rosettes (two are evident in the picture), consist of neoplastic cells arranged around a central lumen and represent important diagnostic features. Retinoblastomas have a tendency to spread along the optic nerves, and the extent of optic nerve invasion should be carefully recorded because it is directly related to prognosis.

5. Correct choice: A

INTRAOCULAR MELANOMA (p. 1094)—The most frequent of adult intraocular tumors develops from melanocytes of the uveal tract. Because uveal melanomas are usually diagnosed by clinical methods (ophthalmoscopy, fluorescein angiography, and ultrasonography), biopsy is seldom performed. Histologically, uveal melanomas can be divided into spindle cell and epithelioid cell types. Indeed, the classification is more complex, recognizing four main cellular morphologic types as highlighted in the question stem. Generally, *spindle cell melanomas* involve the iris and are associated with a better prognosis. Pure *epithelioid cell melanomas* are rare (3% of all cases) and have a worse prognosis. Combinations of the previous patterns are most common, but the presence of an epithelioid component has a negative prognostic impact.

CHAPTER 25

1. Correct choice: E

USUAL INTERSTITIAL PNEUMONIA (UIP; pp. 1113–1115)—UIP may be associated with immune-related conditions, such as rheumatoid arthritis or scleroderma, but most instances are idiopathic or preceded by a viral infection. An immune-mediated pathogenesis is suspected. An uneven distribution of pathologic changes is highly characteristic of UIP. Ultimately, UIP leads to *honeycombing.* Choice A is characterized by prominent intraalveolar mononuclear exudate, even distribution of changes, and positive response to steroid treatment. Choice B is rare, with numerous multinucleate giant cells. Choice C is suggested by prominent lymphocytic infiltration, frequent association with Sjögren syndrome and immune impairment (AIDS), and poor response to steroids. Choice D is a "wastebasket" diagnosis, with variable etiology but usually a good prognosis.

2. Correct choice: B

ASBESTOS BODIES (p. 1115)—In histologic sections, asbestos bodies have a typical clear central core and golden brown and beaded appearance. Special methods of extraction and detection (e.g., electron microprobe analysis) are required for optimal identification and classification. *Ferruginous* bodies can be due to minerals other than asbestos. Asbestos bodies may be present in the lung parenchyma and hilar lymph nodes, but almost never within mesotheliomas. Asbestos bodies should be looked for in any case of idiopathic UIP.

3. Correct choice: A

DESQUAMATIVE INTERSTITIAL PNEUMONIA (DIP; p. 1116)—This form of pneumonia has the same predisposing conditions as UIP, but occurs on average one decade before UIP. The histopathologic hallmark is an intraalveolar accumulation of macrophages, with hyperplasia of type II pneumocytes. DIP may progress to end-stage (honeycomb) lung, but usually responds to steroid treatment; hence, the importance of differentiating DIP in lung biopsies from other forms of interstitial lung disease. UIP

leads to homogeneous pathologic changes, as opposed to the patchy involvement of UIP. *Respiratory bronchiolitis* may mimic DIP, affects smokers preferentially, but is associated with a predominantly peribronchiolar pattern of inflammatory changes.

4. Correct choice: A

EXTRINSIC ALLERGIC ALVEOLITIS (EAA; p. 1122)—This entity is important because progression of lung disease can be halted by preventing further exposure to the inciting agent. Other synonyms for EAA are *farmer's lung, bird-fancier's lung, maple-bark-stripper's lung, humidifier lung,* and so on, depending on the agent. EAA is a form of hypersensitivity pneumonia leading to inflammatory infiltration of the interstitium, alveoli, and terminal airways. The distribution of inflammatory changes is uneven. Cytotoxic T cells and plasma cells are the predominant inflammatory elements, but scattered histiocytes and multinucleated giant cells are present. Eosinophils and neutrophils are infrequent, whereas granulomas may be found in terminal airways.

5. Correct choice: C

PULMONARY EOSINOPHILIC REACTIONS (p. 1124)—This pattern of injury is common to different conditions, all of which result from a hypersensitivity IgE-mediated reaction to fungi, parasites, and occasionally drugs. Aspergillus is the most commonly involved agent, for example, in *allergic bronchopulmonary aspergillosis, bronchocentric granulomatosis* (BCG), and *chronic eosinophilic pneumonia. Wuchereria bancrofti* is responsible for *tropical eosinophilia.* Tissue and blood eosinophilia represent the unifying theme. Pulmonary changes are described as eosinophilic pneumonia, because the intraalveolar protein-rich fluid, along with polymorphonuclear infiltration and edema, imparts an exudative character to the histologic picture. Chronic eosinophilic pneumonia is associated with bronchiolitis obliterans and few eosinophils. NO_2 causes acute noncardiogenic edema known as *silo-filler's disease.*

6. Correct choice: D

BRONCHOCENTRIC GRANULOMATOSIS (pp. 1126 and 1127)—This pulmonary condition is akin to other conditions covered under the umbrella of pulmonary eosinophilic reactions. It is characterized by necrotizing granulomas centered on the walls of small bronchi and bronchioles. Histologic changes may bear a striking similarity to tuberculosis. There is no necrotizing vasculitis or ANCA, but peripheral eosinophilia may not be present. As with other forms of pulmonary eosinophilic syndromes, *asthma* is a frequent manifestation. Wegener granulomatosis limited to the lungs is histologically identical to the more common systemic form.

7. Correct choice: C

BRONCHIOLITIS OBLITERANS–ORGANIZING PNEUMONIA (BOOP; p. 1128)—BOOP is considered a clinicopathologic syndrome resulting from a number of inciting events, including infectious agents, toxic inhalants, drugs, and immune-related collagenopathies. Clinical presentation may be acute (dyspnea, cough, fever) or insidious. Histologically, intrabronchiolar fibrous plugs (*Masson plugs*), interstitial inflammatory infiltration, and endoluminal macrophages lead to consolidation of pulmonary parenchyma. Masson plugs have a characteristic serpiginous shape. A classification of BOOP with respect to underlying etiologies is proposed in the table that follows.

8. Correct choice: B

BALT-ASSOCIATED LYMPHOMA (p. 1135)—This low-grade lymphoma is usually discovered in asymptomatic middle-aged or

Cases in which an underlying cause is apparent	Extrinsic allergic alveolitis Chronic eosinophilic pneumonia Organizing bacterial pneumonia
Cases in which BOOP constitutes the predominant morphologic pattern	Mycoplasma pneumonia Viral pneumonia Toxic fumes (NO₂) inhalation Collagen vascular diseases
Cases in which the underlying condition remains unknown	Approximately 50%

elderly patients. It is sometimes difficult to differentiate a pulmonary lymphoma from benign lymphoid infiltrates such as LIP or pulmonary pseudolymphoma (PL), and probably pulmonary lymphoma arises from progressive degrees of BALT hyperplasia. Features favoring BALT lymphoma include sheets or confluent nodules of uniform small lymphocytes, B-cell composition (in contrast to LIP), characteristic lymphoepithelial lesions (similar to MALT-lymphoma of the GI tract), and spread along lymphatics and blood vessels. The latter feature is referred to as *lymphatic tracking*. The prognosis is excellent.

9. Correct choice: C

LYMPHOMATOID GRANULOMATOSIS (p. 1138)—This condition is a lymphoproliferative disorder characterized by an angiocentric/angiodestructive proliferation of a polymorphic cell population. It can be thought of as a T-cell–rich B-cell lymphoma. Infiltrates consist of mixtures of atypical lymphocytes, histiocytes, plasma cells, and so on, but B lymphocytes are the true neoplastic element. T lymphocytes and other inflammatory cells are reactive. The angioinvasive nature of this process leads to large areas of coagulation necrosis. Lymphomatoid granulomatosis eventually evolves to aggressive lymphoma with a poor prognosis. The EBV genome has been found in up to 70% of cases. Lungs, skin, and the central nervous system are the most commonly involved sites.

10. Correct choice: D

PLASMA CELL GRANULOMA (PCG; p. 1141)—This lesion consists of variable mixtures of plasma cells (polyclonal, nonneoplastic) and spindly cells with features of myofibroblasts. The latter cell component, which may generate confusion with spindle cell neoplasms, expresses vimentin and actin but not CD68 (a histiocytic marker). PCG is usually observed in young people, most of whom are asymptomatic. The lesion that most closely mimics PCG is *mycobacterial pseudotumor*, which can be diagnosed by CD68 immunoreactivity for histiocytes and, most important, stains for acid-fast bacilli. *Pulmonary hyalinizing granuloma* is composed of collagen bands arranged in a storiform pattern and contains scanty lymphocytes and plasma cells.

11. Correct choice: A

IDIOPATHIC HEMOSIDEROSIS (p. 1150)—This case highlights the principal clinical and histopathologic findings of idiopathic hemosiderosis, which manifests in children and young adults with hemoptysis and anemia. Histologically, hemosiderin-laden macrophages, alveolar cell hyperplasia, varying degrees of interstitial inflammatory infiltration, and fibrosis are the main findings. Vasculitis and linear IgG deposits along the alveolar basement membrane are absent. The latter negative findings, as well as absence of renal involvement, distinguish idiopathic hemosiderosis from Goodpasture syndrome.

12. Correct choice: C

PRIMARY PLEXOGENIC HYPERTENSION (PPHT; p. 1152)—This form of primary pulmonary hypertension affects young women. Although plexogenic lesions are the most characteristic, early stages are associated with hypertrophy of vascular media. Intimal hyperplasia and reduplication of the elastic lamina follow, and arteriolar dilatation, plexogenic lesions, and fibrin thrombi occur in late phases. This sequence of events, however, has been questioned. Morphologic changes of PPTH are identical to those due to *secondary* pulmonary hypertension, for example, cases due to cardiac disease with a left-to-right shunt.

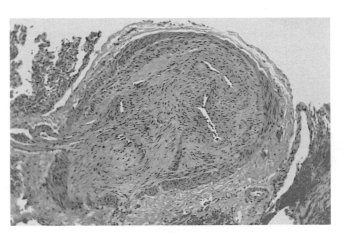

ANSWER 25.12

13. Correct choice: C

PRIMARY LYMPHANGIOMYOMATOSIS (pp. 1156 and 1157)—The defining histopathologic change of this condition is widespread smooth muscle proliferation arising from bronchi, bronchioles, veins, and lymphatics. Grossly, lymphangiomyomatosis may resemble emphysema (early stages) or honeycombing (advanced stages). Cystic spaces are separated by thick septa occupied by fascicles of smooth muscle cells. This condition is usually bilateral and diffuse, and affects women of reproductive age. Some of these patients have tuberous sclerosis, which also leads to the development of angiomyolipomas. A feature common to both angiomyolipomas and lymphangiomyomatosis is immunoreactivity for HMB-45. The main differential diagnosis is with benign metastasizing leiomyomas from the uterus.

14. Correct choice: A

ALVEOLAR PROTEINOSIS (p. 1158)—This clinicopathologic syndrome may be associated with a variety of conditions (e.g., disseminated severe bacterial, fungal or viral infections, leukemia and lymphoma, radiation or chemotherapy) that usually develop in immunocompromised patients. However, most cases are idiopathic. Radiographically, the disease may mimic pulmonary edema. Histologically, the alveolar cavities are filled with granular, PAS-positive homogeneous material, which derives from abnormal precipitation of surfactant apoprotein.

CHAPTER 26

1. Correct choice: D

SQUAMOUS CELL CARCINOMA OF LUNG (p. 1180)—This type of lung cancer usually arises from segmental bronchi (thus perihilar), undergoes central cavitation, is associated with HPV in up to 20% of cases, and does not arise in proximity to pulmonary scars. Most cases of lung cancer associated with peripheral scars are adenocarcinomas. Lambert-Eaton (myasthenic) syndrome is most commonly associated with small cell carcinoma. Hyperparathyroidism is the most common paraneoplastic syndrome associated with squamous cell carcinoma.

2. Correct choice: B

SMALL CELL CARCINOMA: ULTRASTRUCTURAL FEATURES (p. 1186)—Neurosecretory granules are characteristic of cells of neuroendocrine origin, including small cell carcinomas of the lung. These granules range from 100 to 200 nm in diameter, contain a dense osmiophilic core, and usually lie beneath the cell membrane. Other features that may be found in small cell carcinomas include basal bodies, small lumina into which long microvilli project, and scanty intermediate filaments. Choice A is characteristic of adenocarcinoma of the bronchial surface cell type, choice C of Clara cell adenocarcinoma, choice D of mesothelioma, and choice E of type II alveolar epithelial cell-type adenocarcinoma.

3. Correct choice: C

SMALL CELL CARCINOMA AND CARCINOID (p. 1187)—Differentiation between small cell carcinoma and atypical carcinoid tumor may be challenging, because both of these neoplasms may share some features, including peripheral location, nuclear morphology, foci of spindly tumor cells, chromogranin immunoreactivity (which tends to be more diffuse in carcinoid), and neurosecretory granules (which tend to be more numerous and larger in carcinoid). However, necrosis and a high mitotic rate favor small cell carcinoma.

4. Correct choice: C

BRONCHIOLOALVEOLAR CARCINOMA (p. 1189)—According to the revised WHO classification, this type of adenocarcinoma is classified into *nonmucinous*, *mucinous*, and *mixed* subtypes. The mucinous subtype arises from goblet cells and is characterized by mucin-producing columnar cells lining the alveolar walls. The nonmucinous subtype originates from Clara cells or type II pneumocytes; neoplastic cells are cuboidal and have characteristic intranuclear tubular inclusions identifiable by EM. Alpha-1-antitrypsin is a useful marker for Clara cells, and surfactant apoprotein is a useful marker for type II pneumocytes. The nonmucinous subtype of bronchioloalveolar carcinoma has a better prognosis than the mucinous variant and usually presents as a single subpleural nodule.

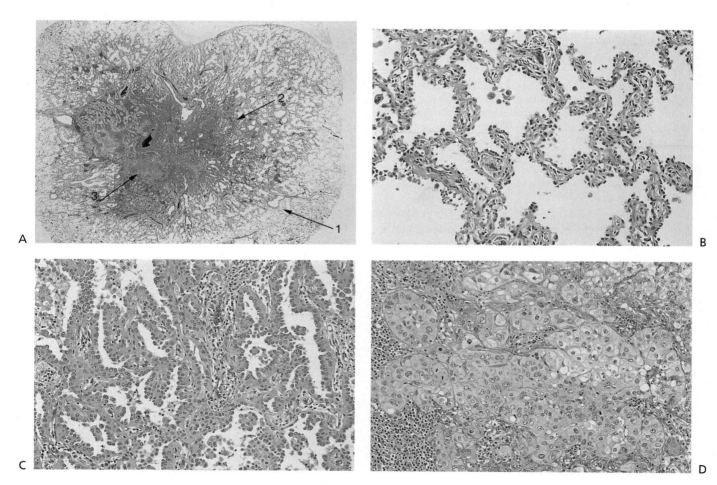

A

B

C

D

ANSWER 26.4

5. Correct choice: A

BLASTOMA (pp. 1201 and 1202)—This malignant tumor resembles Wilms tumor and consists of a glandular component within a cellular mesenchymal component. The former mimics fetal lung in the pseudoglandular stage, whereas the latter may differentiate into muscle, cartilage, or bone. Solid nests of glandular cells with ground-glass nuclei (*morulas*) are common in blastoma, but are also found in fetal adenocarcinoma. Choice B is similar to blastoma in both histology and prognosis (poor), but is distinguished by an admixture of adenocarcinoma and sarcoma in sharply demarcated islands. Choice C is a pulmonary endodermal tumor resembling fetal lung, similar to blastoma in the glandular component, but lacking a mesenchymal component; tubules surrounding morulas are the defining feature.

6. Correct choice: C

BRONCHIAL CARCINOID (pp. 1202 and 1203)—This neoplasm constitutes approximately 1% to 2% of all lung tumors. Most cases are endocrinologically inactive, only infrequently leading to *carcinoid syndrome*. They may be located centrally or peripherally and may be typical or atypical. The central variant is most frequent and grows within a segmental bronchus as a polypoid mass. Its histology is similar to intestinal carcinoids. The peripheral variant is characterized by a spindle cell population (see photo). The atypical variant may be central or peripheral and exhibits pronounced nuclear pleomorphism, mitotic activity, and necrosis. The latter is associated with a high likelihood of lymph node metastases and a poor prognosis.

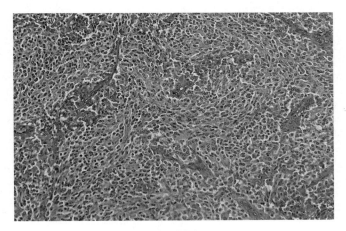

ANSWER 26.6

7. Correct choice: B

ADENOID CYSTIC CARCINOMA OF LUNGS (p. 1204)—Tumors morphologically similar to salivary gland neoplasms are rare in the lungs and usually arise from the major bronchi. Adenoid cystic carcinoma is the most frequent type and exhibits features similar to its salivary gland counterpart. As with adenoid cystic carcinomas of the salivary glands, long-term prognosis is poor because of this neoplasm's propensity to track along nerves and recur many years after complete resection. Mucoepidermoid carcinoma is the next most frequent type.

8. Correct choice: B

CLEAR CELL TUMOR (SUGAR TUMOR) (p. 1206)—This unusual neoplasm presents as a well-demarcated mass composed of clear cells within a fine sinusoidal network. The cytoplasm of neoplastic cells is filled with glycogen-containing lysosomes. The neoplasm is diffusely immunoreactive for HMB-45 and focally positive for S100. Its histogenesis is obscure, but EM shows presence of premelanosomes and, rarely, mature melanosomes. Because of these features, sugar tumors are thought to be of melanocytic origin, perhaps akin to angiomyolipoma.

9. Correct choice: D

SCLEROSING HEMANGIOMA (pp. 1207 and 1208)—This benign slow-growing lesion is usually discovered incidentally in young women. It is a well-demarcated, solid, tan mass composed of polygonal cells arranged in a nesting or papillary pattern. The cells have eosinophilic cytoplasm. Characteristic is a sort of zonal pattern: Peripheral regions show a papillary architecture and increased cellular atypia (which may lead to an erroneous diagnosis of adenocarcinoma), whereas central areas have an angiomatous appearance. Features favoring an origin from type II pneumocytes include immunoreactivity for *surfactant apoprotein*, as well as lamellated bodies and short microvilli on EM (all features of normal type II pneumocytes). Thus, this lesion is not a hemangioma.

10. Correct choice: D

INFLAMMATORY PSEUDOTUMOR (p. 1208)—This condition is a reactive lesion that often affects young adults or children. Its histology varies from case to case, but fascicles of spindle-shaped mesenchymal cells with chronic inflammatory cells are salient features. Vascular proliferation, plasma cell infiltration, collagen formation, hemosiderin deposition, xanthomatous change, and so on, may be seen in various degrees and, depending on whether one or the other of such features predominates, inflammatory pseudotumors may be mistaken for plasmacytoma, hemangiopericytoma, amyloid tumor, carcinoid, and so on. Plasma cells are numerous in lesions affecting adolescents. Occasionally, mycobacteria have been demonstrated.

11. Correct choice: A

PULMONARY HAMARTOMA (p. 1208)—This benign lesion is usually discovered as an incidental finding on chest x-rays. An admixture of cartilage, smooth muscle, epithelium-lined clefts, and adipose tissue is characteristic. In contrast to previous hypotheses, lung hamartoma is an acquired lesion. It probably arises from overgrowth of mesenchymal components of the bronchial walls, with secondary entrapment of bronchial epithelium.

12. Correct choice: C

IMMUNOHISTOCHEMISTRY OF SMALL CELL CARCINOMA (pp. 1211 and 1212)—Immunohistochemical markers of small cell carcinoma (SCC) include amine and peptide hormones and markers of neural differentiation (chromogranin, synaptophysin, neuron specific enolase, etc.). None of these is 100% sensitive or specific, being found in carcinoid tumors as well as in non–small cell carcinomas (NSCC). NSE and the brain isoform of creatine kinase (CK-BB) are found positive in the majority of SCCs, but also in NSCCs. N-CAM has been immunohistochemically identified in the great majority of SCCs and may become the most useful marker of this type of neoplasm.

13. Correct choice: D

SURFACTANT APOPROTEIN (pp. 1212 and 1213)—Immunohistochemistry to identify surfactant apoprotein may be used for the diagnosis of bronchioloalveolar carcinoma of type II alveolar cell origin (the less common form of the *nonmucinous* subtype). Clara cells express alpha-1-antitrypsin.

CHAPTER 27

1. Correct choice: D

REACTIVE MESOTHELIAL CELLS (p. 1223)—Regenerating mesothelium has been shown to derive from subserosal fibroblast-like cells that migrate toward the surface and acquire an epithelial/mesothelial phenotype. Originally such cells express vimentin exclusively, but they retain the ability to express low-molecular-weight keratin and actin in response to noxious stimuli. This phenotypical change has been observed in other serosal sites. A common problem in the differential diagnosis of serosal lesions is distinguishing reactive from neoplastic cells. Keratin-positive reactive cells do not show infiltrative behavior and are arranged in a bandlike fashion parallel to the serosal surface, in sharp contrast to the underlying mesenchymal or neoplastic tissue.

2. Correct choice: E

SOLITARY FIBROUS TUMOR (pp. 1226 and 1227)—The clinical and histologic features are consistent with solitary fibrous tumor (SFT) of the pleura. This usually benign neoplasm has been described in a variety of anatomical sites, including the mediastinum, kidney, sinonasal cavity, soft tissue, meninges, and so on. CD34 immunoreactivity is highly characteristic and allows differentiation from histologically similar tumors. A keloidlike fibrous stroma is a frequent feature of SFT. Recurrence of SFT after excision is approximately 15%; malignant transformation is rare.

3. Correct choice: E

MALIGNANT MESOTHELIOMA (MM; p. 1227)—The main differential diagnosis in this case is with lung adenocarcinoma or metastasis from distant cancer. Features highly suggestive of MM include the following: Alcian blue staining removed by pretreatment with hyaluronidase, absence of PAS staining, and ultrastructural evidence of thin long microvilli devoid of glycocalyx. Keratin immunoreactivity is not specific to MM, but helps in the differential diagnosis with other tumors. There is no specific diagnostic marker, but certain immunohistochemical profiles are more consistent with MM than adenocarcinoma. A list of antibodies for a mesothelioma panel and their reactivity in mesotheliomas versus adenocarcinomas, *although there is variation of specificity and sensitivity in each,* is given in the table below.

4. Correct choice: E

DIFFERENTIAL DIAGNOSIS IN EPITHELIAL MESOTHELIOMA (p. 1231)—The answers include the main entities to consider in the differential diagnosis of the epithelial type of mesothelioma. *Epithelial mesothelioma* is characterized by a tubulopapillary architecture. Neoplastic cells lining the tubules and papillae have a cuboidal, domelike shape, in contrast to adenocarcinomas, where cells have a columnar shape. Epithelioid hemangioendothelioma may rarely mimic the morphologic features of epithelial mesothelioma. Immunohistochemistry for epithelial and endothelial antigens is important in differentiating epithelioid hemangioendothelioma from a poorly differentiated epithelial mesothelioma or metastatic adenocarcinoma.

5. Correct choice: D

FIBROUS MESOTHELIOMA (p. 1232)—Of the main histologic types of mesothelioma (epithelial, fibrous, and mixed), *fibrous mesothelioma* (also known as *sarcomatous mesothelioma*) retains a fibroblast-like appearance, which may resemble fibromatosis in its well-differentiated form. However, focal expression of keratin or other epithelial markers is demonstrable in mesotheliomas but not fibromatosis. A storiform pattern, hemangiopericytoma-like foci, abundant collagen, and bland cytologic appearance can all be found in mesotheliomas. Actin expression, on the other hand, is frequent in fibromatosis, reflecting the myofibroblastic origin of this condition.

CHAPTER 28

1. Correct choice: C

CLINICAL MANIFESTATIONS OF MEDIASTINAL LESIONS: SUPERIOR VENA CAVA SYNDROME (pp. 1253 and 1254)—Mediastinal lesions need not reach a large size to produce symptoms. Chest pain, dyspnea, dysphagia, and cough are the most common symptoms. Less frequently, mediastinal processes cause superior vena cava syndrome. In this case, the most frequent etiologies include lymphomas in both adults and children, metastatic lung cancer in adults, and acute leukemias in children. Occasionally, chronic mediastinitis (caused by mycobacteria, fungi,

Antibodies	
Low-molecular-weight keratins (MABs or cocktails)[a]	
Vimentin[b]	
Epithelial markers[c]	CEA
	Ber-EP4
	BG-8
	Leu-M1 (CD15)
	B72.3
Mesothelial markers[d]	HBME-1
	Calretinin
	CK5/6

[a]Useful particularly in distinguishing sarcomatous MM from sarcoma.
[b]Concomitant expression of vimentin and keratin is more frequent in mesotheliomas than lung adenocarcinoma, but it is seen as well in several adenocarcinomas (e.g., renal, thyroid, and endometrial).
[c]Monoclonal antibodies (MABs) to antigens expressed preferentially by epithelial cells.
[d]Newly developed MABs to antigens preferentially expressed by mesothelium.

nocardia, etc.) or fibrosing mediastinitis may manifest with superior vena cava syndrome.

2. Correct choice: B
THYMIC CYSTS (p. 1256)—In general, *cystic mediastinal lesions* account for 15% of all mediastinal masses. Cystic mediastinal lesions include *thymic cysts*. These manifest within a 20- to 50-year range and may be *unilocular* or *multilocular*. Unilocular cysts are found anywhere along a line drawn from the angle of the mandible to the manubrium of the sternum and are developmental in origin, arising from remnants of the third branchial pouch. Multilocular cysts are probably akin to branchial cleft cysts and cervical lymphoepithelial cysts. They result from an inflammatory reaction leading to cystic transformation of medullary thymic epithelial structures. They have been described in association with Hodgkin lymphoma or dysgerminoma.

Thymic Cysts	Unilocular	Multilocular
Content	Clear	Turbid ("cheesy")
Wall	Thin	Thick, fibrous
Lining	Bland squamoid	Proliferative, micropapillary
Inflammatory infiltrate	Absent	Present
Hassall corpuscles remnants	Absent	Present in up to 50%
Pathogenesis	Developmental	Inflammatory

3. Correct choice: A
BRONCHOGENIC CYST (pp. 1257 and 1258)—In contrast to intrapulmonary bronchogenic cysts, those developing in the mediastinum are not connected with the bronchial tree and are thus asymptomatic. Their wall is composed of respiratory epithelium (at least focally) and islands of mature cartilage. *Cystic hygroma* is a cystic lymphangioma, usually seen in the neck or mediastinum of children. *Enteric cysts* are lined by gastroenteric epithelium and develop in the posterior mediastinum of children. *Pericardial cysts* are mesothelium-lined cysts located at the cardiophrenic angle.

4. Correct choice: B
CYSTIC THERATOMA OF MEDIASTINUM (p. 1261)—This is the most common germ cell–derived tumor of the mediastinum. It usually appears as a multilocular cystic mass in the anterior compartment. It constitutes 10% to 15% of all mediastinal tumors. The presence of immature neuroepithelium (e.g., with rosettelike structures mimicking primitive neural tubules) is virtually the only histologic feature justifying a diagnosis of immature teratoma. However, exceptionally rare examples of immature teratomas have been reported, which contain areas of angiosarcoma, rhabdomyosarcoma, osteosarcoma, chondrosarcoma, or carcinoma.

5. Correct choice: F
THYMOMA, MICROSCOPIC FEATURES (pp. 1263–1265)—The question stem describes some of the most significant histopathologic features of thymoma, which allows distinguishing this tumor from other most common mediastinal neoplasms. Important clues are the rosettelike formation *without* true lumina (carcinoid have similar rosettes, but *with* lumina), perivascular spaces

(serum lakes) filled with lymphocytes and histiocytes, the angular shape of the lobules separated by thick fibrous septa (Hodgkin has rounded lobules), and the nuclear features (seminoma cells have prominent nucleoli).

6. Correct choice: A
THYMOMA: CLASSIFICATION (pp. 1263 and 1264)—The new WHO classification aims at incorporating features of two previous classifications, that is, the one by Lattes and Bernatz (LB: purely descriptive), and the one by Marino, Muller-Hermelink, and colleagues (MMH: supposedly having a functional/anatomic relationship with the normal thymus).

Type A (*atrophic*): The atrophic thymus of adult life is composed of spindly epithelial cells. A-type thymomas, therefore, recapitulate the features of the adult-type inactive thymus and may be considered well differentiated.

Type **B** (*bioactive*): The thymus in fetal and early childhood life is composed of plump, round, or stellate epithelial cells. B-type thymomas, therefore, recapitulate the morphology of the fetal/infantile thymus and are less well differentiated. The number following B relates to the amount of accompanying lymphoid population:

- B1 if the lymphoid population is prevalent
- B2 if epithelial and lymphoid populations are equivalent
- B3 if the epithelial component is prevalent. Because the epithelial component is neoplastic, B1–B3 reflects a progressive increase in malignant behavior.

Type C (*carcinoma*): In this case, histologic and cytologic features are obviously malignant, with marked pleomorphism, mitotic activity, necrosis, and absence of ancillary features of thymic differentiation (e.g., abortive Hassall's corpuscles).

Recent studies suggest that this system has a good prognostic correlation. The spindle cell variant (WHO type A) is the least likely to be associated with myasthenia gravis.

7. Correct choice: E
THYMIC LYMPHOID HYPERPLASIA (pp. 1264 and 1265)—Thymic lymphoid hyperplasia refers to the presence of numerous reactive lymphoid follicles, which may contain germinal centers. The weight of the thymus is usually within normal limits. Thymic lymphoid hyperplasia is found in two-thirds of patients with myasthenia gravis, but may be occasionally seen in association with other immune-related processes such as Addison disease, HIV infection, systemic lupus erythematosus, and so on. It must be distinguished from lymphocyte-predominant thymoma.

8. Correct choice: E
THYMOMA VERSUS LYMPHOID HYPERPLASIA (p. 1265)—Of all patients with myasthenia gravis (MG), 65% will have thymic follicular hyperplasia, 10% a thymoma, and 25% no thymic changes. Lymphoid (follicular) hyperplasia is the morphological feature that correlates best with MG even when a thymoma is found. The listed features help to distinguish lymphocyte-rich thymomas (B1 according to the new WHO classification) from lymphoid hyperplasia. In particular, effacement of thymic architecture is seen in thymoma but not in lymphoid hyperplasia. Medullary differentiation refers to loosely structured aggregates of lymphocytes mimicking thymic medulla. Serum lakes are very important diagnostic clues.

9. Correct choice: A
THYMOMA VERSUS CASTLEMAN DISEASE (p. 1266)—Usually, Castleman disease (also called *angiofollicular lymphoid*

hyperplasia) in the mediastinum affects lymph nodes and not the thymus itself. This case highlights the salient microscopic features of Castleman disease. The main differential diagnosis in the mediastinum is with lymphocyte-predominant thymoma.

10. Correct choice: D
THYMOMA VERSUS LYMPHOBLASTIC LYMPHOMA (p. 1267)—Although LBL occurs at a younger age than LPT, radiologic and clinical features overlap to such an extent that morphologic diagnosis is of crucial importance. CD1, CD3, CD43, CD99, *bcl-2*, and terminal deoxynucleotidyl transferase are often positive in lymphocytes of both tumors. However, cytokeratin immunohistochemistry will highlight a fine meshwork of interconnecting epithelial cells in LPT, thus helping to differentiate it from LBL. Electron microscopy also will demonstrate epithelial features (desmosomes) in LPT but not LBL. Note that, besides LBL, Burkitt-like (small noncleaved) lymphoma may arise in the mediastinum.

11. Correct choice: C
EPITHELIAL SPINDLE CELL THYMOMA VERSUS OTHER SPINDLE CELL TUMORS (pp. 1268 and 1269)—Predominantly epithelial thymomas with a spindle cell appearance (type A of the WHO classification) may display a storiform pattern mimicking fibrous histiocytoma or a staghornlike vascular pattern resembling hemangiopericytoma. Both such tumors express vimentin and lack keratin, whereas spindle cell thymomas express keratin but not vimentin.

12. Correct choice: C
MEDIASTINAL SCHWANNOMA (NEURILEMOMA; p. 1270)—Tumors of peripheral nerves in the mediastinum include schwannoma, neurofibroma, and malignant peripheral nerve sheath tumor (MPNST). Mediastinal schwannomas usually grow to a large size before manifesting clinically. The presence of a capsule is a unique feature compared to schwannomas developing in other sites. Regressive changes are common and include hemorrhages, cystic degeneration, hemosiderin deposition, and vascular wall hyalinization. By the time the tumor is discovered and removed, regressive changes may be so pronounced as to make histologic diagnosis rather difficult (*ancient schwannoma*). The prognosis is excellent.

13. Correct choice: C
THYMIC CARCINOMA AND VARIANTS (pp. 1284 and 1285)—It is now well established that primary thymic carcinoma constitutes a distinctive entity to be separated from thymomas. Grossly, thymic carcinoma usually lacks a capsule and the broad septation characteristic of thymomas. Histologically, the features of malignancy are obvious, such as cellular atypia, necrosis, mitotic activity, intravascular invasion, and so on. The great majority of thymic carcinomas arise *de novo* and not from dedifferentiation of thymomas. Keratin expression and tonofilaments on EM are common to all types. Choice A is characterized by an admixture of neoplastic glandular and squamous components, choice B cells contain clear cytoplasm, choice D is similar to the nasopharyngeal form and associated with EBV, and choice E is a poorly differentiated variant of the keratinizing type.

14. Correct choice: B
THYMIC CARCINOID/NEUROENDOCRINE CARCINOMA (p. 1290)—This unique type of thymic tumor is often confused with thymoma. It is associated with Cushing syndrome in one-third of cases, but never with carcinoid syndrome. Metastatic spread is seen in more than two-thirds of cases. The ribbonlike architecture and presence of rosettes with well-formed

lumina are the most important clues to diagnosis. Synaptophysin immunoreactivity and the ultrastructural finding of dense-core granules may help to confirm the diagnosis of thymic carcinoid. Perinuclear deposits of microfilaments (5 nm) are an additional but rarer feature. Choice A is found in thymoma, choice C in seminoma, choice D in lymphoblastic lymphoma and large cell lymphoma, and choice E in ganglioneuroma and related tumors.

15. Correct choice: D
PARAGANGLIOMA (p. 1292)—This neoplasm is rare in the mediastinum (less than 0.5%), where it includes aorticopulmonary and paravertebral forms. Low-power examination of this lesion allows a presumptive diagnosis on H&E, showing its typical nesting arrangement (often referred to as "zellballen"), in which round nests of neoplastic cells are surrounded by delicate fibrovascular septa. Immunohistochemistry confirms the diagnosis: Neoplastic cells within zellballen are immunoreactive for synaptophysin and similar neural antigens, whereas sustentacular cells around zellballen are positive for S100.

16. Correct choice: D
SETTLE AND CASTLE (p. 1305)—SETTLE occurs in or around the thyroid and affects adolescents and young adults (mostly males). Histologically, its most distinguishing feature is the biphasic pattern similar to *synovial sarcoma*. The long-term prognosis is poor because of late-occurring metastases. CASTLE is a thymic carcinoma developing in a juxtathyroid location. Ectopic cervical thymoma occurs almost exclusively in females around the thyroid and is histologically indistinguishable from its thymic counterpart. *Ectopic hamartomatous thymoma* is a benign tumor developing in the supraclavicular/suprasternal regions and composed of a spindle cell epithelial component amid anastomosing squamous cell strands.

17. Correct choice: A
THYMOMA: PROGNOSTIC FACTORS (pp. 1305 and 1306)—Histologic classification of thymomas has been (and continues to be) one of the most controversial issues in surgical pathology. Regardless of the histologic type, however, the presence and extent of *extracapsular invasion* is the single most important prognostic parameter. Extracapsular invasion is usually assessed by the surgeon at the time of the operation, but histologic typing does have a correlation with neoplasm's biologic behavior. Of histological types, predominantly spindle cell thymoma (WHO type A) has the best prognosis.

CHAPTER 29

1. Correct choice: C
HYPERTROPHIC CARDIOMYOPATHY (p. 1324)—This condition is characterized by asymmetric left ventricular hypertrophy, which results in abnormal thickening of the interventricular septum, decreased compliance, and stenosis of the outflow aortic segment. Histologically, the disarray of myofibers, myofiber hypertrophy, basophilic degeneration, and interstitial fibrosis are characteristic (although nonspecific). A substantial number of cases are due to inherited mutations of genes encoding myofibrillary proteins such as myosin chains. Endomyocardial biopsies do not have a high diagnostic yield, showing myofiber disarray in only one-third of cases.

2. Correct choice: D
ADRIAMYCIN TOXICITY (p. 1327)—The changes described in the question stem are typical (although not pathognomonic) of adriamycin toxicity. It should be emphasized that the evaluation of

a posttransplant rejection and the assessment of adriamycin toxicity are the two most common reasons for performing endomyocardial biopsies. Adriamycin toxicity first manifests with vacuolization of myocytes, which corresponds to *sarcotubular dilatation,* followed by the appearance of typical *adria cells* (basophilic myocytes with loss of myofilaments). Inflammatory infiltration is absent. Grading of adriamycin toxicity is routinely performed.

3. Correct choice: E

MYOCARDITIS (p. 1328)—The *Dallas criteria* for a morphologic diagnosis of myocarditis have been used increasingly since 1984. To establish a definitive diagnosis of myocarditis, inflammatory infiltration must be present in association with myocyte necrosis. Any form of inflammatory infiltrate alone is considered consistent with *borderline* myocarditis. Giant cell myocarditis and necrotizing eosinophilic myocarditis have a higher morbidity and mortality than the usual myocarditis with lymphocytic infiltration.

4. Correct choice: C

RHEUMATIC HEART DISEASE (p. 1330)—Bacterial/parasitic myocarditis usually affect the myocardium by indirect, immune-mediated reactions. The prototypical example is rheumatic heart disease, whose characteristic changes (lymphohistiocytic infiltration with Aschoff bodies) are seen most commonly in the atrial appendages and valves, and occasionally in endomyocardial biopsies as well. *Chagas disease* is caused by *Trypanosoma cruzi,* an intracellular parasite. *Lyme disease* is caused by spirochetes (*B. burgdorferi*): and characterized by plasmacellular infiltration. *RMSF* is caused by

rickettsiae and associated with lymphocytic infiltration. *Toxoplasma myocarditis* is seen in AIDS patients.

5. Correct choice: E

QUILTY LESION (p. 1338)—This change, referred to as a Quilty lesion, is observed in up to 30% of endomyocardial biopsies following transplantation. It does not imply rejection and is not due to drug toxicity. EBV infection, involved in posttransplant lympho-proliferative disorder, does not play a role in Quilty lesions. Quilty lesions may be confined to the endocardial surface or extend to the adjacent subendocardial myocardium. Prior biopsies lead to healing foci of ischemic injury, which should not be confused with acute rejection.

6. Correct choice: B

MYOCARDIAL BIOPSIES (p. 1337)—Grade 1a (Photo A) is a focal infiltrate without necrosis; 1b (Photo B) is a diffuse sparse infiltrate with no necrosis; 2 is a single focus of aggressive infiltrate and/or myocyte damage; 3a (Photo C) is multifocal aggressive infiltrate and/or myocyte damage; 3b (Photo D) is diffuse inflammation and necrosis; and 4 is reserved for those biopsies with diffuse aggressive infiltrates including polys, myocyte necrosis always, and often edema, hemorrhage, and vasculitis.

7. Correct choice: E

RHEUMATIC HEART DISEASE (p. 1343)—*Gross* evaluation of surgical specimens is crucial in the diagnosis of cardiac valvular disease. Commissural fusion is highly characteristic of rheumatic heart disease, giving rise to a "fish mouth" appearance. Myxomatous

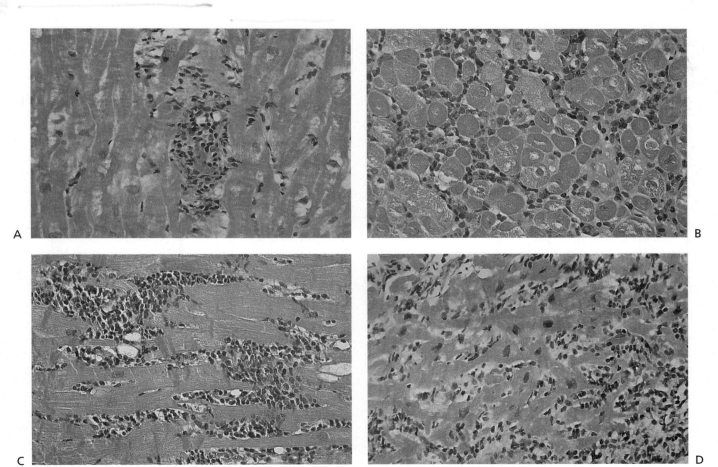

A

B

C

D

ANSWER 29.6

degeneration is associated with the ballooning of leaflets and stretching of chordae tendinae. Left ventricular enlargement leads to widening of the annulus and mitral valve insufficiency. Defects in valve leaflets and the rupture of chordae tendinae are often the results of infective endocarditis.

8. Correct choice: D

CARDIAC MYXOMA (p. 1351)—Myxoma, the most common primary cardiac tumor, is located in the left atrium in 80% of cases. Women are preferentially affected. The clinical presentation may be variable, with an infective endocarditis–like picture, systemic embolism, or mitral valve obstruction. The tumor is composed of stellate cells within an abundant myxoid matrix. However, the microscopic appearance may vary considerably, including calcifications or ossification, superficial thrombosis, glandlike structures, and extramedullary hematopoiesis. The familial form of myxoma is associated with extracardiac anomalies in *Carney syndrome.*

CHAPTER 30

1. Correct choice: A

ENDARTERECTOMY (pp. 1371 and 1372)—Endarterectomy is performed in patients with severe stenotic atherosclerosis at the carotid bifurcation. Clinical studies have shown important therapeutic benefits in patients with symptomatic cerebrovascular disease (such as transient ischemic attacks, or TIAs). An endarterectomy specimen usually reaches the pathology laboratory in a single piece that consists of atheromatous material and the inner layers of intima and media. The main purpose of histologic examination is to define the plane of surgical cleavage within the wall. No more than a few lamellae of elastic tissue should be present.

2. Correct choice: B

ANEURYSMS (p. 1373)—The list of choices includes different conditions associated with different types of aneurysms. Pseudoaneurysms (also called *traumatic aneurysms*) are due to trauma and result from development of a false arterial wall around a hematoma. Choice A is the presumed predisposing condition for the development of *Berry aneurysms,* affecting arteries of the circle of Willis. Choice C names strong predisposing factors for *abdominal aortic aneurysms.* Choice D is most commonly associated with *mycotic aneurysms,* due to seeding of bacteria in the vessel wall. Choice E is associated with aortic *dissecting aneurysms.*

3. Correct choice: A

ABDOMINAL AORTIC ANEURYSM (AAA; p. 1373)—AAA is usually caused by severe atherosclerosis that weakens the media of the artery. This condition leads to progressive dilatation of the aortic wall. Defects in genes coding for collagen or intercellular matrix components may play a contributory role. Complications of AAA include mural thrombosis with partial or complete stenosis of the ostia of branching arteries, and superinfection, commonly due to *Salmonella.* Choice B usually involves the aortic arch and results in aortic dissection. Among infective aneurysms (choice C), a *syphilitic aneurysm* develops in the ascending portion of the aortic arch as a complication of tertiary syphilis. Choice D is a pathogenetic mechanism underlying Berry aneurysms, and choice E may result in pseudoaneurysms.

4. Correct choice: A

GIANT CELL (TEMPORAL) ARTERITIS (p. 1379)—This cause of fever of unknown origin commonly affects the elderly and is often associated with polymyalgia rheumatica. If not promptly treated with high-dose corticosteroids, temporal arteritis may spread to the ophthalmic artery causing visual loss. A bilateral temporal biopsy has a diagnostic yield of up to 90% to 95%. The pathologic changes may be patchy, and therefore biopsy segments of the temporal artery should be as large as possible. Furthermore, multiple levels should be examined histologically. Generalized artery involvement has been reported, including the aortic branches. *Degos disease* leads to a diffuse subendothelial fibrosis of arterial walls, resulting in infarcts, particularly in skin and GI tract. *Hepatitis B* is associated with polyarteritis nodosa, and loss of the radial pulse is characteristic of *Takayasu arteritis.*

5. Correct choice: D

POLYARTERITIS NODOSA (PN; p. 1384)—The classification of vasculitides is based on the size of the involved vessels:

- Large vessels: *giant cell arteritis* and *Takayasu arteritis*
- Medium vessels: *polyarteritis nodosa* (PN) and *Kawasaki disease*
- Small vessels: *microscopic polyangiitis, Churg-Strauss syndrome, Wegener granulomatosis, Goodpasture syndrome, cutaneous leukocytoclastic arteritis, Henoch-Schönlein syndrome.*

PN predominantly affects medium-sized arteries. The skin, kidneys, heart, GI tract, and joints are most frequently involved, but renal pathology is the most important source of morbidity and mortality. Transmural inflammation, fibrinoid necrosis, thrombosis, and scarring are found at different stages in different vessels or within the same vessel. PN derives its name from the nodularity imparted by alternating aneurysms and stenotic segments. Hepatitis B is the most commonly identifiable associated condition. ANCAs are not present in classic PN.

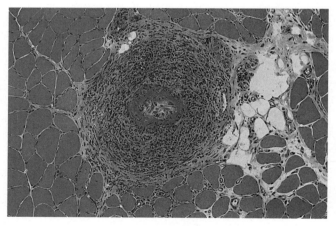

ANSWER 30.5

6. Correct choice B

MICROSCOPIC (PAUCI-IMMUNE) POLYANGIITIS (p. 1385)—Microscopic polyangiitis involves vessels of small caliber, including arterioles, capillaries, and venules. The skin, kidneys, GI tract, brain, and muscles are most commonly involved. Frequently, drugs (such as penicillin) and infectious agents (such as streptococci) are the most commonly identifiable triggering factors. Vascular lesions contain scanty or no immune deposits (*pauci-immune vasculitis*). Most cases are associated with p-ANCA. These autoantibodies react with the *myeloperoxidase* of neutrophils and produce a perinuclear pattern of immunofluorescence staining.

7. Correct choice: B
RENAL ARTERY FIBRODYSPLASIA (p. 1393)—This is a heterogeneous set of conditions including various morphologic patterns. *Medial fibroplasia*, the most common form, is characterized by segmental fibrous thickening of the media alternating with aneurysmal dilatation, which creates the typical "beaded" appearance on angiography. This form accounts for about two-thirds of all cases of renal artery dysplasia, manifests with hypertension, and is more common in women in their 30s and 40s. *Perimedial fibroplasia* is the second most common form (about 20% of cases): it consists of diffuse fibrosis of the media without intervening aneurysmal segments.

CHAPTER 31

1. Correct choice: H
REFLUX ESOPHAGITIS (p. 1401)—Alone, none of the named histological changes represents a reliable diagnostic marker of GERD. Therefore, diagnosis of GERD rests on clinicopathologic correlation. Intraepithelial eosinophilic infiltration is perhaps one of the most specific correlates of GERD, but scattered intraepithelial eosinophils are observed in one-third of esophageal biopsies from patients without GERD, and only up to 55% of patients with clinical GERD have intraepithelial eosinophils. Ballooned cells are swollen epithelial cells with pale cytoplasm. Intraepithelial neutrophils and mucosal ulceration are associated with more severe stages of GERD or severe mucosal insults. The differential diagnosis of GERD-associated changes includes infectious esophagitis and pill-induced esophagitis.

2. Correct choice: B
HSV ESOPHAGITIS (p. 1405)—The photomicrograph shows squamous cells and multinucleated cells containing Cowdry type A inclusions, characteristic of HSV. These are eosinophilic ground-glass inclusions separated by a clear halo from a thickened nuclear membrane. Multinucleated giant cells will also show typical nuclear molding. Three main pathogens can cause infective forms of esophagitis, for example, *candida*, *HSV*, and *cytomegalovirus*. These infections are more frequent in immunocompromised patients.

3. Correct choice: D
BARRETT ESOPHAGUS (p. 1407)—This condition consists of columnar metaplasia of the normal squamous esophageal mucosa. Microscopically, the presence of goblet cells is the most significant feature: Goblet cells contain acid mucin that can be demonstrated by Alcian blue at pH 2.5. In contrast, columnar cells usually contain neutral PAS-positive mucin. Barrett esophagus increases the risk of adenocarcinoma by 20 to 50 times that of the general population.

4. Correct choice: C
DYSPLASIA IN BARRETT ESOPHAGUS (p. 1410)—The picture demonstrates features of high-grade dysplasia, including loss of polarity, severe cytologic atypia, and mitotic figures. Barrett esophagus is an acquired condition resulting from gastroesophageal reflux. The epithelium of the lower esophagus is replaced (in a diffuse, fingerlike, or patchy pattern) by columnar epithelium. There are three main types:

- *Atrophic fundal*, containing parietal and chief cells
- *Junctional* (*cardiac*), with mostly mucous glands
- *Specialized columnar*, consisting of epithelium resembling that of the small bowel, with columnar, goblet, and endocrine cells

The *specialized columnar* type is most frequently associated with progressive dysplasia preceding the development of *Barrett-associated adenocarcinoma*.

5. Correct choice: C
SUPERFICIAL SQUAMOUS CELL CARCINOMA (p. 1419)—Superficial squamous cell carcinoma is infrequent in the United States. Alcohol and smoking are the most important risk factors. It is preceded by progressive dysplastic changes (esophageal intraepithelial neoplasia, or *EIN*) progressive to *in situ* and invasive carcinoma. Spread of *superficial carcinoma* is confined to the submucosa, with or without node metastasis: It is potentially curable and associated with a 65% to 90% 5-year survival.

6. Correct choice: B
BASALOID SQUAMOUS CARCINOMA (pp. 1420 and 1421)—Of the various types of esophageal carcinoma, *basaloid carcinoma* and *small cell carcinoma* are the most aggressive. Basaloid carcinoma has architectural features reminiscent of adenoid cystic carcinoma. It is morphologically similar to homonymous tumors of the upper aerodigestive tract and anal canal. It is a squamous cell carcinoma with glandular differentiation. Round lumina containing basement membrane–like material and peripheral palisading are characteristic. Choice A is a high-grade neoplasm with concomitant squamous and glandular differentiation, choice C is associated with Epstein-Barr virus, and choice E is composed of fronds of extremely well differentiated squamous epithelium.

7. Correct choice: D
ESOPHAGEAL ADENOCARCINOMA (p. 1421)—The incidence of this cancer has been steadily increasing in the United States. It occurs most commonly in white men in their 60s to 70s. The great majority of cases are associated with Barrett esophagus and thus develop in the lower esophagus. Adenocarcinomas of the gastroesophageal junction are actually twice as frequent as those limited to the esophagus. Rarely, adenocarcinoma originates from the upper esophagus, specifically from a small area of gastric heterotopia known as the *esophageal inlet*. The prognosis of esophageal adenocarcinoma is as poor as that of squamous cell carcinoma. Histologically, it is similar to gastric adenocarcinoma.

CHAPTER 32

1. Correct choice: A
INTESTINAL METAPLASIA (p. 1438)—In areas of intestinal metaplasia (IM), the gastric epithelium is replaced by an epithelium that acquires the features and mucin content typical of *small* or *large* bowel epithelium. In *incomplete* IM, columnar cells are still present, but they produce acidic mucin: *sialomucin* in the small-bowel type, *sialomucin* and *sulfomucin* in the large-bowel type. In *complete* IM, the normal epithelium is replaced by goblet cells, which may produce as well sialomucin (small bowel) or sialo/sulfomucin (large bowel). These changes can be identified only by using multiple histochemical stains, better if in combinations (e.g., combined

Alcian blue at pH 2.5 and high-iron diamine). There are, in summary, four types of IM:

a. Small bowel, incomplete: columnar cells producing sialomucin (no goblet cells)
b. Large bowel, incomplete: columnar cells producing sialo/sulfomucin (no goblet cells)
c. Small bowel, complete: goblet cells producing sialomucin
d. Large bowel, complete: goblet cells producing sialo/sulfomucin

In *pyloric metaplasia*, acid-secreting fundic-type mucosa is replaced by mucus-secreting pyloric-type glands, which may lead to reduced gastric output.

2. Correct choice: E

SUPERFICIAL GASTRITIS (p. 1440)—Superficial gastritis is characterized by a *superficial* inflammatory infiltrate limited mostly to the foveolar region of the gastric mucosa. Lymphocytes predominate, but scattered neutrophils and occasional eosinophils may be present. The absence of glandular atrophy is important, because glandular atrophy implies a diagnosis of *atrophic gastritis*, which is usually accompanied by widespread chronic inflammation. *Gastric atrophy* refers to the complete loss of gastric glands.

3. Correct choice: B

H. PYLORI GASTRITIS (p. 1441)—The acute form is rarely seen, but chronic *H. pylori* gastritis is often observed in biopsies. Formation of lymphoid follicles with active germinal centers within the deep mucosa (so-called *follicular gastritis*) is virtually always associated with *H. pylori*. This gram-negative organism can be identified on good H&E sections or on sections stained with modified Steiner, Giemsa, or Leung stains. Neutrophilic infiltration of the epithelium is a sign of active gastritis, which may even result in pit abscesses. Severe atrophic gastritis is seen in the advanced stages of autoimmune gastritis affecting the fundus.

4. Correct choice: B

AUTOIMMUNE GASTRITIS (p. 1443)—Also called *type A chronic gastritis* in the traditional Strickland and MacKay classification, this form of gastritis affects the fundus, but not the antrum, of the stomach. It is associated with diminished peptic acid secretion, elevated blood levels of gastrin, and a high incidence of pernicious anemia. It is related to autoantibodies against various antigens of the gastric epithelium, particularly the molecular components of the gastric pump of parietal cells. All of the remaining factors mentioned previously are important in the pathogenesis of *type B* (*nonimmune*) *chronic gastritis*, which predominantly affects the antral region, but may extend to the fundus. The latter is the form most frequently associated with gastric carcinoma and gastric peptic ulcer.

5. Correct choice: E

MOST COMMON FORMS OF CHRONIC GASTRITIS (p. 1447)—*Reactive gastropathy* was originally described in postgastrectomy specimens. Also called reflux or chemical gastritis, it involves the prepyloric region and results from a nonspecific response to a number of chemical insults, including bile reflux. It can be defined as pit gastritis, because the most significant changes involve the gastric pits. Mucin depletion and hyperplasia of gastric pits are associated with edema and a sparse inflammatory infiltrate. The corkscrew appearance of pits is typical, although gastric glands are normal. *Eosinophilic gastritis* is analogous to eosinophilic enteritis and affects the antrum. *Granulomatous gastritis* is caused by infective and noninfective etiologies (e.g., Crohn

disease). *Lymphocytic gastritis* is characterized by lymphocytic infiltration of the fundic glands (more than 25 lymphocytes/100 epithelial cells), due to a T-cell–mediated reaction to intraluminal antigens.

6. Correct choice: D

GASTRIC POLYPS (p. 1452)—Hyperplastic polyps represent 85% to 90% of all gastric polyps and may occur in any location. Usually, they develop in hypochlorhydric/achlorhydric patients. A central dimple is a typical gross feature. Histologically, they consist of hyperplastic glands without atypia. Progression to malignancy is rare (2% to 3%). *Adenomas* are subdivided into tubular, tubulovillous, and villous, in analogy to colonic adenomas. *Fundic gland polyps* are tiny polyps consisting of dilated fundic glands. *Hamartomatous polyps* have gross and microscopic features similar to those occurring in Peutz-Jeghers syndrome. *Inflammatory fibroid polyps* preferentially affect the antrum and consist of a submucosal overgrowth of fibrous tissue admixed with chronic inflammatory cells and eosinophils.

7. Correct choice: E

ZOLLINGER-ELLISON SYNDROME (p. 1454)—Zollinger-Ellison syndrome (secondary to hypergastrinemia) resembles Ménétrier disease both radiologically and macroscopically. Grossly, there is marked thickening of the gastric mucosal folds, acquiring a cerebriform pattern. Histologically, Zollinger-Ellison syndrome is characterized by glandular hyperplasia with a prominent increase in the number of parietal cells. Ménétrier disease is due to hyperplasia of crypts with cystic dilatation of the glandular component. Gross changes of Ménétrier disease are sharply demarcated and limited to the fundus. Gastric lymphoma is also somewhat similar to Ménétrier disease in its gross appearance.

8. Correct choice: B

INTESTINAL METAPLASIA: RISK FACTOR FOR GASTRIC CANCER (pp. 1456 and 1460)—There is a statistical correlation between the *intestinal type* of gastric adenocarcinoma (histologically similar to colon cancer) and large bowel type incomplete metaplasia (also known as type III metaplasia). There is evidence suggesting that gastric adenocarcinoma arises from a sequence of epithelial changes involving progressive *H. pylori* infection, chronic atrophic gastritis, large bowel type incomplete metaplasia, and increasing degrees of dysplasia. Gastric epithelial dysplasia is further subclassified into adenomatous and hyperplastic variants and, most important, *low grade* and *high grade*. High-grade dysplasia is associated with a strong probability of coexistent cancer (60%) or malignant progression (25% within 15 months), whereas low-grade dysplasia may even regress.

9. Correct choice: C

PROGNOSTIC FACTORS (p.1457)—Stage is the single most important prognostic factor. Staging based on the TNM system should be included in the pathologic report; it is based on evaluation of at least 15 regional nodes. Negative prognostic factors include age greater than 70 years, CEA greater than 10 ng/mL, CA19-9 greater than 37 g/mL. If compared stage by stage, the prognosis is the same for the intestinal and diffuse type.

10. Correct choice: D

SUPERFICIAL SPREADING (EARLY) CARCINOMA (p. 1459)—This carcinoma is limited to the mucosa or mucosa and submucosa with or without involvement of regional lymph nodes. Differentiation is variable, and most cases are classifiable as the *intestinal type* according to the Lauren system. Its prognosis is remarkably good, with a 5-year survival rate in the range of 80% to 93%. Carcinoma limited to the mucosa is referred to as *intramucosal carcinoma*. The detection rate of superficial spreading carcinoma is obviously higher in countries (like Japan) with active screening programs by periodic endoscopy and biopsy.

11. Correct choice: B
GASTRIC ENDOCRINE TUMORS (p. 1460)—Endocrine tumors of the stomach are relatively frequent, accounting for 11% to 41% of all GI neoplasms. They are divided into four main types.

- *Type 1* tumors are the most common and develop in association with achlorhydria: Achlorhydria results in compensatory hypergastrinemia and subsequent gastrin stimulation of fundic ECL-secreting cells. ECL tumors are often multiple. Trabecular and microglandular patterns are most frequent in gastric endocrine tumors.
- *Type II:* solitary, analogous to those in the small bowel, may produce ACTH or serotonin.
- *Type III:* associated with MEN-I syndrome.
- *Type IV:* poorly differentiated, small round cell tumors with a high metastatic potential.

12. Correct choice: C
GASTRIC LYMPHOMAS (pp. 1461–1463)—Lymphomas account for 5% of gastric cancer. Most of these are lymphomas arising from the mucosa-associated lymphoid tissue (MALT) and are characterized by the following: tropism for mucosal sites, especially the GI tract; infiltration and destruction of glands creating so-called *lymphoepithelial lesions*; frequent plasmacytoid differentiation; and PAS-positive intranuclear inclusions known as *Dutcher bodies*. The diagnosis of "MALToma" should always be accompanied by grading. Most cases of MALToma are low grade and have a slow course. Extension to other MALT sites is typical. Large cell lymphoma of the stomach is a high-grade lymphoma expressing BER H2 and Ki-1.

13. Correct choice: A
GASTROINTESTINAL STROMAL TUMORS (p. 1463)—GIST is a category of tumors showing two main cellular patterns: spindle cell and epithelioid. The *spindle cell type* consists of fascicles of spindly cells with cigar-shaped nuclei. The *round cell type* is composed of round cells with artifactual clearing of their cytoplasm. Immunohistochemical and ultrastructural evidence suggests that GIST derives from *GI pacemaker cells*, also known as the *interstitial cells of Cajal*. Both tumor cells of GIST and interstitial cells of Cajal are immunoreactive for CD117, the protein encoded by the KIT protooncogene. The subclassification of GIST based on morphologic or immunohistochemical evidence of neural or smooth muscle histogenesis has been abandoned. Size, mitotic activity, and cellularity are the three most important histologic predictors of malignancy.

CHAPTER 33

1. Correct choice: B
CELIAC SPRUE (p. 1477)—On inspection of a jejunal biopsy under the dissecting microscope, four normal patterns may be observed, that is, villouslike, leaflike, cerebroid, and mosaic. A *flat* pattern is most often pathologic and correlates with the microscopic feature of villous atrophy. The jejunal mucosa in celiac disease undergoes dramatic atrophy of villi, although the thickness of the mucosa itself may appear normal. Lymphoplasmacytic infiltrates expand the lamina propria. The condition resolves following a gluten-free diet, and the diagnosis is confirmed by follow-up biopsies. The condition is diagnosed on the basis of combined clinical, laboratory, and pathologic findings. The laboratory test that proves most reliable is measurement of *IgA-endomysial antibodies*.

2. Correct choice: D
WHIPPLE DISEASE (p.1481)—Whipple disease manifests usually with malabsorption syndrome in men in their fourth decade. This is a systemic infection that may affect the small and large bowel, lymph nodes, central nervous system, heart, lungs, and other organs. The organism cannot be cultured, but it is detectable by electron microscopy (EM). Large clusters of macrophages with their cytoplasm filled with PAS-positive granules are characteristic. Often, optically clear vacuoles containing neutral fat are also seen in biopsies. The main differential diagnosis, especially in AIDS patients, is with mycobacterial and histoplasma infections. Antibiotic treatment is highly effective against this otherwise fatal condition.

3. Correct choice: C
PARASITIC INFESTATIONS (pp. 1483 and 1498)—The picture shows the typical appearance of *Giardia lamblia* trophozoites in duodenal biopsies. They appear sickle-shaped in profile and pear-shaped *en face*. Giardiasis is common in poor countries. In the United States, it is usually diagnosed on stool samples by direct microscopic examination, enzyme-linked immunosorbent assay (ELISA), or indirect immunofluorescence. It manifests with intermittent diarrhea or, in severe cases, malabsorption. *Capillariasis* (due to *Capillaria philippinensis*) and *strongyloidiasis* (usually caused by *S. stercoralis*) may also cause intestinal malabsorption, but they are rarely seen in intestinal biopsies.

4. Correct choice: D
ULCERATIVE COLITIS (p. 1487)—The macroscopic and microscopic features of ulcerative colitis differ significantly between the active and inactive stages of the disease. *Active UC* is associated with superficial ulcers, bleeding, crypt abscesses, mucin depletion, regenerative activity (nuclear enlargement and mitotic figures), and diffuse mixed inflammatory infiltrate involving mucosa and submucosa. These changes will regress during quiescent stages, but the involved mucosa will never appear entirely normal. In clinically *inactive UC* (UC in remission), crypts are shortened, branched, and decreased in number. Paneth cells (normally absent in colonic epithelium) and scattered neutrophils may also be found.

5. Correct choice: C
ACTIVE COLITIS: UC VERSUS CROHN DISEASE (CD; pp. 1488 and 1502)—Crohn disease (CD) and ulcerative colitis (UC) share a spectrum of clinical and histopathologic features referred to as *inflammatory bowel disease*. Both may result in a pattern of active colitis, characterized by inflammatory infiltration of lamina propria, mucosal architectural distortion, crypt abscesses, and mucin depletion. These changes may be diffuse or focal. The *diffuse* pattern is most characteristic of overt UC, whereas the *focal* pattern suggests CD or infectious colitis. Microscopic changes most characteristic of CD include nonnecrotizing, sarcoidlike granulomas (present in two-thirds of cases), transmural inflammatory infiltration, and linear fissures. Furthermore, CD may affect any segment

of the alimentary tract, including the colon and rectum, although the terminal ileum is most commonly involved. Bowel segments affected by Crohn disease are sharply demarcated from the adjacent noninvolved bowel. Pseudopolyps resulting from hyperplasia are common in both CD and UC. Crypt abscesses are common in acute UC and rare in CD.

6. Correct choice: B

COLLAGENOUS AND LYMPHOCYTIC COLITIS (p. 1492)—Biopsy is the only available test for the diagnosis of collagenous/lymphocytic colitis. Colon biopsies show two features: a thick collagenous layer beneath the epithelium, and lymphocytic infiltration in the lamina propria with epithelial lymphocytosis. Additional nonspecific changes are usually present. Collagenous and lymphocytic colitis probably represent different phases of the same condition. Subepithelial collagen thickening is prevalent in collagenous colitis, whereas intraepithelial lymphocytes are more prominent in lymphocytic colitis. The acute stage of bacterial colitis is morphologically similar to ulcerative colitis, but it presents features of focal active colitis.

7. Correct choice: B

COLORECTAL MUCOSAL PROLAPSE SYNDROME (p. 1496)—*Mucosal prolapse syndrome* appears in adults in their 30s or 40s and manifests with constipation and rectal bleeding. Disorders of defecation lead to mucosal prolapse and resultant mucosal injury. Mucosal prolapse syndrome should include all those conditions that share a similar histologic picture, that is, *solitary rectal ulcers* (may be multiple), *inflammatory cloacogenic polyp*, and *colitis cystica profunda*. All of these lesions represent manifestations of the same underlying condition. The defining feature of mucosal prolapse is the presence of lakes of mucin dissecting through the submucosa, which may lead to the erroneous diagnosis of mucinous adenocarcinoma. *Pneumatosis cystoides intestinalis* refers to collections of gas surrounded by giant cell reaction, usually associated with necrotizing enterocolitis.

8. Correct choice: E

CRYPTOSPORIDIOSIS (p. 1499)—Immunocompromised patients are prone to cryptosporidiosis, which may produce a potentially life-threatening diarrheal condition and spread to the extrahepatic and intrahepatic biliary system. Cryptosporidiosis is due to *Cryptosporidium parvum* or *Isospora belli*. In biopsy specimens, *C. parvum* is visible as 2 to 4 μm round bodies attached to the apical surface of epithelial cells, whereas *I. belli* appears as ovoid intracytoplasmic or extracellular coccidia. In both cases, diagnosis is easily made by stool examination. In biopsy specimens, organisms are highlighted by Giemsa staining and negative on acid-free bacillus (AFB) stained sections. Mucosal changes are nonspecific, such as villous atrophy and mild lymphocytic infiltration.

9. Correct choice: D

MICROSPORIDIOSIS (p. 1500)—Microsporidiosis causes up to 50% of cases of intractable diarrhea in AIDS patients. Even if most cases of AIDS-related GI infections due to cryptosporidiosis or microsporidiosis can be diagnosed by stool examination, GI biopsies are often performed. The most frequent pathogenic microsporidia include *Enterocytozoon bieneusi* and *E. intestinalis*. Mature spores appear as minuscule paranuclear dots, whereas nucleated sporonts are basophilic ovoids surrounded by a halo. Sporonts produce characteristic nuclear indentation. *Cryptosporidia* appear as 3 μm round

bodies attached to the apical surface of enterocytes. *Spirochetes* produce accentuation of the brush border of colonic epithelium.

10. Correct choice: B

ISCHEMIC BOWEL DISEASE (p. 1509)—This condition affects predominantly elderly patients with atherosclerosis of the aorta and its branches and/or cardiac disease. In the acute stage, there is a thin superficial coat of fibrin and neutrophils resting on necrotic or ulcerated mucosa. In the healed stage, fibrosis of the lamina propria develops. This condition is sometimes confused with ulcerative colitis (UC) or Crohn disease (CD). Crypt abscesses may also be encountered in ischemic colitis, but are more frequently seen in UC. Linear fissures are characteristic of CD. Single-cell necrosis is seen in graft versus host disease. Volcano-like lesions are frequently seen in pseudomembranous (antibiotic-associated) colitis.

11. Correct choice: A

VASCULAR ECTASIAS (ANGIODYSPLASIA; p. 1513)—This lesion commonly manifests in old age with chronic (occult or clinically evident) intestinal hemorrhage. It is located most frequently in the cecum or ascending colon and may be endoscopically inconspicuous. Diagnosis is established by arteriography in uncertain cases. The lesion is composed of tortuous and dilated submucosal vessels. Bleeding is usually chronic, but may be acute and massive. Colonic varices are associated with portal hypertension. *Cavernous hemangiomas* are rare in the bowel, but often multicentric.

12. Correct choice: B

HIRSCHPRUNG DISEASE (p. 1517)—Hirschprung disease results from the absence of ganglion cells in *both* submucosal (Meissner) *and* intramural (Auerbach) plexuses. Suction biopsies allow evaluation of the submucosal plexus, but not that of the intramural plexus. If submucosa is not present in the specimen, the sample is considered inadequate for diagnosis. Because ganglion cells are less frequent in the submucosal plexus, careful search on multiple step-through sections is indispensable. Periganglionic satellite cells are likewise absent, a feature highlighted by S-100 protein immunohistochemistry. Unmyelinated and cholinergic nerve fibers are often hypertrophic. Acetylcholinesterase histochemistry or immunohistochemistry for axonal markers (neurofilament, tau protein, etc.) may highlight this change. *Ret — has a role*

13. Correct choice: A

IDIOPATHIC RETROPERITONEAL FIBROSIS (pp. 1524 and 1525)—This fibrosing process of obscure pathogenesis involves the retroperitoneum, enveloping the aorta and ureters and producing renal failure. The ureters are displaced toward the midline, in contrast to most retroperitoneal tumors, which displace ureters laterally. Liposarcoma is the most frequent retroperitoneal sarcoma, followed by malignant fibrous histiocytoma and leiomyosarcoma.

CHAPTER 34

1. Correct choice: C

HYPERPLASTIC POLYP (p. 1544)—These nonneoplastic polyps are probably present in up to 50% of the adult population. The glandular epithelium closely resembles the normal colonic epithelium, including the presence of goblet cells. The mucin content is not significantly decreased, and the basement membrane is usually thicker than normal. From low power, the glands have a characteristic serrated profile. In contrast to adenomatous polyps, and similar to normal colonic mucosa, hyperplastic polyps show increased mitotic activity *at the base* of the glands and not at their tips. Atypia is by definition absent. Hyperplastic polyps should not be considered preneoplastic lesions.

2. Correct choice: B

HYPERPLASTIC POLYP (p. 1546)—If the biopsy specimen is not properly oriented, the only histologic clue for a diagnosis of hyperplastic polyp may be the *star-shaped crypts*, as illustrated in the photomicrograph. In a properly oriented specimen, hyperplastic polyps appear to be composed of numerous crypts that have a serrated profile reminiscent of secretory endometrium. *Serrated adenoma* is an uncommon form characterized by a pronounced saw-toothed appearance in which there is increased nuclear atypia relative to hyperplastic polyps but less than seen in adenomas.

3. Correct choice: D

HAMARTOMATOUS POLYPS IN PEUTZ-JEGHERS SYN-DROME (p. 1548)—The most characteristic feature of hamartomatous polyps include a rich branching pattern (likened to a Christmas tree and appreciable on low power) and bundles of smooth muscle in continuity with the muscularis propria. This polyp may be seen sporadically or as part of *Peutz-Jeghers syndrome* (PJS). PJS is autosomal dominant and characterized by skin hyperpigmentation, particularly around orifices, palms, and soles. Patients with PJS have a high rate of cancer, both gastrointestinal and nongastrointestinal. Adenomatous polyps of the colon are seen in *familial polyposis coli*, and brain tumors are seen in *Turcot syndrome* along with colonic polyposis. Osteomas of the mandible, soft tissue tumors, and GI adenomas characterize *Gardner syndrome*.

4. Correct choice: E

JUVENILE POLYP (p. 1550)—This polyp develops from the rectal mucosa and predominantly manifests in the first two decades with bleeding or anal protrusion. Cystically dilated glands and a smooth contour are characteristic. *Familial juvenile polyposis* leads to increased risk of colon cancer, but solitary juvenile polyps are not associated with increased risk of malignancy. *Inflammatory polyp* is secondary to chronic inflammatory bowel disorders such as ulcerative colitis, Crohn disease, and so on. *Inflammatory fibroid polyps* are more common in the stomach and small bowel than the colon and consist of a submucosal mesenchymal nodule with chronic inflammatory infiltration.

5. Correct choice: D

ADENOMAS (p. 1555)—Adenomas are neoplastic polyps that are very frequent in the general population. Up to 60% of adults have large bowel adenomas at autopsy. At least 90% of these are tubular adenomas, whereas the remaining ones are tubulovillous (2% to 4%) or villous (1% to 3%). Tubular adenoma may be sessile or pedunculated. Microscopically, it consists of crowded, variably dysplastic glands with nuclear atypia and increased mitotic activity. The mucin content is decreased, which enhances the contrast with the adjacent normal epithelium. Dysplasia ranges from mild to severe—the latter equivalent to *in situ* carcinoma. Polyps associated with *familial polyposis coli* are morphologically indistinguishable from sporadic tubular adenomas.

6. Correct choice: E

VILLOUS ADENOMAS (p. 1556)—These are the least frequent neoplastic colorectal polyps and tend to occur in elderly people, presenting with watery diarrhea and hypokalemia. Usually located in the rectum, villous adenomas are large soft masses, most of which are sessile. Histologically, the tumor has a typical frondlike pattern, and epithelial cells show mild to severe dysplasia. The majority of villous adenomas will eventually degenerate into invasive carcinoma if not resected. Because most adenomas contain a mixture of tubular and villous pattern, adenomas are arbitrarily called villous adenomas if at least 75% of the tumor has a villous architecture (vice versa for tubular adenomas). Tubulovillous adenomas fall between such cases.

7. Correct choice: E

ADENOMA WITH CANCER (p. 1562)—Adenomas may transform into adenocarcinoma at a rate that depends on size, histologic type, and presence of dysplasia. Invasive cancer is found in

a. 0.5% of adenomas less than 1.0 cm, 5% of adenomas measuring 1.0 to 1.9 cm, and 10% in those greater than 2 .0 cm

b. 2% to 3% of tubular, 6% to 8% of tubulovillous, and 10% to 18% of villous adenomas

Intramucosal carcinoma contains malignant glandular buds extending into the lamina propria. It is essential to distinguish adenomas with cancer from those in which the malignant growth *extends beyond the lamina propria* into the muscularis mucosae: The latter has metastatic potential, but the former does not. *Epithelial misplacement* is a mechanism by which epithelium is misplaced into the submucosa by torsion or trauma, mimicking invasive carcinoma ("pseudoinvasion"). *Flat adenomas* have a tendency to undergo malignant changes and rapid infiltration.

8. Correct choice: E

FAMILIAL ADENOMATOUS POLYPOSIS (p. 1567)—The condition known as *familial adenomatous polyposis* is due to mutations of the *APC gene* and results in the development of hundreds to thousands of adenomas in the colon as well as in the small bowel and stomach. Without treatment, malignant transformation of colonic adenomas is constant. The APC gene encodes a protein that degrades β-catenin, which enters the nucleus and activates growth-promoting factors. Thus, APC mutations lead to increased levels of β-catenin, resulting in excessive growth. Clinically, familial adenomatous polyposis is characterized by the development of hundreds of colorectal polyps (mostly tubular adenomas), which will eventually transform into cancer.

9. Correct choice: D

SMALL BOWEL ADENOCARCINOMAS (p. 1568)—Adenocarcinomas of the small intestine are far less frequent than adenocarcinomas of the colon, representing less than 5% of all GI tract malignancies. Approximately half of the cases occur in the duodenum, particularly around the ampulla of Vater, and most of the remaining cases are located in the jejunum. Brunner gland nodules are hyperplastic/hamartomatous lesions that never evolve to carcinoma. Peutz-Jeghers syndrome, celiac disease, and particularly Crohn disease increase the risk of developing small bowel cancer. Microscopically, they are similar to colonic adenocarcinomas. Lymph node metastasis is an important prognostic factor.

10. Correct choice: C

HISTOLOGIC TYPES OF COLORECTAL CANCER (p. 1569)—The picture shows cells floating in a sea of mucin. This is the extracellular variant of mucinous adenocarcinoma that comprises 10% of all colorectal cancers. The intracellular variant is rare and includes signet ring cell carcinoma, a tumor of highly aggressive behavior. *Adenocarcinoma* is the conventional type of colorectal cancer: It is subclassified into three grades depending on glandular differentiation. All of the other types are rare. *Undifferentiated (medullary) carcinoma* is characterized by a lack of mucin, conspicuous nucleoli, marked lymphocytic infiltration, and, surprisingly, a better prognosis than the conventional adenocarcinoma.

11. Correct choice: A

PROGNOSTIC FACTORS IN COLORECTAL ADENOCARCINOMA (pp.1572–1574)—Although staging evaluated by the Dukes, Astler-Coller, or TNM system is the most important prognostic parameter, other features have been reported to influence prognosis. For example, mucinous adenocarcinoma (defined as a carcinoma in which at least 50% of the tumor mass is represented by extracellular mucin) has a worse prognosis. Other negative prognostic indicators are older age and intravascular/perineurial invasion. Inflammatory infiltration, especially when displaying a *Crohn-like pattern*, imparts a better prognostic outlook. The multiplicity of lesions or size of the tumor does not affect survival rate. Differentiation, ploidy, proliferative, and molecular markers are still under evaluation.

12. Correct choice: E

IMMUNOHISTOCHEMISTRY OF COLORECTAL ADENOCARCINOMA (p. 1575)—The most frequent combination of immunohistochemical markers in colorectal adenocarcinoma includes positive immunoreactivity for type 20 keratin and negative type 7 keratin. The reverse is usually observed in pulmonary adenocarcinoma, which is characterized by immunoreactivity for *TTF-1* (thyroid transcription factor-1). CEA is consistently positive in colon adenocarcinoma. Perinuclear immunoreactivity for type 20 keratin having a dotlike pattern is suggestive of Merkel cell carcinoma. GFAP is a marker of astrocytic differentiation.

13. Correct choice: E

CARCINOID OF APPENDIX (p. 1580)—Small carcinoid tumors of the vermiform appendix are frequent incidental findings (approximately 1 every 300). Most of them are less than 1 cm in main diameter and histologically they display a classic *insular* pattern. Carcinoid syndrome may develop only when liver metastases are present. Adenocarcinoid refers to a carcinoid having a *glandular* pattern and does not imply malignancy. Of the two main types of adenocarcinoid (i.e., *tubular* and *goblet cell* types), the goblet cell type is more aggressive. Chromogranin and similar markers are expressed by this type of adenocarcinoid. Tubular adenocarcinoid may be mistaken for metastatic or primary adenocarcinoma.

14. Correct choice: D

RECTAL CARCINOIDS (p. 1582)—Rectal carcinoids show a ribbonlike arrangement (not the classic insular pattern) and are not associated with carcinoid syndrome. The immunohistochemical reaction for *prostate-specific acid phosphatase* is frequently positive, whereas *prostatic-specific antigen* is negative. The latter feature is important in the differential diagnosis with metastases from prostatic cancer. Rectal carcinoids may produce lymph node metastases, especially when large and aneuploid. Multicentric carcinoids are most frequent with Crohn disease and ulcerative colitis.

15. Correct choice: A

SPORADIC (WESTERN) GASTROINTESTINAL LYMPHOMA (p. 1584)—The *Western type* of MALT lymphoma is the most common intestinal lymphoma. Nodal involvement may be present, but the spleen, liver, bone marrow, and so on should not be involved at the time of presentation for a diagnosis of *primary* gut lymphoma. It may be low grade or high grade. The high-grade form is highly aggressive: It consists of sheets of noncleaved cells with open nuclei, prominent nucleoli, and numerous immunoblasts.

16. Correct choice: E

IMMUNOPROLIFERATIVE SMALL INTESTINAL DISEASE (IPSID; p. 1584)—IPSID is mainly found in Third World countries, affects young adults, and manifests with chronic diarrhea and malabsorption. Intestinal lymphomas in the Middle East are most frequently of the Western variant (MALT associated). IPSID is a low-grade β-cell lymphoma characterized by cytoplasmic deposition of monoclonal heavy chains of the alpha type. Monoclonal α chains can also be detected in the urine and serum. Histologically, it consists of slightly immature lymphocytes with plasma cell differentiation. The condition may arise from a chronic hyperplastic response to antigenic stimuli, perhaps related to recurrent infections.

17. Correct choice: E

ENTEROPATHY-ASSOCIATED T-CELL LYMPHOMA (EATCL; p. 1584)—Patients with malabsorption, and especially those with celiac disease, are at increased risk of developing small intestinal lymphomas. Such lymphomas are usually of T-cell origin. Clinically, these lymphomas manifest after a long latency period (20 or more years) with recurrence of malabsorption despite a gluten-free diet, bowel ulcerations and strictures, and elevated serum IgA levels. Because of the presence of multinucleated RS-like cells, EATCL may lead to a mistaken diagnosis of Hodgkin disease. Hodgkin disease is rare in the small bowel.

18. Correct choice: B

GANGLIOCYTIC PARAGANGLIOMA (p. 1592)—This rare benign tumor is composed of a mixture of neuroendocrine, gangliocytic, and Schwann cells. It occurs in the duodenum, usually around the ampulla of Vater. Immunoreactivity for pancreatic polypeptide is frequent and suggests a possible derivation from the anterior pancreatic bud. The lesion is considered by some to be a hamartoma rather than a neoplasm. *GANT* is a rare spindle cell tumor with ultrastructural features suggesting an origin from the myoenteric plexus.

CHAPTER 35

1. Correct choice: B

ACUTE PANCREATITIS (p. 1607)—Eighty percent of cases are associated with bile stones or alcohol consumption. Small bile stones may impact into the ampulla of Vater, causing backflow of bile into the pancreatic duct, thus initiating intrapancreatic activation of proteolytic enzymes. Alcohol, instead, may cause direct acinar injury. The remaining conditions are rare causes of acute pancreatitis: *Acute ischemia, drugs* (e.g., thiazide diuretics, estrogens), *hyperlipoproteinemia* types I and V, and *infections* (measles virus, coxsackieviruses, and *Mycoplasma pneumoniae* may infect the pancreas; *Ascaris lumbricoides* and *Clonorchis sinensis* may block the pancreatic duct).

2. Correct choice: A

CHRONIC PANCREATITIS (p. 1609)—This condition may result from nonobstructive causes (95% of cases, usually related to *alcoholism*) or obstructive causes (minority of cases, secondary to carcinoma or bile stones). Hyperparathyroidism and autosomal dominant hereditary pancreatitis are uncommon etiologies. In poor countries, protein malnutrition is the most common cause of chronic pancreatitis, referred to as *tropical pancreatitis*. One-third of cases, however, are not associated with any known predisposing factor (idiopathic).

3. Correct choice: E

CHRONIC PANCREATITIS (pp. 1609 and 1610)—The morphologic features are typical of chronic pancreatitis. The great majority of these cases are due to nonobstructive causes, of which alcoholism is the most common factor. Chronic pancreatitis often leads to formation of pseudocysts, but its association with ductal adenocarcinoma is less well established. Florid hyperplasia of islet cells is sometimes found, but this change does not result in development of endocrine neoplasms. Migratory venous thrombosis may be associated with ductal carcinoma (Trousseau syndrome).

4. Correct choice: D

PANCREATIC CARCINOMA (1612)—Ductal adenocarcinoma represents the most common form of pancreatic cancer and the fourth leading cause of cancer-related death. Histologically, the differential diagnosis between adenocarcinoma and chronic pancreatitis is challenging because the two conditions may coexist. Cancer may cause the obstruction of ducts with resultant ductal dilatation, parenchymal atrophy, fibrosis, and so on. At low power, neoplastic glands are irregular in contour and produce a total loss of lobular architecture. At high power, neoplastic cells show nuclear atypia, prominent nucleoli, and mitotic figures. Perineurial invasion is common in pancreatic cancer. Up to one-third of invasive carcinomas are associated with *in situ* carcinoma of adjacent ducts.

5. Correct choice: D

ANAPLASTIC CARCINOMA (p. 1625)—Also referred to as pleomorphic, sarcomatoid, or undifferentiated, this variant of pancreatic carcinoma is characterized by an extremely aggressive behavior, shows a male predilection, and derives (as does the more common adenocarcinoma) from ductal epithelium. It is composed of undifferentiated cells resembling melanoma or sarcoma intermixed with areas of glandular differentiation. Epithelial markers can be demonstrated in the latter areas. The *acinar cell variant* originates from acinar cells and gives a positive butyrate esterase reaction (p. 1623). B: Evidence of neuroendocrine differentiation may be seen in the *small cell variant* (p. 1627).

6. Correct choice: C

SEROUS NEOPLASMS, MICROCYSTIC TYPE (p. 1630)—Most pancreatic serous neoplasms are *serous cystadenomas*. They are usually discovered in elderly individuals, often located in the pancreatic body or tail. One may see two patterns, with cysts that may be minute and regular (the *microcystic* type) or large and irregular. The cut surface is highly characteristic, resembling the spongy appearance of the infantile form of polycystic kidney disease. Whether diagnosed incidentally or manifesting with clinical symptoms, the tumor is associated with a good prognosis. *Mucinous*

tumors (cystadenoma or cystadenocarcinoma) develop in younger individuals.

7. Correct choice: D

PANCREATOBLASTOMA (p. 1634)—Although all types of pancreatic tumors have been reported in the pediatric age, pancreatoblastoma is the most common type. This tumor is composed of uniform small cells arranged into acini, tubules, and solid islands containing *squamoid corpuscles*. Neoplastic cells express keratin, neuroendocrine markers, and CEA. Pancreatoblastoma has been described in association with Beckwith-Wiedemann syndrome and familial adenomatous polyposis. The prognosis is good, with most patients cured by surgical ablation.

8. Correct choice: D

SOLID CYSTIC-PAPILLARY EPITHELIAL NEOPLASM (pp. 1635–1637)—Also known as *Gruber-Franz tumor*, this neoplasm occurs almost exclusively in young females. Neoplastic cells are arranged around small vessels, creating a pseudopapillary pattern. A prominent feature is the presence of eosinophilic, PAS-positive globules immunoreactive for alfa-1-antitrypsin. Clusters of lipid crystals surrounded by foreign-body macrophages are often seen (as in the picture). Curiously, this neoplasm expresses progesterone receptors. Cells are also immunoreactive for keratin, neuron-specific enolase, various endocrine markers, and insulin/glucagon. The prognosis is good, even after incomplete resection.

9. Correct choice: C

INSULINOMA AND ISLET CELL TUMORS (pp. 1637 and 1641)—Insulinoma is the most common type of pancreatic endocrine tumors. Less than 10% of insulinomas are malignant tumors, showing infiltrative and metastatic behavior. It should be noted that purely morphological parameters such as pleomorphism and the mitotic rate are not reliable in predicting tumor behavior. In contrast to insulinomas, most of the other islet cell tumors have a malignant behavior. Electron microscopy may allow presumptive identification of the cell of origin based on cytoplasmic granules: β-cell tumors contain irregular/crystalline granules, whereas α-cell tumors have large granules with peripheral nucleoid.

10. Correct choice: D

NESIDIOBLASTOSIS (p. 1643)—This condition is characterized by hyperplasia of islets of Langerhans connected with the ductular system, forming ductuloinsular complexes. In mild degrees, the condition is present in all infants, but may become particularly pronounced in infants with hypoglycemia, for example, those born to diabetic mothers. Rarely, it is the only pathologic change found in adults suffering from hyperinsulinemic hypoglycemia.

CHAPTER 36

1. Correct choice: E

SURGICAL HEPATITIS (p. 1657)—The liver in subcapsular regions may show nonspecific changes, which are not representative of the real hepatic pathology. Surgical manipulation frequently produces subcapsular inflammation, hepatocellular necrosis, and architectural changes, which are known in the pathologic jargon as "*refractoritis.*" Thus, incisional biopsies should be accompanied by deeper needle biopsies. The remaining choices include the most common causes of intralobular neutrophilic infiltration with or without hepatocyte necrosis.

2. Correct choice: B
EXTRAHEPATIC BILIARY ATRESIA (EBA; p. 1664)—One of the most frequent and important tasks in interpreting liver biopsies from infants with a diagnosis of *neonatal hepatitis* is distinguishing between medical and surgical conditions. Within the first category, the most common disorders include α-1-antitrypsin deficiency, galactosemia, infections, and hereditary fructose intolerance, whereas EBA is the most important member of surgically treatable conditions. EBA is characterized by bile duct proliferation with portal edema and preserved lobular architecture. Bile duct loss follows at about 6 to 7 months of age. Giant cells are nonspecific. The success of surgical repair (portoenterostomy) is more likely when performed early in life.

3. Correct choice: B
EXTRAHEPATIC BILIARY ATRESIA (EBA; p. 1664)—EBA is the most common cause of liver cirrhosis in infants: 90% of cases are due to destruction of all segments of extrahepatic bile ducts including those at the porta hepatis, with no connection between extrahepatic and intrahepatic bile system: From a surgical standpoint, these cases are *noncorrectable*. *Correctable* cases are those (10%) in which the patency of proximal extrahepatic ducts allows biliary enteric anastomosis. The condition is due to *postnatal* inflammatory destruction of the biliary system, resulting in fibrosis. Viral agents may be involved. The great majority of babies with this condition are born with a normal biliary system.

4. Correct choice: E
INTRAHEPATIC BILIARY ATRESIA (p. 1665)—This condition occurs in two settings: syndromic (associated with abnormal facies, vertebral anomalies, and pulmonary stenosis) and nonsyndromic. Loss of interlobular ducts is the cardinal pathologic change, associated with abnormally small portal tracts. Proliferation of bile ductules is inconstant and usually mild. Ductular proliferation and portal edema occurs in extrahepatic biliary atresia. Giant cell transformation and extramedullary hematopoiesis is typical of neonatal hepatitis.

5. Correct choice: E
ALPHA-1-ANTITRYPSIN (AAT) DEFICIENCY (p. 1668)—This autosomal recessive condition is due to the inheritance of alleles that result in abnormally low levels of AAT. The genotype PiZZ leads to levels of ATT that are 10% of normal values. This biochemical defect results in: (i) the progressive accumulation of AAT within hepatocytes, identifiable as diastase-resistant PAS-positive intracytoplasmic globules, with subsequent chronic hepatitis and cirrhosis; (ii) panacinar emphysema. Liver biopsy is intended to confirm a clinical diagnosis (which can be established by laboratory assessment of serum ATT levels) and determine the stage of disease.

6. Correct choice: B
WILSON DISEASE (p. 1671)—The clinical picture is diagnostic of Wilson disease, a hereditary disorder caused by the accumulation of copper. Chronic hepatitis usually leads to cirrhosis and is commonly accompanied by the characteristic Kayser-Fleisher rings. Serum ceruloplasmin is *decreased*, copper urinary excretion is increased, and the copper content in the liver is markedly elevated. Neuropsychiatric manifestations are common in childhood/early adulthood and are mostly due to degeneration of the basal ganglia, especially putamen. The diagnosis is based on the combination of clinical, laboratory, and histologic features. Wilson disease may manifest with acute hepatitis accompanied by hemolysis. EM shows intramitochondrial crystalline inclusions and widely open, "fish-mouth"-like canaliculi.

7. Correct choice: E
PRIMARY SCLEROSING CHOLANGITIS (PSC; p. 1674)—Seventy percent of PSC cases are associated with inflammatory bowel disease (IBD; 95% with UC and 5% with Crohn disease). Conversely, only 5% of patients with IBD will develop PSC. Liver biopsies usually show changes consistent with PSC, including concentric periductal fibrosis resulting in an onionskin pattern. The diagnosis rests on combined clinical, radiological, and pathological findings. Liver biopsy is also used to follow progression of the disease. Segmental obliteration with dilatation of intervening segments imparts a beaded appearance to bile ducts on contrast imaging. PSC predisposes to cholangiocarcinoma.

8. Correct choice: B
PRIMARY BILIARY CIRRHOSIS (PBC; p. 1675)—PBC often affects middle-aged women and manifests with cholestatic jaundice. Morphologically, it leads to chronic hepatitis, which may be indistinguishable from chronic active hepatitis of a different etiology. The early *florid stage* is most characteristic and includes ductule degeneration surrounded by a granulomatous reaction. Antimitochondrial antibodies are present in 95% of patients. Copper accumulation is frequent and favors a diagnosis of PBC over that of chronic hepatitis of an other etiology. The PiZZ genotype is associated with severely reduced levels of ATT, with resultant cirrhosis and emphysema. Choice D is expected in hemochromatosis, and choice E is typical of Wilson disease.

9. Correct choice: A
MEDICATION-INDUCED LIVER DISEASE (p. 1676)—A great number of substances may injure the liver. Morphologic changes related to drugs or toxins are nonspecific. The classification is based on two parameters: (i) *intrinsic* reactions (predictable, dose related) versus *idiosyncratic* reactions (unpredictable, dose unrelated) and (ii) histopathologic changes. The pattern of morphologic changes may suggest the underlying cause. The following are examples:

Pattern of Liver Injury	Causes
Macrovesicular steatosis	Ethanol, amiodarone
Microvesicular steatosis	Tetracyclines, valproate
Centrilobular necrosis	Acetaminophen
Massive necrosis	Acetaminophen, alothane, *Amanita phalloides*
Hepatitis	Isoniazid, methyldopa
Granulomatous inflammation	Sulfonamides, methyldopa
Cholestasis	Anabolic steroids, oral contraceptives, chlorpromazine

10. Correct choice: B
HEPATITIS B VIRUS INFECTION (p. 1678)—Approximately 50% of the 2,000 cases of FHF recorded in the United States yearly are due to hepatitis B virus (HBV). However, FHF is a relatively rare complication, occurring in about 1% of all cases of acute hepatitis B. It is an important cause of liver-related mortality and accounts for 10% of liver transplantation in the United States. HBV is similar to HIV in routes of transmission: blood transfusions, intravenous

drug abuse, sexual contact, dialysis, maternal–neonatal transmission, and accidental needle-sticks. Drugs are the most important causes of nonviral FHF.

11. Correct choice: C
HEPATITIS C VIRUS INFECTION (p. 1680)—Viral diseases represent a major risk associated with transfusion of whole blood or blood components. Hepatitis C virus (HCV) accounts for approximately 90% of transfusion-related cases of hepatitis. Conversely, of all cases of hepatitis due to HCV, 4% are attributable to blood transfusion and 50% to intravenous drug abuse. The source of infection remains unknown in a high number of cases. Transmission of HCV from mother to neonate and by sexual contact is infrequent. Acute infection with HCV is usually asymptomatic, but it progresses to chronic hepatitis in 80% of cases. HAV transmission is by the *fecal-oral* route. HBV is transmitted through blood and all other bodily fluids.

12. Correct choice: D
GRADING OF CHRONIC HEPATITIS (p. 1681)—In the evaluation of chronic hepatitis, *grade* refers to the degree of necrosis and inflammatory activity and *stage* to the extent of fibrosis. As of now, there is no universally accepted grading/staging system for chronic hepatitis, but the one proposed by Scheuer has gained widespread acceptance. This system recognizes five stages:

- Grade 0 corresponds to absent or minimal periportal inflammation, with no lobular necrosis and no fibrosis.
- Grade 4 is virtually equivalent to cirrhosis and thus encompasses the typical histopathologic changes seen in this condition, that is, lobular necrosis of the *bridging* type and usually marked periportal inflammation.
- Grades 1, 2, and 3 have intermediate morphologic changes, with grade 3 showing bridging fibrosis but no obvious cirrhosis.

13. Correct choice: B
AUTOIMMUNE (LUPOID) HEPATITIS (p. 1690)—The morphologic features are consistent with chronic hepatitis of moderate severity (grade 2 to 3 according to the Scheuer scheme). Laboratory tests are consistent with *type I* lupoid hepatitis, a form of liver disease mostly affecting young women. Morphologic features are nonspecific (similar to chronic hepatitis C), but laboratory tests are highly informative. In type I lupoid hepatitis, the most specific autoantibodies are those against *smooth muscle actin*. Antimitochondrial and antinuclear antibodies are also often detected. Two more variants have been described:

- Type II, associated with anti–liver-kidney microsomal (LKM) antibodies and affecting children
- Type III, associated with antisoluble liver protein (SLP) antibodies

14. Correct choice: D
HUMORAL REJECTION (p. 1694)—This unusual event occurs within hours after transplantation, manifesting with rapidly progressive liver dysfunction. Histologically, it is characterized by coagulative necrosis of liver parenchyma with neutrophilic infiltration. Platelet and fibrin microthrombi are seen in the hepatic small vessels.

15. Correct choice: A
ACUTE (CELLULAR) REJECTION (p. 1694)—This problem usually manifests itself 5 to 30 days after liver transplantation. The reaction has two main epithelial cell targets: *bile ducts* and *endothelial cells*. Picture A shows the features of bile duct damage, with an interlobular bile duct surrounded by a mixed inflammatory infiltrate of lymphocytes and neutrophils. Picture B is an example of endothelialitis, where lymphocytes insinuate themselves into the subendothelial space. Vascular damage may lead to hepatocyte necrosis. Rejection should be graded as mild, moderate, or severe.

16. Correct choice: B
CHRONIC (DUCTOPENIC) REJECTION (p. 1695)—Obliterative arteritis, as shown in the picture, is the hallmark of chronic rejection. It is characterized by accumulation of foamy histiocytes within arterial walls, which results in ischemic necrosis of hepatocytes. In addition, there is progressive bile duct loss (*vanishing bile duct syndrome*), even though the degree of inflammation gradually decreases. Obliterative arteritis and bile duct loss usually coexist. It is not clear whether they represent different forms of chronic rejection.

17. Correct choice: B
WORKUP OF LIVER BIOPSIES (p. 1697)—Liver biopsies are often performed in the diagnostic workup of patients with acute or chronic hepatitis of unknown origin. The "usual suspects" in such cases include viral hepatitis, autoimmune hepatitis (AH), primary biliary cirrhosis (PBC), primary sclerosing cholangitis (PSC), steatohepatitis (SH), Wilson disease (WD), and drug reaction (DR). Examination of these biopsies should be performed through sequential steps, examining the features listed in the table below.

Pattern of involvement	Uneven	PBC, HCV, SH
	Even	AH, PSC, WD
Portal infiltrate	Plasma cells + eosinophils	AH, PBC
	Exclusively lymphocytes	HCV
	Scanty or no infiltrate	WD
Bile ducts	Loss of interlobular ducts	PBC, PSC
	Focal damage	HBV, HCV, AH, SH, DR
	No damage	WD
Lobular alterations	Marked steatosis	SH
	Severe necrosis	AH
	Sinusoidal infiltrate	HCV, PBC
	Unremarkable	PSC, WD
Special features	Granulomas	PBC
	Ground-glass hepatocytes	HBV
	Copper accumulation	WD, PSC, PBC
	Mallory bodies	In all

The following changes are most characteristic of specific entities:

- Exclusively lymphocytic portal infiltrate: *HCV*
- Scanty or no portal infiltrate, and no bile duct damage: *Wilson disease*
- Marked steatosis: *steatohepatitis*
- Severe lobular necrosis: *autoimmune hepatitis*
- Granulomas: *primary biliary cirrhosis*
- Ground-glass hepatocytes: *HBV*

CHAPTER 37

1. Correct choice: A
HEPATIC AMEBIASIS (p. 1709)—Hepatic "abscesses" are observed in up to 9% of amebic infections. The term "abscess" is incorrect because no neutrophils are seen in the cystic fluid. *Entamoeba histolytica* trophozoites are similar to histiocytes, but have a small round nucleus with a distinct karyosome. Trophozoites are recovered in greater number from the periphery of the cyst, but they are rare in the central region. *biliary cystadenoma* is usually of the mucinous type and multilocular. *Echinococcus cysts* contain typical *protoscolices*. *Pyogenic abscesses* contain foul-smelling neutrophil-rich fluid; *E. coli* is the most frequent agent. A *solitary unilocular cyst* is a common incidental autopsy finding. For the differential diagnosis of liver cysts, see Table 37-3, Cystic Masses of the Liver (p. 1709).

2. Correct choice: D
HEPATOCELLULAR ADENOMA (p. 1715)—This lesion usually develops in women taking oral contraceptives or in persons treated with anabolic steroids. It may regress following discontinuation of treatment. The histologic picture is characterized by well-differentiated hepatocytes arranged in sheets and cords without identifiable portal tracts or central veins. Hemoperitoneum is the most important complication, occurring in one-third of cases. Aflatoxin and hepatitis B virus are risk factors for hepatocellular carcinoma. *B. Henselae* is the etiologic agent of *peliosis hepatis* in immunocompromised patients. Thorotrast exposure is associated with liver angiosarcoma and bile duct carcinoma.

3. Correct choice: B
FOCAL NODULAR HYPERPLASIA (FNH; p. 1718)—FNH is frequently asymptomatic or associated with pain or abdominal discomfort. Arteriographic examination yields a typical centrifugal pattern. The characteristic gross appearance is that of a nonencapsulated nodule containing a central scar with radiating fibrous septa. Occasionally, the central scar may be absent. All of the normal histologic components of the liver are present in FNH, so that on biopsy the morphologic features may resemble focal cirrhosis. Hepatocytes may show fatty change, glycogen accumulation, and/or alpha-1-antitrypsin globules. Morphological variations include cases where bile ductule proliferation is pronounced or dilated vessels are particularly abundant (the latter is seen in the *telengiectatic* variant).

4. Correct choice: E
NODULAR REGENERATIVE HYPERPLASIA (NRH; p. 1721)—Changes due to NRH in liver biopsies are often nondiagnostic. However, curvilinear areas of congestion and difficulty in identifying central veins are highly suggestive. NRH has been seen in association with a variety of diseases leading to arteriolar and/or venular damage, such as vasculitis, collagen vascular diseases, rheumatoid arthritis, and so on. Postmortem cases are definitely more frequent than clinically overt cases. The common pathogenetic mechanism is probably an injury to portal venules and/or arterioles, resulting in heterogeneity of blood supply. Zones of ischemia develop, with ensuing multifocal atrophy of liver parenchyma and secondary regenerative nodules. Reticulin stain facilitates diagnosis by demonstrating the abnormal reticulin network. The absence of fibrosis helps in distinguishing NRH from cirrhosis and FNH.

5. Correct choice: E
FACTORS IN THE PATHOGENESIS OF HCC (p. 1726)—The great majority of cases of HCC develop in cirrhotic livers. Alcohol, hepatitis B virus, and hepatitis C virus are the most important etiologic factors worldwide. Several conditions may lead to HCC without causing cirrhosis. Among these are hypercitrillunemia (a high rate of association with HCC), glycogen storage disease (an intermediate rate), and several others with a low rate of association with HCC (e.g., oral contraceptive use, hereditary fructose intolerance, etc.).

6. Correct choice: D
HEPATOCELLULAR CARCINOMA (HCC; p. 1732)—HCC is composed of neoplastic hepatocytes in a trabecular (most common), tubular, glandular, or papillary pattern. Endothelial-lined sinusoidal spaces between cords of neoplastic cells constitute a crucial histologic feature in the differential diagnosis from similar tumors. The most specific immunohistochemical marker is CEA staining in a *sinusoidal* pattern, which, however, is most common in well-differentiated tumors. Neoplastic cells express keratin 8, 18, and 19 (the molecular forms recognized by CAM 5.2), but usually not keratin forms recognized by the AE1 antibody. Cholangiocarcinoma, on the contrary, shows cytoplasmic immunoreactivity for AE1, CAM 5.2, and CEA. Bile formation can be seen in different liver neoplasms.

7. Correct choice: C
FIBROLAMELLAR CARCINOMA (p. 1739)—Although the most important risk factors for the conventional histologic type of hepatocellular carcinoma (HCC) include hepatitis B virus infection and cirrhosis, the fibrolamellar variant develops in young patients (between 20 and 40) with an otherwise normal liver. The presence of thick fibrohyaline bands dividing the tumor in nodules is the salient morphological feature. Neoplastic cells have large nuclei with prominent nucleoli. Viral hepatitis is not a recognized risk factor. Alpha-fetoprotein (AFP) levels are markedly elevated with HCC, but not with the fibrolamellar type. This type is associated with a far better prognosis than classic HCC. It must be differentiated from the *scirrhous variant* of HCC, which has a central scar without fibrous bands and consists of small cells without prominent nucleoli.

8. Correct choice: C
HEPATOBLASTOMA (p. 1743)—This malignant tumor may be considered the hepatic counterpart of Wilms tumor. It probably arises from a precursor that differentiates along epithelial and mesenchymal lines. Thus, variably immature (small) hepatocytes represent the main histologic component, but this may be associated with a mesenchymal component with bone or muscle formation. A typical *light/dark pattern* on low power (as seen in the picture) is due to the uneven distribution of glycogen-rich and glycogen-depleted areas. The prognosis depends on the stage and degree of differentiation of the epithelial component. *Malignant mesenchymoma* is an infantile hepatic sarcoma with giant cells and PAS-positive globules. *Mesenchymal hamartoma* is an infantile hepatic neoplasm with histology strikingly similar to breast fibroadenoma.

9. Correct choice: C
BILE DUCT HAMARTOMA (BDH; p. 1747)—Also called *von Meyenburg complex*, this benign condition may mimic metastatic carcinoma on the cut surface. It results from developmental anomalies of the ductal plate and is usually an incidental autopsy

finding. Occasionally, owing to the multifocal nature of the nodules, BDH is sometimes mistaken for metastases or granulomas. *Bile duct adenoma* is a well-circumscribed wedge-shaped nodule usually in a subcapsular position, composed of well-differentiated small tubules. *Mesenchymal hamartoma* is a rare infantile lesion of the liver, histologically similar to breast fibroadenoma.

10. Correct choice: B

INTRAHEPATIC CHOLANGIOCARCINOMA (ICC; p. 1749)—ICC raises the differential diagnosis with hepatocellular carcinoma (HCC). ICC shows the following features: Often multicentric, it develops in noncirrhotic livers, affects elderly patients, is composed of small tubular structures with marked cytologic variability, and is immunoreactive with antibodies to both low- and high-molecular-weight keratin and CEA. CEA immunoreactivity is cytoplasmic in ICC, whereas it shows a canalicular pattern in HCC. Perineural invasion is frequent in ICC, but vascular invasion is more typical of HCC. Bile production is found in HCC but not in ICC, whereas mucin production is frequent in ICC.

11. Correct choice: D

ANGIOSARCOMA (p. 1756)—This malignant vasogenic neoplasm is rare in the liver, but it is inordinately more common in workers who suffered chronic exposure to vinyl chloride (the PVC industry). Vinyl chloride exposure does not increase the risk of hepatocellular or bile duct carcinoma. Anabolic steroid treatment is known to increase the risk of a variety of liver neoplasms, including bile duct carcinoma (but not angiosarcoma). Cirrhosis is associated with an increased risk of hepatocellular carcinoma *and* angiosarcoma, but not bile duct carcinoma. Clonorchis infestation may lead to bile duct carcinoma. Thorotrast exposure is associated with increased prevalence of *both* bile duct carcinoma *and* angiosarcoma.

12. Correct choice: B

EPITHELIOID HEMANGIOENDOTHELIOMA (p. 1759)—This malignant vascular tumor may develop in the liver, usually in women. There is a positive correlation with oral contraceptives. The tumor is often multifocal. Vascular channels are often inconspicuous. Neoplastic endothelial cells resemble epithelial cells and infiltrate veins, thus producing intravascular tufts. The surrounding fibrous stroma may show focal metaplasia. The endothelial origin of this neoplasm is supported by immunohistochemistry and ultrastructural studies. Epithelioid hemangioendothelioma has a better prognosis than angiosarcoma. The latter is characterized by more pronounced cellular atypia.

CHAPTER 38

1. Correct choice: A

ACUTE CHOLECYSTITIS (p. 1781)—The great majority of cases of acute cholecystitis are associated with the presence of gallstones. Bacterial contamination is usually caused by gallstone occlusion of the cystic duct. Repeated infections by *Ascaris lumbricoides* and liver flukes (*Clonorchis*, etc.) are conditions predisposing to the development of *brown pigment stones*, consisting of a core of mucoprotein and a mixture of bilirubin, calcium, and cholesterol. Chronic hemolysis leads to the formation of *black pigment stones*, composed of bilirubin. Acalculous acute cholecystitis is rare, but it has been reported in AIDS, in which case it is due to opportunistic agents such as cytomegalovirus (CMV).

2. Correct choice: A

GALLBLADDER CARCINOMA (p. 1796)—All of the named conditions predispose to this cancer, but cholelithiasis has the strongest association. Up to 90% of gallbladders removed because of carcinoma contain stones; however, 1% to 3% of patients with gallstones develop gallbladder carcinoma. Older people are most commonly affected. Native Americans have an uncommonly high incidence. Histologically, this tumor is usually an adenocarcinoma. Typically, it appears well differentiated on low power (with well-developed glandular structures), but poorly differentiated cytologically (with anaplastic cuboidal cells in a single or double row). Concentric desmoplastic reaction around neoplastic glands is frequent. Intestinal metaplasia is commonly found in areas adjacent to the tumor. The prognosis is poor, with a 5-year survival of 5%, but tumors limited to mucosa and muscularis can be cured by simple cholecystectomy.

3. Correct choice: C

CHOLEDOCHAL CYST (p. 1804)—This anomaly consists of a fusiform dilatation of the common bile duct, whose wall undergoes calcification. It is the most common cause of cholestatic jaundice in children after the first year of life. Choledochal cysts predispose to the development of gallstones and carcinoma. *Caroli disease* refers to multiple cysts of the intrahepatic ducts. *Phrygian cap* is a clinically silent deformity of the fundus of the gallbladder.

CHAPTER 39

1. Correct choice: C

ANAL CARCINOMA (p. 1833)—This squamous cell carcinoma occurs most commonly along the pectinate line and in association with human papillomavirus (HPV). The old classification of squamous and basaloid (cloacogenic) carcinoma has been abandoned, but it is well recognized that this tumor tends to manifest features of adnexal differentiation, thus resembling basal cell carcinoma of the skin. Peripheral palisading and a plexiform pattern of tumor nodules are characteristics frequently seen. Similar tumors may be observed in the upper aerodigestive tract. Other microscopic types of cancer in the anal canal include *small cell, mucinous* (choice A), *sarcomatoid* (choice B), and *verrucous* (choice E).

CHAPTER 40

1. Correct choice: E

RENAL TUBULAR DYSGENESIS (p. 1850)—This uncommon cause of neonatal oliguria is due to aberrant development of renal tubules. It is inherited as an autosomal recessive condition (family counseling) or in association with prenatal exposure to several drugs, notably ACE inhibitors and cocaine; a similar renal abnormality has been linked to *in utero* exposure to NSAIDs. *Congenital hydronephrosis* is due to congenital obstruction at the ureteropelvic junction. In *renal dysplasia*, there is an abnormal organization of metaphrenic elements, usually associated with other congenital anomalies of the urinary tract. *Renal hypoplasia* may be sporadic, due to chromosomal deletion syndromes, or associated with Down syndrome (15% of cases).

2. Correct choice: E

RENAL SEGMENTAL ATROPHY (p. 1851)—Segmental or lobar atrophy is an acquired condition due to vesicoureteral and intrarenal reflux. Vesicoureteral reflux, however, is not always demonstrable in all cases. The salient macroscopic feature is a shrunken lobe with effacement of the cortex and medullary pyramid. In affected lobes, the cortex is virtually devoid of glomeruli: It contains dilated tubules with intraluminal casts, and the medulla contains few ducts. The remaining renal parenchyma undergoes hypertrophy and often develops focal segmental glomerulosclerosis. Hypertension is the most frequent initial sign.

3. Correct choice: D

AUTOSOMAL RECESSIVE POLYCYSTIC KIDNEY DISEASE (p. 1852)—AR-PKD is a hereditary condition characterized by congenital cystic anomalies of the kidneys and liver. The gene is located on the short arm of chromosome 6; *fibrocystin* is the protein involved. Renal cysts derive from dilated collecting ducts, whereas hepatic cysts develop from abnormal bile ducts. In the liver, cystically dilated bile ducts are associated with portal fibrosis, which progresses with time to a picture mimicking micronodular cirrhosis and leading to portal hypertension. Hepatic abnormalities become increasingly severe with age. Cerebellar/retinal angiomas and pancreatic cysts are seen in *von Hippel-Lindau syndrome;* angiomyolipomas and cardiac rhabdomyomas are seen in *tuberous sclerosis.*

4. Correct choice: A

ADULT (AUTOSOMAL DOMINANT) POLYCYSTIC KIDNEY DISEASE (p. 1854)—About 90% of AD-PKD cases are due to mutations of a gene on chromosome 16 that encodes *polycystin-1*, involved in cell–matrix interactions. A minority of cases are due to mutations involving two other genes, one of which is on chromosome 4 (coding for *polycystin-2*), whereas the other has not yet been mapped. The disease manifests in the fourth or fifth decade with hypertension, microhematuria, and/or enlarged kidneys. Renal cysts derive from virtually all segments of the nephron. Their wall is lined by a hyperplastic micropapillary epithelium. Papillary formations cause luminal obstruction and cause or facilitate cyst development. Only 20% of the nephrons are affected. The remaining ones suffer from cyst compression, but are structurally normal. Lithiasis and infections are common in AD-PKD. Pyelocaliceal occlusion and ureteral agenesis are usually associated with *renal dysplasia*, suggesting that urinary obstruction plays a pathogenetic role.

CHAPTER 41

1. Correct choice: B

DIFFUSE (INTRACAPILLARY) PROLIFERATIVE GLOMERULONEPHRITIS (p. 1867)—The history suggests a nephritic syndrome secondary to streptococcal infection. Subepithelial deposits of electron-dense material, called *humps*, are characteristic of this glomerulonephritis. On light microscopy, this condition is characterized by hypercellular glomeruli due to increased mesangial and intracapillary (inflammatory) cells. The disease resolves spontaneously with supportive treatment. A useful algorithm for the diagnosis of glomerular diseases is proposed (Algorithm of Morphologic Interpretation of Glomerular Patterns on p. 1864). Increased glomerular cellularity is usually consistent with *glomerulonephritis* (GN). Intracapillary hypercellularity

with obliteration of the capillary lumina, if diffuse, suggests postinfectious GN or membranoproliferative GN. Extracapillary hypercellularity is diagnostic of *crescentic* GN.

2. Correct choice: A

MEMBRANOPROLIFERATIVE GLOMERULONEPHRITIS (MPGN), TYPE I (p. 1869)—Clinical presentation (nephritic syndrome with or without nephrotic syndrome) and progression are similar for all three types of MPGN. MPGN may manifest at all ages. Most cases are idiopathic, but some occur in association with certain systemic conditions (hepatitis B, lupus erythematosus, sickle cell disease, etc.). The microscopic features outlined in the question stem are characteristic of MPGN type I, especially the *tram-track* appearance of GBM, which is due to the interposition of mesangium between the glomerular basement membrane (GBM) and the endothelium. Pronounced lobularity may mimic diabetic nodular glomerulosclerosis. Immunofluorescence (IF) usually shows mesangial deposits of C3 and IgG.

3. Correct choice: C

MEMBRANOPROLIFERATIVE GLOMERULONEPHRITIS, TYPE II (p. 1871)—The diagnostic feature of type II MPGN is the presence of electron-dense deposits within the GBM. Such deposits produce a ribbonlike thickening of the glomerular basement membrane, which can be appreciated on silver/PAS stains. IF shows continuous staining for C3 and properdin along the capillary membrane and around the GBM deposits. Seventy percent of patients with DDD have circulating *C3 nephritic factor* (C3NeF). This autoantibody binds C3 convertase and leads to persistent activation of the alternative complement pathway, thus decreasing complement levels. It is unclear how C3NeF activity relates to glomerular damage.

4. Correct choice: E

EXTRACAPILLARY PROLIFERATIVE (CRESCENTIC) GLOMERULONEPHRITIS (p. 1873)—At least 50% of glomeruli must show crescents for a diagnosis of RPGN. Crescents are masses of cells and fibrin accumulating into and obliterating the urinary space of the Bowman capsule. They originate from the rupture of the GBM and the subsequent extravasation of inflammatory cells (monocytes and neutrophils) and the subsequent hyperplasia of visceral and parietal cells. Most cases are idiopathic. The IF pattern recognizes three different forms:

- Minimal or no immune deposits (*pauci-immune*), often associated with circulating anti-neutrophil cytoplasmic autoantibodies (ANCAs). Idiopathic or associated with Wegener's granulomatosis, microscopic polyangiitis, and so on. This is the most common form of RPGN.
- Linear deposition of anti-GBM IgG and C3. Idiopathic or associated with *Goodpasture syndrome.*
- Granular deposition of immune complex. Idiopathic or associated with postinfectious glomerulonephritis, Henoch-Schönlein syndrome, systemic lupus erythematosus (SLE), IgA nephropathy, and so on.

The prognosis of RPGN depends on the extent of crescents and the IF type.

5. Correct choice: A

MINIMAL CHANGE DISEASE (p. 1879)—This is the most common cause of nephrotic syndrome in children, usually presenting before 6 years of age. On light microscopy, glomeruli look virtually normal, but EM reveals diffuse effacement (detachment and fusion) of epithelial foot processes. Immunofluorescence is usually *negative*. The disease commonly resolves with steroid treatment, but relapses may occur, and only infrequently does the disease progress to chronic renal failure. Continuous granular C3 deposition along the capillary wall is seen in *type II MPGN* (dense deposit disease). Granular IgG/C3 deposits along GBM are found in various glomerular diseases, for example, membranous glomerulonephritis and postinfectious glomerulonephritis. Linear IgG deposition along GBM is pathognomonic of *Goodpasture syndrome*. Mesangial IgA deposits are associated with *Berger disease* (IgA nephropathy).

6. Correct choice: B

FOCAL SEGMENTAL GLOMERULOSCLEROSIS (FSGS; p. 1882)—FSGS is currently the most common glomerular pattern seen in adults with idiopathic nephrotic syndrome. It is characterized by the collapse of glomerular basement membrane with the deposition of hyaline material (sclerosis) in a segmental and focal distribution. Lipid droplets and foam cells are characteristic. It may be idiopathic or associated with other conditions such as heroin abuse, HIV infection, obesity, sickle cell disease, and renal ablation.

7. Correct choice: C

HIVAN (p. 1886)—This AIDS-associated complication is particularly prevalent in African-American males. Although FSGS is the predominant pattern of glomerular involvement, there are specific clinical and morphologic features suggesting that HIVAN may be a unique entity. Among the morphologic changes characteristic of HIVAN are the collapse of glomerular loops, interstitial fibrosis with chronic inflammation, and *tubuloreticular inclusions* in endothelial cells (identifiable by EM). Furthermore, podocytes become conspicuously hypertrophic, resulting in crescentlike formations. Resorption droplets are particularly abundant. HIVAN causes rapidly progressive renal failure.

8. Correct choice: D

MEMBRANOUS GLOMERULONEPHRITIS (p. 1887)—The subepithelial deposits detected on EM between the basement membrane and visceral epithelium consist of antigen-antibody complexes, which are highlighted by IF. In most cases, they result from *in situ* production. The basement membrane extensions between such deposits are stained by silver methods, resulting in the characteristic spiked appearance, as shown in the picture. Most cases are idiopathic, but some are associated with infections (hepatitis B and syphilis), SLE, drugs/toxins (mercury exposure), or cancer (e.g., renal cell carcinoma). About *one-third* of idiopathic cases progress to chronic renal failure, whereas the secondary forms usually abate on elimination of the inciting factors. Staging does not have prognostic significance.

9. Correct choice: E

DIABETIC NEPHROPATHY (p. 1890)—This is the most common cause of end-stage renal disease (ESRD) in the United States. Thickening of the glomerular and tubular basement membranes has been observed as early as 1 to 2 years following the onset of diabetes. It appears before the second most frequent glomerular change, that is, the expansion of the mesangial matrix (*diffuse glomerulosclerosis*). *Nodular glomerulosclerosis* (Kimmelstiel-Wilson disease) is less commonly associated with, but more specific of, diabetic nephropathy and consists of spherical deposits of PAS-positive material within the peripheral mesangium. *Insudative lesions*,

including fibrin caps and capsular drops, are less specific and result from exudation of plasma proteins and lipids.

10. Correct choice: B

IgA NEPHROPATHY p. 1894)—Berger disease is related to the mesangial deposition of IgA. It is probably the most common form of glomerulonephritis worldwide. Recurrent hematuria, often discovered incidentally, is the most frequent presentation, sometimes associated with mild proteinuria. IgA deposits can be demonstrated by IF in the mesangium. Overproduction of IgA in response to infectious agents is the most likely underlying mechanism. Episodes of hematuria manifest transiently following respiratory or gastrointestinal infections. Light microscopic alterations are highly variable, but mesangial expansion and hypercellularity without interstitial changes represent the earliest stage. Most cases tend to have a remission/relapsing course, but approximately 30% will eventually progress to renal failure over a 20-year period. Glomerular changes of *Henoch-Schönlein purpura* are indistinguishable from those of Berger disease.

11. Correct choice: E

THIN BASEMENT MEMBRANE DISEASE (p. 1896)—Clinical symptomatology and ultrastructural findings are consistent with *thin basement membrane disease*. Note that GBM thickness varies with age and sex: A value of 300 to 480 nm is considered normal in adults. Some authors suggest using a value of 264 nm as a low cutoff for diagnosis of thin basement membrane disease. This condition is benign and does not progress to renal failure. No associated extrarenal abnormalities have been reported. Alport syndrome initially manifests with ultrastructural features of thin basement membrane disease.

12. Correct choice: A

ALPORT SYNDROME (p. 1898)—This syndrome includes several hereditary conditions, the most frequent of which (the *classic* form) is inherited as an X-linked dominant disorder (thus, females may manifest the disease). The most characteristic glomerular alterations are visualized by EM: *splitting* and variable *thickening* of the GBM. GBM changes lead to recurrent hematuria (similar to thin basement membrane disease). The classic (X-linked) form is due to mutations of the genes encoding α-3, α-4, and α-5 chains of type IV collagen. Immunostaining with antibodies to these collagen chains is absent in Alport syndrome. Ocular defects, leiomyomatosis, and blood cell anomalies occasionally coexist.

13. Correct choice: C

CRYOGLOBULINEMIC GLOMERULONEPHRITIS (p. 1903)—This condition is due to the formation of cryoglobulins, which precipitate at 4° C and become soluble at 30° C. One-third of cases are idiopathic, whereas the remaining cases are associated with various conditions (collagen vascular diseases, liver disease, lymphomas, etc.). The acute manifestation consists of an acute syndrome characterized by purpura, joint inflammation, hepatosplenomegaly, and lymphadenopathy. Intracapillary proliferative GN may develop in the acute phase or years thereafter. Cryoglobulin thrombi are evident within the capillary lumen on PAS staining. EM demonstrates subendothelial accumulation of fibrillary material showing a microtubular/cylindrical substructure often described as a *fingerprint-like* pattern.

14. Correct choice: A

AMYLOIDOSIS (p. 1905)—Amyloid deposition within the glomeruli may develop in various forms of systemic amyloidosis, particularly as a result of chronic inflammatory conditions such as rheumatoid arthritis, collagen vascular diseases, bronchiectases, and so on. This form is due to accumulation of *AA* (amyloid-associated) protein, which can be demonstrated by Congo red staining. Glomerular disease due to amyloidosis usually manifests with nephrotic syndrome.

15. Correct choice: D

LUPUS NEPHRITIS (p. 1909)—Glomerular pathology is extremely common and morphologically variable in SLE. The WHO classification divides SLE-associated glomerular disease into six classes (I-VI), which have important prognostic implications. Class I and II nephritis (choices A and B, respectively) need follow-up but no treatment. Class III and IV nephritis (choices C and D, respectively) require immunosuppressive treatment. Class V nephritis (choice E) requires immunosuppression if associated with proliferative lesions (class III and IV). Class IV nephritis is the most frequent: Mesangial and capillary endothelial proliferation, viral-like inclusions in endothelial cells, fingerprint-like deposits in the subendothelial space, and severe C1q mesangial deposition are all present in various combinations. Class VI (choice F) is referred to as *chronic sclerosing GN* and is associated with irreversible renal failure.

16. Correct choice: D

LIGHT CHAIN NEPHROPATHY (p. 1915)—This condition may produce glomerular changes extremely similar to those associated with diabetes mellitus (diffuse and nodular glomerulosclerosis). Arteriolosclerosis is absent in light chain disease (LCD). LCD is caused by the accumulation of kappa light chains in a nonfibrillary (nonamyloidotic) form, which results in a PAS-positive mesangial deposit. Electron-dense subendothelial deposits are seen on EM. In two-thirds of cases, multiple myeloma or analogous lymphoplasmacellular proliferation occurs concomitantly with LCD or develops later. Sometimes, there is no evidence of plasma cell dyscrasia.

17. Correct choice: C

CHRONIC PYELONEPHRITIS (p. 1919)—This condition is caused by recurrent insults to the pelvicaliceal system secondary to causes that can be *obstructive* (i.e., urolithiasis) or *nonobstructive* (i.e., vesicoureteral reflux with infection). Grossly, the kidneys show irregular scarring, blunted papillae, and dilated calices. Histologically, there is interstitial chronic inflammation and fibrosis, tubular atrophy or dilatation, accumulation of inspissated protein within tubular lumina, interstitial deposits of Tamm-Horsfall protein, and periglomerular fibrosis. Widespread dilatation of the tubules containing eosinophilic material may mimic thyroid tissue (*thyroidization*). A diagnosis of chronic pyelonephritis cannot be made solely on microscopic examination.

18. Correct choice: E

UNDERLYING CAUSES OF ESRD: EPIDEMIOLOGY (p. 1931)—The three most common underlying causes of ESRD in the United States include diabetes (44%), hypertension, and glomerulonephritis. Diabetes is the prevalent cause among whites, hypertension among blacks. Chronic interstitial nephritis and AD-PKD are important but less frequent causes of ESRD.

19. Correct choice: E

HYPERACUTE RENAL REJECTION (p. 1933)—This is a rare complication because cross-matching techniques have become routine before renal transplantation. It is due to preformed circulating antibodies against allograft antigens. Such antibodies develop in the recipient because of prior immunological exposure, which may

result from past pregnancies, blood transfusions, or transplantation. A few minutes or hours following transplantation, the patient develops a sudden decrease in urine output. The recipient's antibodies react with endothelial cells, triggering thrombosis and rapid failure of the graft. Infarction of renal parenchyma, fibrin thrombi, and extensive leukocytic infiltration is seen histologically.

20. Correct choice: C

ACUTE INTERSTITIAL (CELLULAR) REJECTION (p. 1934)—This is the most frequent form of rejection and develops typically days to weeks after transplantation (rarely after months). It is mediated by T lymphocytes and characterized by interstitial mononuclear inflammatory infiltrate. Lymphocytes permeate through the tubular epithelium resulting in tubulitis, the morphologic hallmark. Features of acute cellular rejection are usually combined with those of acute humoral rejection (endothelial damage). The reports on renal biopsies for follow-up of transplant patients should quantify the relative degrees of both acute humoral and cellular rejection patterns. Acute cellular rejection is highly responsive to appropriate treatment.

21. Correct choice: D

ACUTE VASCULAR (HUMORAL; p. 1936)—This type of rejection usually manifests two weeks after transplantation, but it may also occur anytime thereafter. The humoral form is mediated by the recipient's antidonor antibodies targeting endothelial cells. Therefore, acute humoral rejection is a *vascular* rejection. In milder forms, endothelial cells undergo swelling and detachment with subendothelial lymphocytic infiltration. Severe forms lead to vasculitis with fibrinoid necrosis and thrombosis. Acute humoral rejection is less responsive to immunosuppressive therapy than acute cellular rejection. The possibility of acute or chronic rejection can be reduced by careful cross-matching between donor and recipient, but not entirely eliminated as with hyperacute rejection.

22. Correct choice: C

CHRONIC REJECTION (p. 1938)—This is the most common cause of long-term failure of renal allografts. It manifests clinically with progressive renal insufficiency, often associated with proteinuria and hypertension. The most distinctive histopathologic change consists of fibrointimal sclerosis of arteries and arterioles mimicking arteriolosclerosis. This complication may arise from recurrent episodes of acute rejection and is not per se a unique immunologic pattern of rejection. It always progresses to irreversible renal failure. Mesangial prominence with GBM "tram-tracking" refers to *transplant glomerulopathy*, a glomerular change mimicking membranoproliferative GN and occurring in 25% of long-term renal transplants.

23. Correct choice: C

NEPHROTOXICITY OF CALCINEURIN INHIBITORS (p. 1940)—Effects of calcineurin inhibitors such as *cyclosporine* and *FK506* (tacrolimus) include:

- *Acute functional:* manifests with rapid decline in renal function; there are no morphologic changes.
- *Acute tubular:* dose-related but infrequent since adoption of lower dosages; epithelial cells of the proximal convoluted tubules develop isometric vacuolation and inclusion bodies (the latter are giant mitochondria).
- *Chronic vascular interstitial:* the most important form, which manifests with progressive interstitial fibrosis, arteriolosclerosis, and tubular atrophy.

CHAPTER 42

1. Correct choice: D
GRADING OF RCCs (p. 1957)—The Fuhrman system is based entirely on nuclear and nucleolar features. Nuclear size should be evaluated. In practice, grading can be performed as follows:

Grade 1: Nucleoli are inconspicuous (examined at 400x)
Grade 2: Nucleoli are visible (examined at 400x)
Grade 3: Nucleoli are large (visible at 100x)
Grade 4: Nucleoli are large (visible at 100x), and nuclei measure greater than 20 microns.

2. Correct choice: D
CONVENTIONAL (CLEAR CELL) CARCINOMA AND CYTOGENETIC ABNORMALITIES (p. 1958)—The majority of cases of the *conventional* type of renal cell carcinoma show abnormalities of the short arm of chromosome 3. These anomalies result in loss of the region containing the *VHL* (von Hippel-Lindau) gene. In the majority of cases, the nondeleted allele of the VHL gene is found to be inactivated by mutations or hypermethylation. Thus, the VHL gene is thought to act as a tumor suppressor gene. This genetic abnormality occurs in both familial and sporadic forms of the clear cell type of renal carcinoma, but not in the papillary type or the chromophobe type.

3. Correct answer: E
DIFFERENTIAL DIAGNOSIS IN RENAL CELL CARCINOMA (RCC; p.1959)—*Granular* and *sarcomatoid* tumors are indeed morphologic variants of specific renal neoplasms. Conventional (clear cell) RCC is often composed of a mixture of clear and granular cells. A granular cell pattern can be found in chromophobe RCC, oncocytoma, and papillary RCC. A *sarcomatoid* pattern can be seen in conventional (clear cell) RCC, chromophobe RCC, collecting duct carcinoma, and so on.

4. Correct choice: A
PAPILLARY RENAL CELL CARCINOMA (p. 1963)—This variant accounts for 10% to 15% of all renal cancers. It is composed of a predominantly papillary or papillary-solid growth. The most common genetic abnormalities include trisomies 7, 16, and 17, and loss of chromosome Y. The prognosis is better than that of conventional (clear cell) carcinoma. The origin and other features of the most common renal neoplasms are summarized in the following table:

5. Correct choice: C
CHROMOPHOBE CELL CARCINOMA (pp. 1967–1969)—The tumor consists of sheets of cells with sharp cytoplasmic borders, pale cytoplasm, and frequent perinuclear halos. Characteristically, large cells are clustered around vessels. Neoplastic cells contain acid mucin, which accounts for the characteristic positivity for colloidal iron. EM reveals innumerable cytoplasmic vesicles. Like oncocytoma, from which it must be differentiated, chromophobe carcinoma is thought to arise from intercalated cells of the collecting ducts. Hypodiploidy and various chromosome losses are detectable in these tumors.

6. Correct choice: B
CHROMOPHOBE CELL CARCINOMA (p. 1967)—This variant constitutes approximately 5% to 10% of renal cell carcinomas. It is characterized by an excellent prognosis compared to the more frequent clear cell and papillary types. The age of presentation is similar to the clear cell type (55 to 60 years).

7. Correct choice: C
ONCOCYTOMA (p. 1971)—This benign tumor accounts for 5% to 10% of all resected renal neoplasms. It is derived from the intercalated duct and composed of uniform cells with intensely eosinophilic granular cytoplasm. The nuclei are monotonous and have a central nucleolus. Mitotic activity is inconspicuous. Architectural patterns may be variable, for example, tubular-acinar, solid sheets, and biphasic. The gross appearance is highly characteristic because the tumor shows a mahogany-brown color and, when large, a central stellate scar. The latter feature is infrequent in tumors measuring less than 5 cm in main diameter. Choice A is characteristic of *collecting duct carcinoma*, choice B of *medullary carcinoma*, choice D of *papillary carcinoma*, and choice E of *chromophobe cell carcinoma*.

8. Correct choice: D
MEDULLARY CARCINOMA (p. 1977)—This type of renal carcinoma is rare, but shows a striking propensity to affect young people with sickle cell trait, whether of African-American or Mediterranean descent. It is probably a variant of collecting duct carcinoma, with which it shares histologic and histogenetic features.

9. Correct choice: C
METANEPHRIC ADENOMA (p. 1984)—This tumor is invariably located in the cortex and represents a frequent incidental finding. Histologically, it consists of uniform bland cells arranged in papillary or tubular formations. Cells have eosinophilic cytoplasm (not clear) and lack 3p deletions. A papillary architecture may pose a diagnostic challenge in distinguishing metanephric adenoma from papillary carcinoma. *Papillary carcinoma* contains foamy histiocytes within fibrovascular cores and is frequently multifocal.

10. Correct choice: D
ANGIOMYOLIPOMA (p. 1985)—Angiomyolipoma is a neoplasm of probable hamartomatous (developmental) genesis, seen in approximately 40% of patients with tuberous sclerosis (TS). TS causes various developmental anomalies including cortical tubers (consisting of dysplastic neocortex), skin angiofibromas,

Tumor Type	Cells of Origin	Cytogenetics	Overall 5-Year Survival
Conventional	Proximal convoluted tubule	3p-	62%
Papillary	Distal convoluted tubule	7+, 6+, 17+, Y-	79%–92%
Chromophobe	Intercalated cells of cortex	1-, Y-	94%
Oncocytoma	Intercalated cells of cortex	1-, Y-	100%
Collecting duct	Collecting ducts	1-, 6-, 14-, 15-, 22-	Virtually 0%
Medullary	Collecting ducts	Unknown	Virtually 0%

cardiac rhabdomyomas, and so on. HMB-45 immunoreactivity is also found in similar hamartomatous TS-related lesions, such as lymphangiomyomatosis. *Beckwith-Wiedemann syndrome* is associated with omphalocele-macroglossia and Wilms tumor. Renal *medullary carcinoma* is associated with sickle cell trait. Von Hippel-Lindau syndrome is associated with *conventional* (clear cell) RCC.

CHAPTER 43

1. Correct choice: C
SIGNIFICANCE OF RENAL SINUS IN STAGING OF WILMS TUMOR (p. 2002)—The *renal sinus* is the concave region of the kidney containing major vascular and pelvicaliceal structures. Here, tumor invasion may gain access to blood and lymphatic vessels and spread to distant sites. Vascular invasion within the renal sinus is a primary discriminant between stage I and stage II. If resection margins are involved or there is peritoneal spread, but the tumor is still confined within the abdomen, the tumor is in stage III. Hematogenous spread corresponds to stage IV, and bilateral tumors to stage V.

2. Correct choice: E
WILMS TUMOR (p. 2005)—Ninety percent of Wilms tumors occur before the age of 6 years. Staging is the most important prognostic factor. However, diagnosis before the age of 2 years is associated with a better survival. Furthermore, tumor size has prognostic implications in stage I. The extent of epithelial and muscle differentiation has no apparent prognostic implications.

3. Correct choice: A
MESOBLASTIC NEPHROMA (p. 2016)—This congenital neoplasm represents 3% of childhood renal tumors and usually becomes apparent in the first 3 months of life. It is a well-circumscribed mass often located near the renal sinus. It consists of a monotonous mesenchymal growth of fibroblast-like spindly cells; this is referred to as the *classic pattern*. The *cellular pattern* is more common and is similar to fibrosarcoma, with high cellularity and numerous mitoses. The tumor often shows focal myofibroblastic, smooth muscle, or cartilage differentiation. It is a benign tumor, which infrequently displays local infiltrative behavior or metastatic spread. *Cystic nephroma*, a rare variant of Wilms tumor, is characterized by multiple cysts lined by tubular epithelium.

4. Correct choice: A
CLEAR CELL SARCOMA (p. 2019)—This highly malignant renal tumor has a controversial histogenesis, but is distinct from that of Wilms tumor. Despite its name, the clear cell appearance is seen in a minority of cases. It consists of uniform cells arranged in nests and cords separated by fibrovascular septa. The nesting or trabecular pattern is characteristic and results from a chicken-wire network of thin intersecting vascular septa. Other morphological patterns are epithelioid, spindled, and myxoid. Helpful diagnostic features include extreme uniformity of gross and microscopic features, *negative immunostains* except for vimentin, a characteristic scalloped edge, and the propensity of this tumor to metastasize to bones and brain (utterly unusual for other childhood renal tumors). The prognosis is poor, but it has recently improved thanks to the use of doxorubicin. Metastases often manifest a long time after the initial diagnosis.

CHAPTER 44

1. Correct choice: E
CYSTITIS GLANDULARIS/CYSTICA (p. 2037)—This pattern of reaction may be due to a number of chronic stimuli, such as recurrent cystitis, neurogenic bladder, bladder exstrophy, and so on. Nests of urothelium (*Von Brunn nests*) grow inward and undergo metaplastic changes (*cystitis glandularis*) and/or cystic dilatation (*cystitis cystica*). This change is unlikely to predispose to adenocarcinoma. *Mesonephroid metaplasia* also occurs in response to various irritative stimuli: It consists of papillary or sessile masses composed of tubules lined by cuboidal cells. *Follicular cystitis* refers to chronic cystitis associated with the formation of lymphoid follicles.

2. Correct choice: C
INTERSTITIAL CYSTITIS (p. 2039)—Also referred to as *Hunner ulcer*, this form of cystitis is probably of autoimmune nature. Cultures are usually negative. The condition is most commonly seen in women with systemic lupus erythematosus or other autoimmune disorders. A chronic inflammatory infiltrate of mucosa and submucosa with numerous mast cells is the typical morphologic substrate. Mucosal fissures are frequent.

3. Correct choice: E
URETHRAL CARUNCLE (p. 2039)—This benign lesion manifests characteristically as a small, friable, raspberry-like mass that protrudes from the meatus. It occurs exclusively in elderly women and is probably reactive. It is composed of highly vascular and chronically inflamed granulation tissue with accompanying islands of metaplastic squamous epithelium. The latter may mimic a malignant growth. *Urethral carcinoma* develops in the region of the meatus, is associated with HPV infection, and has a predilection for elderly women. *Mesonephric adenoma* (also called nephrogenic adenoma) is a reactive lesion morphologically similar to the homonymous lesion in the bladder.

4. Correct choice: B
MALAKOPLAKIA (pp. 2042 and 2043)—This reaction is characterized by multiple yellow nodules and plaques in the trigone region that may be mistaken for cancer on cystoscopy. Microscopically, the lesion consists of macrophage collections. *Michaelis-Guttmann bodies* are frequently identified in the cytoplasm of macrophages and in the interstitium. They consist of concentrically layered corpuscles that contain iron and calcium. Malakoplakia probably results from the deficient phagocytic function of macrophages and is more common in immunodepressed patients. *E. coli* and less frequently *Proteus* are frequently involved. It may also develop in the kidneys, colon, lung, prostate, and other sites.

5. Correct choice: B
BLADDER CARCINOMA AND RISK FACTORS (pp. 2044 and 2045)—Cigarette smoking is probably the most important risk factor in transitional cell carcinoma in industrialized countries. Arylamine exposure was an important risk factor when aniline dyes (2-naphthylamine) were used extensively as coloring agents in the food industry. Cyclophosphamide causes hemorrhagic cystitis and increased risk for urinary bladder cancer following long-term administration. The association between HPV and bladder cancer is at best controversial. *Schistosoma hematobium* is an important risk factor for squamous cell (less frequently transitional) carcinoma of the urinary bladder in regions where this infection is endemic.

6. Correct choice: A
STAGING OF BLADDER TCC (p. 2045)—Staging is the most important prognostic factor in TCC of the bladder. The system developed by Jewett and Strong in 1946 is similar to that proposed by the American Joint Committee on Cancer (AJCC). Clinical staging is highly inaccurate, and thus pathologic staging acquires a great importance. Crushing and cautery artifact, biopsy orientation, and distortion due to prior biopsy all account for difficulty in evaluating invasion of the lamina propria. Important parameters in assessing lamina propria invasion include the following: pattern of infiltrating cells; continuity of basement membrane; stromal reaction; retraction artifact around tumor cells; *paradoxical differentiation* of infiltrating cells, which shows better differentiation compared to the primary focus. T1 tumors (with invasion of the lamina propria) have a significantly worse prognosis than T0 tumors (*in situ*).

7. Correct choice: B
TRANSITIONAL CELL TUMOR (TCC; p. 2048)—*Pathologic staging* is the most powerful determinant of metastatic potential and survival in TCCs. The 5-year survival rate is 75% for tumors infiltrating no deeper than the lamina propria, 50% for those infiltrating the muscularis propria, and 20% for those invading perivesical fat.

TCCs account for 90% of urothelial neoplasms. According to the grading/classification system developed by a joint committee of the WHO and the International Society of Urological Pathology (*WHO-ISUP*), transitional cell neoplasms can be classified as follows:

- *Papilloma* and *inverted papilloma:* entirely benign tumors
- *Papillary tumor of low malignant potential:* papillary neoplasm lined by well-differentiated urothelium with no or minimal atypia but increased cell layers. Prone to recurrence, usually with same histology, rarely as invasive TCC
- *Low-grade TCC:* papillary growth, urothelium with disordered orientation and mild/moderate nuclear atypia, and infrequent invasion of deep layers. Frequent recurrence but infrequent (5%) malignant progression
- *High-grade TCC:* often solid, broad based, shows marked cytologic and architectural atypia, and invades the deep layers of the bladder wall. It shows malignant progression in 15% to 40% of cases.

8. Correct answer: C
UROTHELIAL CARCINOMA *IN SITU* (p. 2054)—Urothelial carcinoma *in situ* (CIS) refers to areas of bladder mucosa where the normal urothelium has been replaced by neoplastic epithelium that does not invade through the basement membrane. CIS is a recognized precancerous lesion, but is usually asymptomatic (the presentation in the question stem is rare). It is usually detected in association with other urothelial neoplasms or in patients with a history of prior bladder tumors, and the presentation described here is rare. To make a diagnosis of urothelial CIS, one should remember that:

- Cytologic atypia need not be full thickness
- CIS cells may have a pagetoid spread
- A high nuclear to cytoplasmic ratio is not a constant feature of CIS
- Umbrella cells may still be present
- The degree of cytologic atypia is variable

9. Correct choice: A
ADENOCARCINOMA OF THE BLADDER (p. 2060)—This tumor represents 2% of all bladder cancers, but it constitutes the great majority of those associated with bladder exstrophy. It usually grows as a polypoid mass in the trigone. Sometimes, it behaves like a signet ring carcinoma, with diffuse infiltration of the bladder wall. Urachal remnants and bladder diverticula are other anatomic abnormalities that predispose to the development of adenocarcinoma of the bladder. Cigarette smoking is associated with an increased risk of transitional cell carcinoma. Mesonephric rests may be related to some cases of the *mesonephric type* of adenocarcinoma (*clear cell* type). *Schistosoma hematobium* infection is most frequently associated with *squamous cell carcinoma*. The coexistence of *cystitis glandularis/cystica* and adenocarcinoma is frequent but probably coincidental.

10. Correct choice: D
RHABDOMYOSARCOMA OF THE BLADDER (pp. 2068 and 2069)—This constitutes the most common bladder malignancy in pediatric age. The *botryoid* subtype is the most frequent. This presents as a large polypoid mass that protrudes above the trigone underneath an atrophic mucosa. The so-called *cambium layer* is a highly characteristic histologic feature. Cross-striations and muscle markers are identifiable in the better differentiated cells. The prognosis is poor. Leiomyosarcoma is the most common bladder *sarcoma* in adults.

11. Correct choice: E
POSTOPERATIVE SPINDLE CELL NODULE (p. 2070)—This small nodular lesion may develop after transurethral surgical interventions and has been reported in the vagina as well. It may generate confusion with sarcoma because of its high proliferative rate and immunoreactivity for actin. A delicate vascular network, scattered inflammatory cells, and a myxoid matrix favor a benign lesion. An *inflammatory pseudotumor*, also of a reactive nature, develops most commonly in children and is composed of spindly cells within a myxoid background and a chronic inflammatory infiltrate. *Postoperative granuloma* may develop as a result of surgery.

CHAPTER 45

1. Correct choice: A
PROSTATIC HYPERPLASIA VERSUS ADENOCARCINOMA (p. 2083)—The features listed in choices B through E are variably present in prostatic hyperplasia, but nucleoli of epithelial cells remain inconspicuous. Prostatic adenocarcinoma, on the contrary, is composed of cells that usually show prominent nucleoli (larger than 1 micron). Squamous metaplasia is often present in the foci of healed prostatic infarcts.

2. Correct choice: D
RISK FACTORS FOR PROSTATIC CARCINOMA (p. 2089)—Of the previously mentioned factors, only age and race seem to affect the risk of developing prostatic carcinoma. By the age of 50, up to 34% of men will have *occult* foci of prostatic carcinoma, a rate that increases to 70% by the age of 70. The age-adjusted incidence (cases/100,000) rate varies dramatically among different ethnic groups: 3 to 4 for Japanese men, 50 for American Caucasian men, and higher rates for blacks. Environmental influences are suspected of playing a role in the development of this cancer, but no specific toxin has been identified. The role played by fat

consumption and vitamin A intake is currently under investigation. Prostatic hyperplasia, although often associated with cancer, does not predispose to cancer according to most studies.

3. Correct choice: B

PROSTATE CANCER SCREENING (p. 2090)—PSA levels with or without TRUS are the mainstay of most screening programs. TRUS alone has a low sensitivity, for example, 60%. Methods to increase the sensitivity and specificity of PSA measurement include the following:

- Determination of the PSA index: PSA/gram of tissue determined by TRUS
- Age-specific reference ranges
- Percentage of free PSA. Free PSA is released predominantly by hyperplastic tissue, whereas the complex form of PSA is released mainly by cancer

Core needle biopsies may be performed by transrectal or, seldom, transperineal route. The latter is less sensitive, but it is rarely associated with tumor seeding through the needle track. Overall, the false-negative rate of core needle biopsies by the transrectal route is 25%.

4. Correct choice: C

GLEASON GRADING (pp. 2091 and 2092)—This widely used grading system is based on architectural features evaluated on low power. Two main patterns are identified, the *dominant* pattern (to which a score from 1 to 5 is assigned), and a subdominant pattern (to which another score of 1 to 5 is applied). The Gleason score is determined by adding the two scores. If only one pattern is identifiable, its score is doubled. The photomicrograph shows a pattern 3; thus, in this example, the Gleason score is 6.

5. Correct choice: H

PROSTATE CANCER DIAGNOSIS IN CORE BIOPSIES (p. 2094)—One of the most difficult problems is diagnosing prostatic cancer in biopsies where the amount of neoplastic tissue is scanty. This problem is obviously more frequent in needle biopsies than in transurethral resection (TUR) material. In these cases, one should not rely on a single parameter (e.g., nuclear enlargement or macronucleoli), but rather on the full spectrum of cytological changes. Cytological features are more important than architectural ones in needle biopsy specimens. Atrophic glands and seminal vesicles are two of the most common sources of diagnostic difficulties in needle biopsies.

6. Correct choice: A

DIFFERENTIAL DIAGNOSIS: ADENOSIS VERSUS ADENOCARCINOMA (p. 2096)—Distinguishing between adenosis and low-grade adenocarcinoma of the prostate is particularly challenging with TUR specimens. Adenosis may show atypical features, such as minimal infiltration at the periphery, occasionally prominent nucleoli, and back-to-back crowding of glands. Adenosis, however, is composed of glands with a lobular configuration, whereas in adenocarcinoma the glands are arranged haphazardly. Furthermore, in adenosis there is a gradual transition with adjacent normal-appearing glands. Immunolabelling with basal cell–specific antibodies (e.g., 34 βe12) may help in the differential diagnosis.

7. Correct choice: C

FEATURES DIAGNOSTIC OF PROSTATIC CANCER (p. 2098)—The three morphological features virtually diagnostic of prostatic cancer include perineural invasion, mucinous fibroplasia,

and glomerulations. Adenosis may show small crowded glands arranged in a back-to-back configuration, contain intraluminal crystalloids, and occasionally display medium-sized nucleoli. Perineural *invasion* should not be confused with perineural *indentation*, which may be produced by normal glands.

8. Correct choice: D

PROSTATE CANCER MIMICKERS (p. 2099)—In needle biopsies, seminal vesicles may result in the overdiagnosis of prostatic adenocarcinoma. Seminal vesicles are often seen at the edge of the tissue sample and appear as glands arranged around a central lumen. Their lipofuscin pigment is a helpful diagnostic feature. Atrophic glands may produce a seemingly infiltrative pattern, but they appear more basophilic than carcinoma. *Cowper glands* consist of ducts surrounded by mucinous glands. *Verumontanum glands* are located beneath the urethra and contain pale red concretions and corpora amylacea.

9. Correct choice: C

PROSTATIC INTRAEPITHELIAL NEOPLASIA (PIN; p. 2103)—PIN refers to the presence of cytologically atypical cells lining architecturally normal acini or ducts. It can be low or high grade, and the distinction between the two grades relies on the presence of prominent nucleoli (e.g., visible at 20x magnification). High-grade PIN is found in approximately 5% of prostate needle biopsies. When high-grade PIN is diagnosed on biopsy, there is a 23% to 35% probability of finding prostate cancer on a subsequent biopsy. Glands in PIN are architecturally similar to benign glands, but more basophilic owing to hyperplasia, nuclear enlargement and hyperchromasia, and amphophilic cytoplasm. The *tufting* pattern is the most common type of high-grade PIN, with papillary tufts lined by atypical cells.

10. Correct choice: C

STAGE II PROSTATIC CARCINOMA (p. 2107)—Clinically, stage II cancer is palpable but it does not spread outside the prostate. Histologic evaluation shows that 50% of these cases have a microscopic extracapsular extension, thus becoming stage III. Extracapsular extension occurs in the posterolateral region. The tumor is grossly evident in up to 85% of specimens. Capsular invasion is frequent, but it should not be confused with extracapsular extension, that is, infiltration of extraprostatic tissues. Perineural infiltration is a common finding in prostatic adenocarcinoma and correlates with the likelihood of extracapsular extension; however, it is not an independent prognostic factor.

CHAPTER 46

1. Correct choice: E

VASITIS NODOSUM (p. 2145)—This condition is a benign granulomatous reaction around the vas deferens, which most commonly arises following vasectomy or herniorrhaphy. Proliferative funiculitis is a peculiar entity histologically identical to proliferative fasciitis. It constitutes a frequent incidental finding in hernia sacs. Lipomas are the most common neoplasms of the spermatic cord.

2. Correct choice: A

NONSPECIFIC GRANULOMATOUS ORCHITIS (p. 2154)—This condition is thought to result from an autoimmune reaction against testicular antigens, perhaps unmasked by traumatic injury.

Indeed, history of trauma can be elicited in a significant number of cases. It usually presents in middle-aged or elderly men in a manner simulating carcinoma. Histologically, it may be confused with *malakoplakia*.

CHAPTER 47

1. Correct choice: D
INTRATUBULAR GERM CELL NEOPLASIA (IGCN; p. 2171)—IGCN refers to the presence of germ cells with enlarged nuclei, prominent nucleoli, and PAS-positive/diastase-sensitive clear cytoplasm. Cells of IGCN, unclassified (IGCNU) are also positive for placental alkaline phosphatase (PLAP). Patients with a diagnosis of IGCN eventually develop germ cell tumors in 50% of cases. IGCN is most commonly found in cryptorchid patients, patients with infertility, and in the testis contralateral to a testis affected by a germ cell tumor. IGCN may be seen in association with virtually all germ cell tumors except spermatocytic seminoma. Likewise, spermatocytic seminoma is the only germ cell neoplasm reported not to occur in an undescended testis. The association of IGCN with prepubertal yolk sac tumor is controversial.

2. Correct choice: D
SEMINOMA (p. 2173)—This represents 50% of germ cell tumors in its pure form. It is composed of two cell types, neoplastic germ cells with central conspicuous nucleoli and reactive lymphocytes within the stroma. The architectural features may vary from the classic multinodular pattern, to a cordlike, tubular or pseudomicrocystic pattern. It is important to differentiate these neoplasms from embryonal carcinoma and spermatocytic carcinoma. Embryonal carcinoma displays more severe pleomorphism and high mitotic activity and retains an epithelial-like appearance even in the most anaplastic types. Positive keratin immunoreactivity favors embryonal carcinoma.

3. Correct choice: D
SPERMATOCYTIC SEMINOMA (pp. 2176–2178)—Spermatocytic seminoma occurs in patients over 50 years of age. Variability in cell size is a peculiarity of this neoplasm, which consists of round small- and medium-sized cells with scattered multinucleated giant cells. The cytoplasm is scanty and eosinophilic without glycogen vacuoles. Tumor cells are usually negative for PLAP, CEA, AFP, LCA, human chorionic gonadotropin (hCG), and keratin. Electron microscopy may show evidence of spermatocytic differentiation, that is, a meiotic-like chromosome. This slowly growing tumor rarely metastasizes and is thus associated with a good prognosis. Orchiectomy alone is usually curative.

4. Correct choice: C
EMBRYONAL CARCINOMA (p. 2179)—This malignant tumor is composed of pleomorphic epithelial-like cells that consistently express keratin but less often PLAP. Mitotic activity is brisk, and tumor giant cells are frequent. Neoplastic cells are arranged in glandular or solid patterns. In its pure form, it is rare (less than 5% of all testicular neoplasms), but embryonal carcinomas mixed with either choriocarcinoma or yolk sac tumor are common. Note that patients with embryonal carcinoma are on average 10 years younger than those with seminoma. In contrast to seminoma, embryonal carcinoma is treated with orchiectomy and chemotherapy. The overall survival rate is about 80%.

5. Correct choice: E
YOLK SAC TUMOR (pp. 2183 and 2184)—Yolk sac tumor is the most common, whereas teratoma is the second most common testicular tumor in children less than 3 years old. The cut surface of yolk sac tumor has a spongy appearance due to numerous microcysts. Eleven microscopic patterns have been described, but commonly several of these patterns are present in various combination within the same tumor. Typically, yolk sac tumor has an organoid architecture characterized by cuboidal cells arranged in glandular, alveolar, and papillary formations, admixed with mesenchymal components. *Schiller-Duval bodies* are diagnostic features. Cells express AFP and keratin and are aneuploid. In adults, yolk sac components are most often seen in mixed germ cell tumors. The *hepatoid* pattern (more common in ovarian tumors) has a striking resemblance to hepatocellular carcinoma.

6. Correct choice: C
TERATOMA (pp. 2188 and 2189)—Teratoma is the second most common testicular tumor in children (after yolk sac tumor). The pure form is usually found in children but is distinctly rare in adults, in whom it is usually associated with other forms of germ cell neoplasms. Paradoxically, mature teratomas are more frequent in children than in adults. Childhood teratomas behave as benign tumors treatable with simple orchiectomy, whereas adult teratomas have a higher propensity for metastatic spread. Association with IGCNU is another important feature, present in adult cases but absent in prepubertal cases. *Dermoid cysts* are a rare form of testicular mature teratoma.

7. Correct choice: A
CHORIOCARCINOMA (p. 2193)—In its pure form, choriocarcinoma is found in 1 of 300 testicular neoplasms, but it is present in 15% of mixed germ cell tumors. Its hemorrhagic appearance and propensity for cerebral metastatic spread is highly characteristic. The classic histologic pattern of this tumor is that of a combination of cytotrophoblastic cells with pale cytoplasm capped by multinucleated syncytiotrophoblastic cells with dark cytoplasm. Neoplastic cells express hCG (whose plasma levels are usually elevated as well), keratin, epithelial membrane antigen (EMA), and sometimes PLAP. The most important differentials in orchiectomy specimens include testicular torsion and infarction.

8. Correct choice: D
LEYDIG CELL TUMOR (pp. 2198 and 2199)—Although so-called *Reinke crystalloids* are found in only 40% of Leydig cell tumors, they constitute a virtually pathognomonic feature. Neoplastic cells produce androgens and estrogens. These tumors occur in children as well as in adults: Children usually manifest sexual precocity, whereas adults present with a testicular mass and, occasionally, gynecomastia. Histologically, they are composed of sheets of polygonal cells with sharp borders and eosinophilic cytoplasm. The differential diagnosis is with Leydig cell hyperplasia (interstitial growth pattern), malakoplakia (Michaelis-Gutman bodies), and nodules associated with adrenogenital syndrome (multifocal, without Reinke crystalloids).

9. Correct choice: E
SERTOLI CELL TUMOR (p. 2200)—This rare testicular neoplasm is composed of neoplastic Sertoli cells that form solid cords resembling primitive seminiferous tubules. Each cord is

surrounded by an artifactual, but diagnostically significant, separation from the adjacent stroma. These tumors may produce estrogens and manifest with gynecomastia without associated virilism (in contrast to Leydig cell tumors). Approximately 10% are malignant.

10. Correct choice: C
LYMPHOMA OF TESTIS (p. 2206)—This represents approximately 5% of all testicular tumors, and it is the most frequent testicular neoplasm over the age of 60. Not uncommonly, testicular involvement is the first manifestation of disease, but in most cases lymphoma is widely disseminated when the testicular tumor becomes clinically apparent. Testicular biopsies are thus used for staging purposes. Most cases are high-grade, usually diffuse large cell lymphomas. An interstitial growth pattern with relative sparing of tubules is the most important low-power clue to diagnosis of testicular lymphoma. Primary lymphoma of the testis has a 60% 5-year survival.

11. Correct choice: A
ADENOMATOID TUMOR (p. 2213)—This tumor is also commonly seen in the spermatic cord, fallopian tube, and uterus. It is thought to be of mesothelial origin and usually presents with a painless testicular mass. Histologically, it is composed of tubular structures lined by cuboidal cells with large cytoplasmic vacuoles. Long, slender apical microvilli of the mesothelial type are detected on ultrastructural examination. *Lipoma* is the most common tumor of the spermatic cord. *Melanotic neuroectodermal tumor* is similar to the homonymous tumor of the jaw. *Papillary cystadenoma* is characterized by papillary structures lined by clear cells within cystic spaces, often associated with von Hippel-Lindau syndrome. *Rhabdomyosarcoma* is the most common malignant tumor of the spermatic cord.

CHAPTER 48

1. Correct choice: D
FOURNIER GANGRENE (p. 2236)—Fournier gangrene is a necrotizing fasciitis of the genitalia. Dartos and penile fascia are preferred sites of involvement. Predisposing factors are local or perineal trauma, burns, or anorectal disease added to debilitating conditions such as diabetes, leukemia, and alcoholic cirrhosis.

Streptococci and staphylococci are the most common causative agents in children, as gram-negative bacilli and anaerobic bacteria are in adults.

2. Correct choice: C
GRANULOMA INGUINALE (p. 2237)—This infection manifests with slowly enlarging painless perianal nodules that become ulcerated. The etiologic agent is *Calymmatobacterium granulomatis (donovanii)*. On tissue sections or scrapings, it is identifiable as *Donovan bodies* by Giemsa or Wright staining. These are intracytoplasmic deeply staining bodies contained within a cystic structure in large histiocytes. The incidence of this sexually transmitted disease has been increasing. Clinically, the lesions are often interpreted as carcinoma. *B. henselae* is the etiologic agent of *cat-scratch disease*, *C. trachomatis* of *lymphogranuloma venereum* as well as nongonococcal urethritis, *H. ducreyi* of *chancroid*, and *T. pallidum* of *syphilis*.

3. Correct choice: B
PRECANCEROUS LESIONS OF PENILE CARCINOMA (p. 2242)—*Erythroplasia of Queyrat* and *Bowen disease* refer to *in situ* carcinoma: Erythroplasia of Queyrat involves the glans, whereas Bowen disease involves the skin of the shaft. Acanthosis with spotty proliferation of atypical cells is seen in *bowenoid papulosis*. Koilocytotic atypia is commonly associated with the warty type of penile carcinoma. Superficial spreading is the most frequent pattern of squamous cell carcinoma of the penis, analogous to the horizontal phase of the growth of melanoma.

CHAPTER 49

1. Correct choice: A
COMPLETE MOLE (p. 2279)—This complication arises from androgenesis due to fertilization of an empty ovum by one X-sperm that undergoes duplication, thus resulting in a 46,XX karyotype (90% of cases); 10% have a 46,XY phenotype due to dispermy. Histologically, *all* villi undergo hydropic degeneration and contain few or no blood vessels. There is variable trophoblastic hyperplasia. The uterus becomes enlarged, and levels of hCG rise above normal limits by the third month of pregnancy. Often, signs of toxemia manifest early in pregnancy. This form is associated with a 2% risk of choriocarcinoma. The differential diagnosis between complete and partial moles and hydropic abortus is presented in the table that follows.

	Hydropic Abortus	**Partial Mole**	**Complete Mole**
Gross swelling	Absent	Present, affects a proportion of villi	Present, affects all villi in varying degrees
Microscopy	Attenuated trophoblast	Moderate trophoblastic hyperplasia	Marked trophoblastic hyperplasia
	Central vessels present	Central vessels present	Central vessels absent
Cytogenetics	Variable	69,XXX or 69,XXY	46,XX (90%) or 46,XY
Pathogenesis	Depends on underlying cause of miscarriage	Fertilization of ovum by one or two sperm: paternal and maternal DNA	Fertilization of empty ovum by one or two sperm: no maternal DNA
Fetal parts	May be present	May be present	Absent
Risk of persistent GTD	0%	5%	Up to 30%
Risk of choriocarcinoma	None	Minimal	Significant (2%)

Abbreviation: GTD, gestational trophoblastic disease.

2. Correct choice: B
EXAGGERATED PLACENTAL SITE (p. 2284)—Often an incidental microscopic finding, this benign change is simply an exaggeration of a physiologic process involving intermediate-type trophoblastic cells. It has also been known as syncytial endometritis. Morphologically, it overlaps with *placental-site trophoblastic tumor*, also of intermediate trophoblastic origin.

3. Correct choice: E
GESTATIONAL CHORIOCARCINOMA (p. 2287)—Approximately half the cases follow a molar pregnancy (almost always complete mole), one-fourth ectopic pregnancy, and one-fourth a normal pregnancy. This aggressive cancer is highly responsive to chemotherapy (methotrexate, actinomycin D, and chlorambucil). It consists of a mixture of extremely pleomorphic cytotrophoblastic and syncytiotrophoblastic cells. It is richly vascularized and often leads to hemorrhage. The metastatic spread to the lungs and brain is common. One of the most unusual features of this neoplasm is its relationship with blood group type. Women with group A married to men with the same group have the highest risk.

4. Correct choice: E
PLACENTAL SITE TROPHOBLASTIC TUMOR (PSTT; p. 2290)—PSTT is a rare tumor that originates from the intermediate trophoblastic cells of the implantation site. It occurs usually in parous women, sometimes long after the last known pregnancy. Its usual location is in the fundus, where it infiltrates the endometrium and myometrium up to the serosa. PSTT is composed of intermediate trophoblastic cells that display a marked propensity to invade vessel walls. Vascular invasion is associated with fibrin deposition (as shown in the picture). Usually a self-limited disease, cured by curettage alone, PSTT is malignant in approximately 10% to 15% of cases. In *choriocarcinoma,* there is a combination of mononucleate trophoblastic cells and syncytiotrophoblast, accounting for a biphasic pattern. An e*pithelioid trophoblastic tumor* is also of intermediate trophoblastic origin, but it resembles a squamous cell carcinoma. An *exaggerated implantation site* overlaps morphologically with PSTT, from which it is difficult to differentiate in curettage specimens. A *placental site nodule* is usually an incidental finding in an endometrial biopsy or curettage samples.

CHAPTER 50

1. Correct answer: E
OLIGOHYDRAMNIOS (p. 2302)—Oligohydramnios indicates an abnormally reduced volume of amniotic fluid. The reduced available space leads to fetal deformities as well as to umbilical cord compression. In these cases, meconium discharge is usually associated.

2. Correct choice: A
ABRUPTIO PLACENTAE (p. 2302)—The most typical histopathologic correlates of abrutpio placentae include intravillous and intervillous hemorrhage. Intravillous hemorrhage is the most specific change, but identifiable in only 15% of cases. The presence of hemorrhage and myocytes between basal decidual cells is suggestive of *placenta accreta.*

3. Correct choice: E
MATERNAL FLOOR INFARCTION (pp. 2309 and 2310)—*Maternal floor infarction* is characterized histologically by massive perivillous fibrin deposition and hyperplasia of X (intermediate) cells. These changes involve the basal decidua to a depth of 0.4 cm.

Studies show that 50% of women with this complication have suffered from previous abortions or stillbirths. Association with maternal antiphospholipid antibody syndrome has been described. Maternal serum *major basic protein* is typically elevated.

4. Correct choice: E
CHORIOAMNIONITIS (p. 2316)—Group B streptococci are the most frequent etiologic agents of severe fetal/neonatal sepsis. The infection, as in most cases of chorioamnionitis, results from ascending spread from the birth canal. Clinical criteria for a diagnosis of chorioamnionitis include maternal fever during labor, leukocytosis, uterine tenderness, and maternal or fetal tachycardia. The clinical diagnosis must be confirmed by microscopic evidence of placental/chorioamnionic inflammation. Placental infection by group B streptococci is usually associated with mild or no signs of chorioamnionitis, as with group A streptococci, *S. pneumoniae,* and herpes simplex virus.

5. Correct choice: C
VILLITIS OF UNKNOWN ETIOLOGY (p. 2319)—This change is found in approximately 4% of all placentas. It has been observed with increased frequency in small for gestational age newborns and in an association with intrauterine growth retardation. Chronic inflammatory cells infiltrating the villi derive from both the fetus and the mother. VUE is probably caused by viruses or fastidious microorganisms.

6. Correct choice: E
MECONIUM STAINING (p. 2321)—Passage of meconium *in utero* at the time of delivery is a frequent, probably physiologic event. It may occur as a response to acute hypoxic events or chronic hypoxia. By itself, meconium is toxic to the fetus, as it contains vasoconstrictive substances that cause tissue hypoperfusion. Furthermore, aspiration of meconium can cause inflammatory pneumonitis, surfactant inactivation, and airway obstruction. This is the basis of *meconium aspiration syndrome,* a potentially severe condition that occurs in approximately 5% of meconium-exposed newborns. Pathological changes correlate with the time of antenatal exposure to meconium.

a. 2 to 3 hours: meconium-laden macrophages are found within the fetal-placental chorionic plate
b. 6 to 12 hours: numerous meconium-laden macrophages are seen in the extraplacental membranes
c. 24 to 48 hours: necrosis of umbilical vessels, with occasional umbilical ulcerations

7. Correct answer: A
CHORANGIOSIS (p. 2324)—Normally, each chorionic villus contains no more than five capillary lumina. In chorangiosis, there are at least ten capillary lumina per villus. For a diagnosis of chorangiosis, such a change must be demonstrated in at least ten different regions of the placental disc. This condition is thought to derive from protracted fetal-placental hypoxia, which hypothesis is consistent with the high incidence of chorangiosis and chorangioma in pregnant mothers living at high altitudes. Fetal nucleated red blood cells are also a consequence of fetal-placental hypoxia.

CHAPTER 51

1. Correct choice: B
VULVAR CYSTS (p. 2335)—Epidermoid cysts are the most common vulvar cysts. They are usually located in the anterior half of

the labia majora. Hymenal cysts are the most common type in newborns. Vulvar cysts other than epidermoid are listed in the following table.

Type	Origin	Lining
Bartholin duct cyst	Bartholin duct	Transitional
Pilonidal cyst	Hair follicle	Squamous
Hymenal cyst	Hymen	Squamous
Skene duct cyst	Skene duct	Transitional
Cyst of canal of Nuck	Processus vaginalis	Mesothelium
Mucinous cyst	Minor vestibular glands	Mucus secreting
Gartner duct cyst	Mesonephric/wolffian	Non–mucus secreting cuboidal
Fox-Fordyce disease	Apocrine glands	Hair follicle wall
Endometriotic cyst	Endometrotic foci	Endometrium

2. Correct choice: E

CONDYLOMA LATUM (p. 2236)—*Condyloma latum* is a manifestation of secondary syphilis and develops 4 to 6 weeks following primary infection. It consists of gray-white soft papules or plaques, which histologically are composed of plasma cell infiltration and obliterative endarteritis. *Calymmatobacterium granulomatis* causes *granuloma inguinale*. Serotypes L1 to L3 of *C. trachomatis* cause *lymphogranuloma venereum*, and serotypes D to K cause sexually transmitted diseases. *Haemophilus ducreyi* is the etiologic agent of the rare *chancroid.*

3. Correct answer: A

AGGRESSIVE ANGIOMYXOMA (p. 2342)—This tumor arises in the perineal region, most commonly in the vulva or scrotum. The paucicellular nature of the myxoid background and dilated vessels are the most important features in distinguishing this lesion from other entities (e.g., fibroepithelial polyp and angiomyofibroblastoma). Cells display immunohistochemical features of myofibroblasts, including expression of actin, desmin, and vimentin; they are also frequently positive for the endothelial marker CD34. The lesion frequently recurs after surgical removal, in contrast to angiomyofibroblastoma.

4. Correct choice: A

VULVAR INTRAEPITHELIAL NEOPLASIA (VIN; p. 2345)—Bowenoid papulosis is a form of *vulvar intraepithelial neoplasia* (*VIN*). VIN has variable gross manifestations, such as velvety plaques, scaly plaques, or condyloma-mimicking lesions. VIN may or may not be associated with *dystrophic conditions*, such as lichen sclerosus and squamous cell hyperplasia. VIN III is the type most frequently detected. It progresses to squamous cell carcinoma in approximately 10% of cases. HPV 16 is most frequently associated with this lesion. Bowenoid papulosis manifests as pigmented papules around the vulva in young women, is usually associated with low-grade VIN, and progresses to invasive carcinoma less frequently than classic VIN. VIN is currently subdivided into two morphological types:

a. *Warty* (bowenoid): condylomatous appearance, associated with HPV, most common in younger women
b. *Basaloid:* smooth surface, not associated with HPV, most common in elderly women.

5. Correct choice: B

SQUAMOUS CELL CARCINOMA OF VULVA (p. 2347)—There are three main types, *keratinizing, warty,* and *basaloid.* The keratinizing type is shown in the picture. It occurs usually in elderly women (sixth to seventh decade) and is rarely associated with HPV or VIN; squamous hyperplasia is detected adjacent to keratinizing carcinoma in 83% of cases. In contrast, warty and basaloid carcinomas tend to affect younger women and are usually associated with the presence of type 16 or 33 HPV. In 77% of cases, VIN of the warty or basaloid type is observed adjacent to warty or basaloid carcinomas. Finally, 40% of women with warty or basaloid carcinoma of the vulva develop neoplastic changes in the cervix, whereas cervical neoplasia is found in 4% of those with the keratinizing type.

6. Correct choice: A

VULVAR PAGET DISEASE (p. 2353)—Vulvar and mammary Paget disease are very similar, macroscopically and histologically. The clear cells spreading through the epidermis are immunoreactive for both apocrine and epithelial markers, which lends support to their presumed *apocrine* origin. Virtually all cases of *mammary* Paget disease are accompanied by an underlying breast carcinoma, whereas *vulvar* cases result from the following:

- Intraepithelial malignancy arising from adnexa or mammary-like glands: most common
- Pagetoid or metastatic spread from adenocarcinoma of the cervix, Bartholin glands, or transitional cell carcinoma

Furthermore, approximately 29% of patients with vulvar Paget disease have some unrelated malignancy in the breast, urogenital tract, or gastrointestinal tract.

7. Correct choice: C

HIDRADENOMA PAPILLIFERUM (p. 2354)—This benign tumor is sometimes clinically mistaken for a malignant tumor because of its tendency to undergo ulceration. It is thought to originate from either apocrine glands or ectopic breast tissue in the vulvar region. It is strikingly similar to intraductal papilloma of the breast. Similar to the latter, it consists of glandular papillary fronds lined by a two-cell epithelial layer. Often, signs of apocrine differentiation are seen in epithelial cells.

8. Correct choice: B

VAGINAL ADENOSIS (pp. 2355 and 2356)—This condition is found in 2% of women unexposed to *diethylstilbestrol* (DES) and consists of müllerian-type epithelium within the vaginal mucosa. The epithelium may be of the endocervical (mucus-producing) type or tubal/endometrium (clear cell) type. The form associated with *in utero* DES exposure is similar to that unassociated with *in utero* DES exposure. Rarely, vaginal adenosis progresses to cancer, and usually it is gradually replaced by squamous metaplasia. Microglandular hyperplasia develops in foci of vaginal adenosis, especially after oral contraceptive use. Microglandular hyperplasia may be confused with clear cell adenocarcinoma (also DES associated). Vaginal adenosis appears as red nodules on inspection and manifests with excessive mucous discharge in postpubertal age.

9. Correct choice: C
RHABDOMYOMA (p. 2361)—It is important to distinguish this benign tumor, which usually occurs in adult patients, from botryoid rhabdomyosarcoma, which affects children under the age of 5 years. Rhabdomyoma is composed of very large strap cells with evident cross-striations. Cross-striations are difficult to identify in rhabdomyosarcoma of the embryonal type (botryoid). The latter exhibits a characteristic accumulation of neoplastic cells underneath the epithelium, a feature known as the *cambium layer. Mixed tumor of the vagina* is composed of basophilic cells arranged in cords, glandular structures, and squamous nests. *Stromal polyp* is a pedunculated polyp composed of a dense fibrovascular core covered by intact epithelium.

10. Correct choice: E
SQUAMOUS CELL CARCINOMA OF VAGINA (p. 2362)—This rare tumor preferentially involves the upper anterior portion of the vagina. Because cervical carcinoma tends to spread to the upper third of the vagina, care should be taken not to diagnose a cervical cancer with vaginal extension as a vaginal carcinoma. HPV has been implicated in the pathogenesis of vaginal carcinoma analogously to tumors of the cervix. A morphologic precursor named *vaginal intraepithelial neoplasia* (VAIN) has been identified in some cases. Most of these tumors are squamous cell carcinomas. Variants include verrucous, sarcomatoid, transitional, and lymphoepithelioma-like carcinomas.

11. Correct choice: D
CLEAR CELL (MESONEPHROID) ADENOCARCINOMA (p. 2363)—This neoplasm develops in children and adolescents with a history of prenatal exposure to *diethylstilbestrol* (DES), previously used for treatment of threatened abortion. Morphologically, the tumor resembles analogous uterine or ovarian neoplasms arising in elderly women. It is composed of cells with clear glycogen-filled cytoplasm, which acquire a hobnail appearance when lining papillary structures. Neoplastic cells contain glycogen but not mucin. This may indicate that the tumor originates from adenosis of the tuboendometrial type and not the mucinous type. *In utero* DES exposure leads most commonly to vaginal adenosis or anatomical abnormalities such as mucosal membranes, apical narrowing, vaginal septa, and so on. (p. 2356).

CHAPTER 52

1. Correct choice: A
CHLAMYDIA TRACHOMATIS INFECTION (p. 2377)—This is the most common sexually transmitted disease in industrialized countries. Morphologic changes detected in cervical biopsies are nonspecific and consist of chronic inflammatory infiltration with occasionally prominent lymphoid follicles (*follicular cervicitis*). Follicular cervicitis is not diagnostic of *Chlamydia*, but it is more often associated with positive cultures. The organism can be demonstrated by immunohistochemistry but not on histologic sections. An ulcer should suggest the possibility of *herpes simplex virus* (HSV): Look for multinucleated cells with smudged chromatin and intranuclear inclusions.

2. Correct choice: E
SQUAMOUS CELL NEOPLASIA OF CERVIX (p. 2378)—The greater part of cervical SSC results from progression of a squamous intraepithelial lesion (SIL). HPV types 16 and 18 genomes have been detected in most cases, whereas types 6 and 11 are most often associated with low-grade dysplasia and condyloma acuminatum. Two HPV proteins, E6 and E7, interact with p53 and, respectively, Rb gene products, thus leading to their inactivation and genomic instability. These molecular events are crucial in the progression of cervical carcinogenesis. In contrast to other human cancers, p53 is rarely mutated in cervical SCC. Neoplastic cells express keratin and frequently CEA, blood group antigens, and progesterone receptors. Although low-grade lesions tend to be euploid or polyploid, invasive SCC is consistently aneuploid. The basaloid type is very aggressive.

3. Correct choice: C
LOW-GRADE SQUAMOUS INTRAEPITHELIAL LESION (LSIL; p. 2380)—The photomicrograph shows acanthosis and minimal parabasal atypia without atypical mitotic figures. By definition, in LSIL, cytologic atypia is limited to the lower third of the epithelium. Koilocytotic changes, which are cytopathic effects due to HPV infection, are present in the upper two-thirds. Morphologically, there are three types of LSIL:

a. *Exophytic* LSIL (*condyloma acuminatum*): characterized by exophytic growth and papillomatosis, usually associated with low-risk HPV types
b. *Flat* LSIL (*flat condyloma*): flat lesion without papillomatosis, more often associated with high-risk HPV types
c. *Immature condyloma* or *papilloma* (previously known as *papillary immature metaplasia*): immature cells with a high nucleocytoplasmic ratio and prominent chromocenters lining filiform papillae. Associated with low-risk HPV types

The latter type is important because it may easily be mistaken for high-grade SIL, or vice versa.

4. Correct choice: C
HIGH-GRADE SQUAMOUS INTRAEPITHELIAL LESION (HSIL; p. 2382)—A diagnosis of HSIL implies that dysplastic changes are present in the lower and upper epithelial cell layers. It includes both cervical intraepithelial neoplasia (CIN) II and CIN III of the old classification. The list of choices reflects the range of lesions to be considered in the differential diagnosis of HSIL (see p. 2388). Morphologic variants of HSIL include the following:

a. *Keratinizing/koilocytotic HSIL:* there is superficial keratinization in addition to atypia
b. *HSIL with immature metaplastic differentiation:* combines features of immature metaplasia with those of HSIL
c. *Stratified mucin-producing intraepithelial lesion:* characterized by the presence of mucin droplets along with immature metaplasia, suggesting adenosquamous differentiation

5. Correct choice: C
NONNEOPLASTIC STROMAL CHANGES (p. 2390)—The finding of multinucleated giant cells in the endocervical stroma is relatively common and is probably the result of a nonspecific reaction to various stimuli. It is also seen in other mucosal sites (oral, anal, etc.). A decidual reaction is also known as an *Arias-Stella reaction.* Necrobiotic granuloma may occur after a surgical procedure, analogous to the prostatic form. A *placental implantation site* is an eosinophilic nodule composed of cytotrophoblast immunoreactive for keratin and PLAP. Choices A, C, and D may be confused with cancer, whereas choice B suggests infection.

6. Correct choice: C

MICROINVASION (pp. 2391 and 2392)—Superficially invasive carcinomas (less than 5 mm in depth) represent 20% of all newly diagnosed cervical cancers. Microinvasion is usually associated with stromal desmoplastic response, blurring of the epithelial/stromal interface, and loss of nuclear polarity at the infiltrating border. Mimics of microinvasion include the following:

a. Tangentially cut crypts involved by HSIL
b. Cautery/crush artifact
c. Reparative changes in SIL
d. Blurring of stromal/epithelial interface by inflammation
e. Placental implantation site

7. Correct choice: C

MICROGLANDULAR HYPERPLASIA (p. 2405)—This frequent condition is often discovered incidentally in women using oral contraceptives, but is also found in women of postmenopausal age. It is benign, but it may be misdiagnosed as carcinoma when some atypia or mitotic activity (both features usually absent or minimal) is present. It consists of clusters of small glandular structures lined by cuboidal or flat epithelial cells. CEA immunohistochemistry is negative, in contrast to squamous cell and adenocarcinoma of the cervix. An *Arias-Stella reaction* is a decidual reaction that occurs during pregnancy: Hypersecretory glands show strikingly enlarged and pleomorphic epithelial cells without mitotic figures.

8. Correct choice: E

ADENOCARCINOMA *IN SITU* (ACIS; p. 2411)—The picture shows some of the defining features of ACIS: hyperchromatic, crowded, enlarged nuclei, with mitotic figures and apoptotic bodies. This is a recognized precursor of invasive cervical adenocarcinoma. HPV is present in nearly 90% of cases. In approximately 30% to 60% of ACIS, there is coexistent SIL. ACIS must be differentiated from tubal metaplasia and nonspecific glandular atypia. Immunostains for Ki-67, CEA, and p16 are helpful in the differential diagnosis.

9. Correct choice: A

ADENOMA MALIGNUM AND OTHER VARIANTS (p. 2416)—Also called *minimal deviation adenocarcinoma*, this variant represents approximately 10% of cervical adenocarcinomas. It is a well-differentiated tumor that can be diagnosed mostly thanks to architectural disorganization, infiltrative behavior, and surrounding stromal response. CEA immunoreactivity is positive and helps to differentiate this tumor from microglandular hyperplasia. Although well differentiated, it has a worse prognosis than the classic type. *Adenosquamous carcinoma* has a characteristic biphasic pattern. *Clear cell carcinoma* is analogous to vaginal clear cell adenocarcinoma and is associated with DES exposure; the prognosis is good. *Glassy cell carcinoma* is a variant of adenosquamous that occurs in younger women and is composed of cells with glassy eosinophilic cytoplasm with an eosinophil-rich infiltrate; the prognosis is poor. The *villoglandular papillary* variant has a good prognosis.

CHAPTER 53

1. Correct choice: A

EMB VERSUS D AND C (p. 2435)—D and C requires anesthesia and may result in complications such as uterine perforations and Asherman syndrome (secondary amenorrhea due to postoperative adhesions). Hysteroscopy and directed biopsy are the best techniques to detect and extirpate endometrial polyps.

2. Correct choice: D

ARIAS-STELLA REACTION (p. 2448)—The Arias-Stella reaction is an exaggerated hypersecretory response of the endometrium to hCG stimulation, which may be observed in normal or ectopic pregnancy, gestational trophoblastic disease, exogenous administration of hormones, as well as in foci of endometriosis. Because of its striking nuclear pleomorphism, it may be mistaken for adenocarcinoma. In the Arias-Stella reaction, the nuclei contain smudged chromatin (vs. coarse chromatin in adenocarcinoma) and mitoses are rare. *No desmoplasia, No infiltrative growth*

3. Correct answer: D

CHRONIC ENDOMETRITIS (p. 2450)—This condition is most often associated with IUD use and pelvic inflammatory disease (PID, of which *Chlamydia* and gonococcus are the most frequent etiologic agents). Although lymphocytes and lymphoid follicles are found in the normal endometrium, plasma cells are abnormal and represent the essential criterion for a diagnosis of chronic endometritis. Glandular disarray usually accompanies chronic endometritis and makes *dating* of the endometrium not feasible. Cytomegalovirus is the most common cause of viral endometritis.

4. Correct choice: A

DUB (pp. 2451 and 2452)—DUB includes all cases of abnormal uterine bleeding not related to organic conditions (i.e., tumors, endometriosis, fibroids, etc.). DUB can be differentiated into two groups based on the presence or absence of ovulation. Although the majority of cases fall into the *anovulatory cycle* group, the cases in which ovulation occurs have a more varied etiology. The anovulatory forms lead to constant estrogenic stimulation of the endometrium, which eventually responds with hyperplastic changes. From a morphologic standpoint, an anovulatory endometrium can be identified on biopsy by identifying the endometrium in the proliferative phase when it should have already developed secretory changes.

5. Correct choice: B

DISORDERED PROLIFERATIVE ENDOMETRIUM (p. 2455)—This change is found most commonly in association with anovulatory cycles in women of perimenarchal and perimenopausal age. It is due to desynchronization of glandular maturation. The gland-to-stroma ratio is approximately 1, but glands vary in size and shape. Some glands are markedly dilated, whereas others show budding. There is no increased risk of uterine carcinoma.

6. Correct answer: C

ENDOMETRIAL HYPERPLASIA (p. 2456)—This common alteration is most often associated with anovulatory cycles, because the resultant protracted estrogenic stimulation fosters the proliferation of the endometrium. *Simple* hyperplasia consists of an increased number of cystically dilated endometrial glands. *Complex* hyperplasia consists of back-to-back endometrial glands with frequent *budding*; both these forms are then divided into two subgroups *with* or *without* atypia. Cystic dilation is more frequent in simple or mild hyperplasia, whereas severe hyperplasia with atypia is characterized by nuclear crowding, loss of polarity, an increased nuclear-cytoplasmic ratio, and prominent nucleoli. Complex hyperplasia with atypia is associated with a 20% to 30% risk of cancer.

7. Correct choice: A

ENDOMETRIAL POLYPS (p. 2459)—The great majority of endometrial polyps are found in association with endometrial hyperplasia and probably represent a focal exaggeration of such a process. The appearance of the stroma helps distinguish endometrial hyperplasia from polyps in fragmented biopsy specimens. In polyps, the stroma is composed of mitotically inactive fibroblast-like cells with abundant extracellular matrix and *dilated thick-walled vessels*. Occasionally, polyps may develop in women taking tamoxifen. In these patients, decidual changes may be present.

8. Correct choice: E

ENDOMETRIOID CARCINOMA (p. 2460)—This is the most frequent morphologic type of endometrial cancer. The FIGO grading system is based on assessment of architectural features (i.e., solid vs. glandular growth) and nuclear atypia. Because endometrioid adenocarcinoma often contains villous and papillary projections, this feature does not by itself warrant the diagnosis of *papillary serous carcinoma*, which is a very aggressive subtype characterized by extreme cellular pleomorphism. Estrogen/progesterone receptors are present in the majority of endometrioid carcinomas. It should be emphasized that the FIGO grading system does not apply to special variants of uterine cancer such as papillary serous carcinoma and clear cell carcinoma (by definition clinically high grade) and secretory carcinoma (by definition low grade).

9. Correct choice: D

ENDOMETRIAL METAPLASIA (p. 2476)—A wide range of metaplastic changes may develop in the endometrium, the most frequent of which is squamous metaplasia. Focal collections of squamous (nonkeratinizing) cells scattered in the endometrium are called *morules*. Although a benign change per se, endometrial metaplasia is often associated with varying degrees of hyperplasia, and it is therefore statistically more prevalent in areas of a high incidence of endometrial carcinoma. On the other hand, knowledge of this common morphologic change is necessary to avoid erroneous diagnoses of cancer. For example, clear cell metaplasia must be distinguished from clear cell adenocarcinoma. *Tubal metaplasia* is frequently associated with disordered proliferative endometrium.

10. Correct choice: D

PAPILLARY SEROUS CARCINOMA (p. 2482)—This highly aggressive tumor resembles ovarian papillary serous carcinoma. It has a predilection for women older than 60 years. In contrast to the endometrioid type, it is not associated with clinical or morphologic evidence of hyperestrinism (anovulatory cycles or endometrial hyperplasia). The tumor arises on a background of atrophy. It is very important to differentiate this type from an endometrioid carcinoma with a prominent villous/papillary component. *Clear cell carcinoma* also affects elderly women and is characterized by hobnail cells lining well-differentiated glandular and tubular structures. Unlike the analogous vaginal/cervical tumor, this subtype of ovarian carcinoma is not associated with *in utero* DES exposure and is characterized by an aggressive course.

11. Correct choice: A

ADENOFIBROMA (p. 2491)—This benign tumor consists of a well-differentiated endometrial stromalike component with scattered glandular structures having an architectural arrangement similar to that seen in phylloides tumors. Similarly, adenofibroma has a malignant counterpart, that is, *müllerian adenosarcoma*, in which the mesenchymal component is malignant but the epithelial component is not. *Benign leiomyoblastoma* is a variant of leiomyoma and composed of clear cells with well-defined borders. *Endolymphatic stromal myosis* is also known as low-grade stromal sarcoma. In *mixed müllerian tumor*, both epithelial and mesenchymal components are malignant. *Symplasmic leiomyoma* is a leiomyoma with numerous bizarre tumor cells.

12. Correct choice: B

MALIGNANT MIXED MÜLLERIAN TUMORS (p. 2494)—These highly aggressive neoplasms consist of two histological components: epithelial (carcinoma similar to endometrioid/papillary serous) and mesenchymal. The sarcomatous component imparts the additional qualification of *homologous* (if the stromal tissue looks like endometrial stroma or smooth muscle) or *heterologous* (if there is bone, cartilage, fat, or skeletal muscle differentiation). The great majority of cases arise in women of postmenopausal age. The carcinomatous component is the one that usually metastasizes. Their prognosis is worse than the most aggressive of endometrial carcinomas.

13. Correct answer: C

ENDOMETRIAL STROMAL TUMORS (p. 2497)—This category comprises tumors that resemble the endometrial stroma and includes three types: *endometrial stromal tumors, low-grade stromal sarcoma*, and *high-grade stromal sarcoma*. The resemblance to the normal endometrial stroma is the common histologic feature. Furthermore, they all show a propensity to invade lymphatic and blood vessels, have prominent vascularity (mimicking hemangiopericytoma), and form perivascular concentric arrangements. Endometrial stromal tumors are well demarcated, mitotically inactive, and associated with a good prognosis. Sarcomas are poorly circumscribed infiltrating tumors. The dividing line between low-grade and high-grade stromal tumors is arbitrarily defined by the mitotic count, higher than 10/10 high-power fields (hpf) in the high-grade type. Otherwise, the histological features are similar. High-grade stromal tumors often metastasize to the lungs.

14. Correct choice: C

UTERINE LEIOMYOSARCOMA (p. 2520)—As with smooth muscle tumors arising in other sites, uterine leiomyosarcomas are often histologically similar to leiomyomas except for a high mitotic rate. In fact, a mitotic count of 10/10 hpf is used as a conventional discriminatory parameter between benign and malignant tumors. Other criteria have also been proposed, including necrosis, degree of cellular atypia, size of tumor, and so on, but the mitotic count appears the most reliable. Leiomyosarcomas may occur in women of both premenopausal and postmenopausal age, with a peak incidence between 40 and 60 years. They frequently metastasize to the lungs, bone, and brain. Development from a preexistent leiomyoma is exceptional. Choice B refers to malignant leiomyoblastoma.

CHAPTER 54

1. Correct choice: C

OVARIAN TUMORS (p. 2543)—There is an important correlation between age and certain types of ovarian tumors, which may help in the differential diagnosis. Most ovarian tumors affecting women younger than 45 are benign, and the percentage of malignant tumors increases with age. Borderline surface epithelial tumors occur frequently in the fourth decade.

2. Correct choice: E
SEROUS TUMORS OF THE OVARY (p. 2546)—This category accounts for approximately 40% of all ovarian tumors. One-third are bilateral, and they are most commonly malignant. The benign variant (*serous cystadenoma:* about 70%) consists of a large cyst lined by columnar ciliated cells similar to tubal epithelium. The borderline variant (5% to 10%) has areas of cytologic and architectural atypia without stromal invasion. The malignant variant (*serous cystadenocarcinoma:* 20% to 25%) is solid/cystic and is the most common primary malignant tumor of the ovary. It consists of an anaplastic epithelium with stromal invasion. Benign, borderline, and malignant serous tumors develop at progressively increasing ages.

3. Correct choice: A
MUCINOUS TUMORS OF THE OVARY (p. 2554)—This group constitutes approximately 15% of all ovarian tumors. Benign mucinous tumors of the ovary are lined by a single layer of nonciliated mucus-producing cells similar in appearance to endocervical or intestinal epithelium. They develop in middle-aged or elderly women, rarely in those of younger age. Most tumors are large multilocular cysts filled with mucinous fluid. Of all ovarian mucinous tumors, approximately 75% are benign, 10% are borderline, and 15% are carcinomas. Grossly, they appear as multilocular cysts, whereas serous tumors are usually unilocular.

4. Correct choice: A
MUCINOUS BORDERLINE TUMOR (MBT; p. 2555)—In MBTs, the epithelium shows cytologic atypia and architectural disorganization but no stromal invasion. Areas of nodularity or increased thickness in the cyst wall should be carefully evaluated for stromal invasion. MBTs may be classified further into those with epithelium of the endocervical or intestinal type. Most MBTs are of the intestinal type. In mucinous cystadenocarcinoma, on the other hand, there is unequivocal stromal invasion.

5. Correct choice: B
ENDOMETRIOID CARCINOMA (p. 2559)—This tumor represents approximately 15% of ovarian tumors. Its light microscopic features are very similar to endometrial adenocarcinoma of the uterus: glandular structures with tall pseudostratified epithelial cells and centrally placed nuclei. Currently, it is believed that most endometrioid tumors derive *indirectly* from surface epithelium, through malignant transformation of adenofibromas or endometriotic foci. Hyperestrinism plays a role in the malignant transformation of endometriosis. Tubular glands of endometrioid carcinomas may mimic the tubules of Sertoli cell tumor or Call-Exner bodies of granulosa cell tumors.

6. Correct choice: A
CLEAR CELL CARCINOMA (pp. 2564 and 2565)—Clear cell carcinoma accounts for 5% of ovarian cancers and is the neoplasm associated with endometriotic foci more frequently than any other ovarian tumor, including endometrioid carcinoma. Also, clear cell carcinoma gives rise to paraendocrine hypercalcemia more frequently than any other ovarian neoplasm, excluding *small cell carcinoma of the hypercalcemic type.* Histologically, clear cell carcinoma is composed of clear cells lining tubules, papillae, or cystic spaces. Neoplastic cells typically acquire a *hobnail* appearance. Clear cell carcinoma may mimic dysgerminomas and yolk sac tumors.

7. Correct choice: C
BRENNER TUMOR (p. 2568)—This relatively uncommon ovarian tumor (2% to 3% of all ovarian neoplasms) is histologically similar to transitional epithelium. Nests of cells are surrounded by a dense fibrous stroma and contain scattered microcystic cavities filled with brown fluid. Their histogenetic origin is the surface epithelium, not transitional epithelium nor, as previously believed, Walthard cell nests. They are usually benign tumors, but rare borderline or frankly malignant variants do occur.

CHAPTER 55

1. Correct choice: A
GRANULOSA CELL TUMOR (GCT; p. 2579)—GCTs are divided into two types, *juvenile* (JGCT) and *adult* (AGCT). AGCT may have diffuse (the most common), microfollicular, or macrofollicular patterns. The most typical features of AGCT include rudimentary follicles known as *Call-Exner bodies* (as seen in the picture) and grooved nuclei. In JGCT, the follicles are more irregular in shape and size, and nuclei lack their characteristic grooves. Furthermore, mitotic activity and nuclear atypia are more pronounced in JGCT compared to AGCT. Approximately 75% of GCTs secrete estrogens, thus giving rise to isosexual pseudoprecocity in prepubertal girls. Cells of GCT, as in all other sex cord–stromal tumors, express *inhibin.*

2. Correct choice: A
FIBROMA (p. 2583)—The syndrome of ovarian fibroma, right pleural effusion, and ascites is known as *Meigs syndrome.* Ovarian fibromas are benign tumors composed of well-differentiated fibroblasts arranged in densely packed fascicles with a storiform arrangement. Meigs syndrome resolves once the ovarian neoplasm is excised. The tumor develops most commonly in women of reproductive age and is not associated with endocrine manifestations. In contrast, *thecoma* produces estrogens and develops in women of postmenopausal age. Thecomas show a characteristic yellow cut surface owing to their rich steroid content. Histologically, thecomas consist of spindle-shaped cells with vacuolated cytoplasm that stains with oil red-O.

3. Correct choice: B (A)
STEROID CELL TUMORS AND LEYDIG CELL TUMOR (2593)—Steroid cell tumors are rare ovarian neoplasms composed of cells resembling lutein, Leydig, or adrenocortical cells. When a steroid cell tumor contains *crystals of Reinke*, it is by definition a Leydig cell tumor. Leydig cell tumors usually originate in the ovarian hilus and manifest with hirsutism or virilization in postmenopausal women. *Stromal luteoma* is another form of steroid cell tumor, composed of luteinized cells and androgenic in 60% of cases. When a steroid cell tumor lacks features characteristic of stromal luteoma or Leydig cell tumor, it is diagnosed as *steroid cell tumor, not otherwise specified* (NOS). Currently, steroid cell tumors NOS constitute the majority of tumors in this category.

4. Correct choice: D
OVARIAN DYSGERMINOMA (pp. 2595–2597)—This tumor is analogous to testicular seminoma. The histology is therefore identical, characterized by an admixture of PLAP-positive large cells with clear cytoplasm and prominent nucleoli, and nonneoplastic lymphocytes. Often, dysgerminomas are admixed with yolk sac or choriocarcinomatous foci. Yolk sac components are positive for keratin and AFP, and choriocarcinoma is immunoreactive for HCG. Positivity for keratin may be strongly enhanced in early carcinomatous differentiation (also referred to as anaplastic

dysgerminoma). Ovarian dysgerminomas are often large tumors with a convoluted, cerebroid surface.

5. Correct choice: A
OVARIAN YOLK SAC TUMOR (pp. 2597–2599)—This tumor develops usually in children/adolescents, as do all germ cell tumors of the ovary. The histologic appearance is comparable to testicular yolk sac tumor. *Schiller-Duval bodies* are pseudopapillary structures consisting of a central small vessel surrounded by a double layer of cuboidal cells, which contain intracytoplasmic and extracellular PAS-positive globules. Cells with yolk sac differentiation express both AFP and keratin. This immunohistochemistry pattern is useful in identifying yolk sac elements in *mixed* germ cell tumors, the most common of which is dysgerminoma plus yolk sac tumor.

6. Correct choice: D
TERATOMA OF THE OVARY (p. 2602)—This neoplasm of germ cell origin consists of tissues originating from ectoderm, mesoderm, and endoderm. Thus, a bewildering array of different tissue, sometimes in an organoid arrangement, may be found. Typically, teratomas develop in children or adolescents. *Mature* teratomas consist of well-differentiated elements, whereas *immature* teratomas include atypical components with a propensity for metastatic spread. The glial component (identifiable with GFAP immunohistochemistry) is one of the most common neoplastic elements in immature teratomas. This may spread to the peritoneal cavity, creating implants of glial tissue that are referred to as *gliomatosis peritonei.*

7. Correct choice: A
GONADOBLASTOMA (p. 2609)—This very rare tumor is the most common ovarian neoplasm in individuals with abnormal sexual development, especially in association with gonadal dysgenesis. It may occur, however, in otherwise normal females as well. Histologically, it consists of a combination of germ cells and sex cord cells.

CHAPTER 56

1. Correct choice: E
SMALL CELL CARCINOMA, HYPERCALCEMIC TYPE (p. 2619)—This rare tumor has the usual features of small cell carcinomas, including evidence of neuroendocrine differentiation. The presence of scattered follicle-like microcysts may mimic the Call-Exner bodies of granulosa cell tumors. Two-thirds of cases are associated with hypercalcemia. Most cases occur between in patients 15 and 25 years of age.

2. Correct choice: A
PRIMARY VERSUS METASTATIC TUMORS (p. 2623)—Gross and microscopic patterns that favor *metastases* include bilateral involvement, multiple nodules, hilar location, prominent vascular invasion, single cell infiltration, surface mucin, and signet-ring cells. Features favoring *primary* tumors include expansile growth, a complex papillary architecture, and large size (greater than 10 cm). The following are the most common sources of ovarian metastases:

- Stomach: This organ is the most frequent source of *Krukenberg tumors.*
- Uterus-fallopian tubes: Ovarian involvement is around 40% at autopsy, 15% at surgery.

- Breast: One-third of patients develop ovarian metastases (particularly lobular carcinoma) during the course of the disease.
- Large bowel: Two percent to 10% of patients develop ovarian metastases.
- Other less frequent sites: These include the vermiform appendix, carcinoid tumors, pancreas-gallbladder, kidney, adrenal glands, and melanoma.

Ovarian involvement by endometrial carcinoma has been reported in 34% to 40% of autopsy cases and 5% to 15% of surgical specimens.

3. Correct choice: D
KRUKENBERG TUMORS (p. 2623)—This designation applies to the occurrence of bilateral nodular masses in the ovaries secondary to the metastatic spread of a *signet-ring carcinoma.* Neoplastic cells may be arranged as nests, glands, or tubules, or distributed as single cells within a cellular stroma. Gastric carcinomas are the most common source, but Krukenberg tumors have been described in association with other intraabdominal signet-ring cancers (colon, etc.). Primary Krukenberg tumors are exceedingly rare.

4. Correct choice: C
OVARIAN INFECTIONS (p. 2630)—Most cases of ovarian infection are due to the ascending spread of PID. The long-term result is a *tuboovarian abscess,* usually bilateral. Actinomycotic ovarian infections are rare, but usually due to the use of IUDs.

5. Correct choice: A
HYPERREACTIO LUTEINALIS (p. 2634)—This condition usually occurs in association with disorders leading to high levels of hCG, that is, gestational trophoblastic disease, multiple pregnancies, or fetal hydrops. It is characterized by bilateral multiple luteinized follicle cysts. It manifests with pain and/or a pelvic mass and may complicate with torsion or cyst rupture. Both *ovarian decidual reaction* and *pregnancy luteoma* develop during pregnancy, and both of them are probably related to abnormal endocrine influences. *Massive edema* is usually seen in young women and manifests with pelvic pain, a palpable mass, and menstrual irregularities. Stromal hyperplasia and hyperthekosis is common in perimenopausal women, but usually asymptomatic; in younger women it may cause hypertension, virilization, glucose intolerance, and obesity.

6. Correct choice: A
POLYCYSTIC OVARIAN DISEASE (p. 2635)—This condition affects up to 7% of the female population. Anovulatory cycles and increased luteinizing hormone (LH) secretion are crucial pathophysiologic elements. The ovaries have numerous follicle cysts, prominent luteinization of the theca interna, and stromal hyperplasia with variable hyperthekosis. Corpora lutea are absent in typical cases. Most commonly, patients are in their 30s and present with oligomenorrhea, infertility, and hirsutism (rarely virilization). Unopposed hyperestrinism leads to endometrial hyperplasia.

CHAPTER 57

1. Correct choice: A
SALPINGITIS ISTHMICA NODOSA (p. 2656)—Despite its designation (due to old pathogenetic hypotheses), salpingitis isthmica nodosa is probably analogous to uterine adenomyosis. The

glandular structures are thought to derive from the tubal epithelium extending into the tubal wall. It is usually bilateral and associated with sterility. *Endosalpingiosis* is the condition in which the tubal epithelium is found outside the fallopian tube and is thus analogous to endometriosis.

2. Correct choice: D

FALLOPIAN TUBE CARCINOMA (pp. 2663–2663)—This rare neoplasm is usually diagnosed when metastatic spread or spread through the peritoneum has already occurred. Histologically, most tumors resemble papillary serous carcinoma of the ovary. Fallopian tube carcinoma, however, is ten times less common than its ovarian counterpart. Thus, a diagnosis of primary *tubal* carcinoma is justified only when finding cancer predominantly involving the fallopian tube, with grossly normal ovaries and uterus.

3. Correct choice: D

FEMALE ADNEXAL TUMOR OF PROBABLE WOLFFIAN ORIGIN (p. 2668)—This tumor is usually localized in the broad ligament, occurs at a mean age of 47 years, and may manifest with abdominal pain and swelling. Microscopically, it consists of cells arranged in solid sheets or in a characteristic sievelike pattern, as shown in the picture. Most cases are benign, but rare malignant forms have been reported.

CHAPTER 58

1. Correct choice: D

FOREIGN MATERIALS IN THE PERITONEUM (p. 2677)—A Maltese-cross pattern is characteristic of starch (specifically cornstarch), which is used for surgical gloves and has replaced talc. Cellulose from disposable gowns is another potential peritoneal contaminant. All of the named materials may induce a granulomatous reaction mimicking infection or Crohn disease.

2. Correct choice: E

WELL-DIFFERENTIATED PAPILLARY MESOTHELIOMA (WDPM) (p. 2684)—This uncommon benign lesion of the peritoneal mesothelium usually represents an incidental finding at surgery or autopsy and occurs most commonly in women of reproductive age. A WDPM may be solitary or multiple. It appears as a vascularized nodule composed of papillary structures lined by a single layer of cuboidal cells resembling choroid plexus. *Adenoma-*

toid tumor is much more common in the genital tract. *Gliomatosis peritonei* is due to peritoneal dissemination of glial tissue from an ovarian teratoma. *Localized fibrous tumor* has been reported in the peritoneum. *Müllerian metaplasia* occurs in women and leads to foci of endometrium, tubal epithelium, or reactive decidua in the pelvic peritoneum.

3. Correct choice: B

INTRAABDOMINAL DESMOPLASTIC SMALL ROUND CELL TUMOR (p. 2686)—This small cell tumor of young adults arises from the peritoneal serosa, frequently in the pelvic region. The reciprocal translocation between chromosomes 11 and 22 involves, in contrast to (PNETs) and Ewing sarcoma, not only the EWS gene, but also the WT1 gene.

4. Correct choice: D

PSEUDOMYXOMA PERITONEI AND APPENDICEAL TUMORS (p. 2689)—*Pseudomyxoma peritonei* consists of the accumulation of mucinous fluid and microscopic fragments of neoplastic glandular epithelium within the peritoneal cavity. Floating neoplastic fragments seed the peritoneal cavity, producing macroscopically identifiable nodules. The patient will develop intestinal obstruction, infective peritonitis, and other complications resulting from the invasion of pelvic organs. Mucinous appendiceal tumors, most commonly a mucinous cystadenoma, represent the most common cause, although occasionally ovarian cystadenoma/cystadenocarcinoma may be the source. Coexisting appendiceal and ovarian mucinous tumors are seen in some of these cases, which raises the question as to which of the two neoplasms is the primary tumor.

5. Correct choice: D

ENDOMETRIOSIS (p. 2690)—In addition to changes related to the duration of disease, the histology of endometriotic foci varies in response to endogenous or exogenous hormonal influences. The example shown here is characterized by endometrial glands with a proliferative appearance. During pregnancy, stromal cells are decidualized whereas the glandular epithelium is flat. Menopause leads to glandular atrophy. Estrogen replacement therapy may cause a variety of hyperplastic changes similar to those in the uterus. Atypical hyperplasia in endometriosis has the same potential for malignant transformation. Most cases of endometriosis-related carcinomas are *clear cell* and *endometrioid* carcinomas. The ovary is by far the most common site of endometriosis-related cancer, followed by the rectovaginal pouch.